TEXTBOOK of RADIOLOGY
Musculoskeletal Radiology

TEXTBOOK of RADIOLOGY
Musculoskeletal Radiology

Editors

Hariqbal Singh MD DMRD
Professor and Head
Department of Radiology
Shrimati Kashibai Navale Medical College and General Hospital
Pune, Maharashtra, India

Shrikant Nagare DNB (Radiology)
Consultant
Department of Radiology
Shrimati Kashibai Navale Medical College and General Hospital
Pune, Maharashtra, India

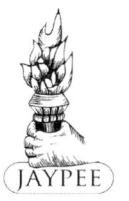

JAYPEE *The Health Sciences Publisher*

New Delhi | London | Philadelphia | Panama

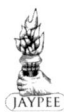 **Jaypee Brothers Medical Publishers (P) Ltd.**

Headquarters
Jaypee Brothers Medical Publishers (P) Ltd
4838/24, Ansari Road, Daryaganj
New Delhi 110 002, India
Phone: +91-11-43574357
Fax: +91-11-43574314
E-mail: jaypee@jaypeebrothers.com

Overseas Offices

J.P. Medical Ltd
83, Victoria Street, London
SW1H 0HW (UK)
Phone: +44 20 3170 8910
Fax: +44 (0)20 3008 6180
E-mail: info@jpmedpub.com

Jaypee-Highlights Medical Publishers Inc.
City of Knowledge, Building 235, 2nd Floor
Clayton, Panama City, Panama
Phone: +1 507-301-0496
Fax: +1 507-301-0499
E-mail: cservice@jphmedical.com

Jaypee Medical Inc.
325, Chestnut Street
Suite 412, Philadelphia,
PA 19106, USA
Phone: +1 267-519-9789
E-mail: support@jpmedus.com

Jaypee Brothers Medical Publishers (P) Ltd
17/1-B, Babar Road, Block-B, Shaymali
Mohammadpur, Dhaka-1207
Bangladesh
Mobile: +08801912003485
E-mail: jaypeedhaka@gmail.com

Jaypee Brothers Medical Publishers (P) Ltd
Bhotahity, Kathmandu, Nepal
Phone: +977-9741283608
E-mail: kathmandu@jaypeebrothers.com

Website: www.jaypeebrothers.com
Website: www.jaypeedigital.com

© 2016, Jaypee Brothers Medical Publishers

The views and opinions expressed in this book are solely those of the original contributor(s)/author(s) and do not necessarily represent those of editor(s) of the book.

All rights reserved. No part of this publication may be reproduced, stored or transmitted in any form or by any means, electronic, mechanical, photocopying, recording or otherwise, without the prior permission in writing of the publishers.

All brand names and product names used in this book are trade names, service marks, trademarks or registered trademarks of their respective owners. The publisher is not associated with any product or vendor mentioned in this book.

Medical knowledge and practice change constantly. This book is designed to provide accurate, authoritative information about the subject matter in question. However, readers are advised to check the most current information available on procedures included and check information from the manufacturer of each product to be administered, to verify the recommended dose, formula, method and duration of administration, adverse effects and contraindications. It is the responsibility of the practitioner to take all appropriate safety precautions. Neither the publisher nor the author(s)/editor(s) assume any liability for any injury and/or damage to persons or property arising from or related to use of material in this book.

This book is sold on the understanding that the publisher is not engaged in providing professional medical services. If such advice or services are required, the services of a competent medical professional should be sought.

Every effort has been made where necessary to contact holders of copyright to obtain permission to reproduce copyright material. If any have been inadvertently overlooked, the publisher will be pleased to make the necessary arrangements at the first opportunity.

Inquiries for bulk sales may be solicited at: jaypee@jaypeebrothers.com

Textbook of Radiology: Musculoskeletal Radiology

First Edition: **2016**

ISBN: 978-93-86056-73-3

Printed at Sanat Printers

Dedicated to

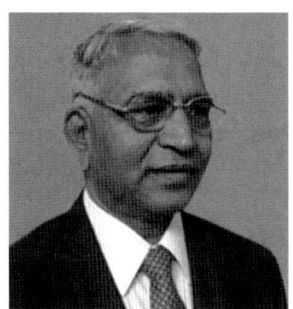

Arvind V Bhore
Director
Shrimati Kashibai Navale Medical College and General Hospital
Pune, Maharashtra, India
An ardent, zealous and holistic educationalist and administrator,
guru and mentor to many scholars.

Saying

*Radiology is a kindergarten
of logical rational coherent exploration and balanced learning
and not dexterous adroit smugness or learning egotism
cultivated by fake self-centeredness and egoism.*

—Hariqbal Singh

Contributors

Aditi Dongre MD (Radiology)
Associate Professor
Department of Radiology
Shrimati Kashibai Navale Medical
College and General Hospital
Pune, Maharashtra, India

Hariqbal Singh MD DMRD
Professor and Head
Department of Radiology
Shrimati Kashibai Navale Medical
College and General Hospital
Pune, Maharashtra, India

Santosh Konde MD (Radiology)
Associate Professor
Department of Radiology
Shrimati Kashibai Navale Medical
College and General Hospital
Pune, Maharashtra, India

Shrikant Nagare DNB (Radiology)
Consultant
Department of Radiology
Shrimati Kashibai Navale Medical
College and General Hospital
Pune, Maharashtra, India

Sikandar Shaikh DMRD DNB EDiR (European Board of Radiology)
Consultant
Department of Radiology and PET-CT
Yashoda Hospital
Hyderabad, Telangana, India

Subodh Laul DNB (Radiology)
Consultant
Shrimati Kashibai Navale Medical
College and General Hospital
Pune, Maharashtra, India

Varsha Rangankar MD (Radiology)
Professor
Shrimati Kashibai Navale Medical
College and General Hospital
Pune, Maharashtra, India

Preface

Textbook of Radiology: Musculoskeletal Radiology is a succinct, concise, short and snappy, laconic, and to-the-point book, which provides the most imaging solutions on musculoskeletal system routinely required at any imaging establishment, and will be a handy reference.

The book does not cover the entire musculoskeletal system but has been structured such that the student is adequately prepared to undertake the postgraduate examination, in a relatively short timeframe; a considerable number of images have been incorporated to give a better grasp over the subject. It covers a few number of questions asked or likely to be asked during the examination.

As today's radiology occupies an important place in concluding the diagnosis, it will be a great advantage for postgraduate students to undertake the examination not only in radiology but also for other clinical subjects. It will be a valuable order for all residents and general practitioners as well as for medical colleges, institutional and departmental libraries.

Hariqbal Singh
Shrikant Nagare

Acknowledgments

We thank Professor MN Navale, Founder President, Sinhgad Technical Educational Society, and Dr Arvind V Bhore, Director, Shrimati Kashibai Navale Medical College and General Hospital, Pune, Maharashtra, India, for their kind acceptance in this endeavor.

We profusely extend our gratefulness to the radiology consultants (Shrimati Kashibai Navale Medical College and General Hospital), Anand Kamat, Prashant Naik, Manisha Hadgaonkar, Pooja Shah, Rajlaxmi Sharma, Yasmeen Khan, and Vivek Chaudhari, for their genuine help in building up this educational entity.

We are obliged and appreciate, Swati Shah (PC Resident) of this institute for helping in development of the chapter on 'Breast'.

We thank the postgraduate residents, Vikram Shende, Jarvis Pereira, Punit Agrawal, Prasad Patil, Swapnil Raut, Priya Bhole, Amar Sangapwad, and Prajakta Jagtap, for their hand which facilitated especially during correction phase of the manuscript.

Our gratitude to Anna Bansode, Sachin Babar, Deepak Shinde, Adinath Sonawane, Shankar Gopale, and Tushar Girme for their clerical help.

We are thankful and grateful to God Almighty and mankind, who have allowed us to have this wonderful experience.

Contents

1. Congenital Skeletal Anomalies and Dysplasia — 1
Preaxial and Postaxial Polydactyly *1*; Ectrodactyly Ectodermal Dysplasia Cleft Lip Syndrome *1*; Madelung's Deformity *1*; Congenital Hip Dislocation *2*; Osteopetrosis *2*; Sprengel Deformity *3*; Macrodystrophia Lipomatosa *3*; Multiple Epiphyseal Dysplasia *3*; Cleidocranial Dysostosis *4*; Holt-Oram Syndrome *5*; Fibrous Dysplasia *6*; Fibrodysplasia Ossificans Progressiva *7*; Mucopolysaccharidoses *7*; Perthes Disease *10*; Congenital Bifid Sternum *10*; Bone Island or Enostosis *11*

2. Trauma — 12
Patterns of Fracture *12*; Healing of Fracture *12*; Fall on Outstretched Hand *14*; Fracture *16*; Stress Fracture *18*; Segond Fracture *19*; Avulsion Fracture *20*; Fracture Scaphoid *21*

3. Metabolic and Endocrine Disorders — 22
Rickets *22*; Renal Rickets *23*; Osteoporosis and Osteomalacia *24*; Acromegaly *25*; Fluorosis *26*; Resorption of Terminal Tufts *26*; Expansile Lesions of Metaphysis *27*; Hand as an Index of Disease *29*

4. Infections — 32
Periosteal Reaction (Periostitis) *32*; Osteomyelitis *32*; Sequelae to Septic Arthritis *36*; Tuberculous Arthritis *36*; Congenital Syphilis *37*; Infectious Arthritis *37*; Sacroiliitis *38*

5. Noninfective Inflammatory Arthritis — 41
Seronegative Spondyloarthropathy *41*; Hypertrophic Osteoarthropathy *42*; Ankylosing Spondylitis *44*; Psoriatic Arthritis *44*

6. Joints — 46
Anatomy Shoulder Joint *46*; Avulsion of Greater Tuberosity *47*; Acromioclavicular Degeneration *48*; Spinoglenoid Cyst *49*; Glenoid Labrum Tear *50*; Tuberculous Arthritis Right Shoulder *50*; Rotator Cuff Tears *52*; Anatomy Hip Joint *52*; Osteoid Osteoma *54*; Avascular Necrosis *56*; Septic Arthritis *58*; Anatomy Knee Joint *58*; Cruciate Ligaments *63*; Collateral Ligaments *63*; Menisci *65*; Pigmented Villonodular Synovitis *69*; Osteomyelitis *69*; Rheumatoid Arthritis *69*; Neuropathic Arthropathy *71*

7. Bone Tumors — 72
WHO Classification of Bone Tumors *72*; Aneurysmal Bone Cyst *73*; Osteoid Osteoma *74*; Osteochondroma *75*; Diaphyseal Aclasis (Chondromatosis) *76*; Tallus Chondroblastoma *77*; Giant Cell Tumor *77*; Hemangioma *78*; Lipoma *78*; Adamantinoma *79*; Fibrolipomatous Hamartoma Median Nerve *80*; Plasma Cell Tumor *81*; Plasmacytoma *82*; Multiple Myeloma *83*; Pigmented Villonodular Synovitis *84*; Fibrous Dysplasia *86*; Polyostotic Fibrous Dysplasia *87*; Ameloblastoma *89*; Loose Bodies in Shoulder Joint *90*; Osteochondritis Dissecans *90*; Odontogenic Fibromyxoma of the Maxilla *90*; Osteosarcoma *90*; Ewing's Sarcoma *96*; Osseous Lymphoma *96*; Liposarcomas *98*; Sacrococcygeal Teratoma *99*; Skeletal Metastasis *99*

8. Soft Tissues — 101

Classification of Soft Tissue Tumors *101*; Subcutaneous Lipoma *101*; Macrodystrophia Lipomatosa *103*; Liposarcoma *105*; Fibrolipomatous Hamartomas of Median Nerve *105*; Baker's Cyst *106*; Complete Tear Tendo-Achilles *106*; Neurogenic Tumors *106*; Bilateral Nasolabial Cyst *109*; Soft-tissue Calcifications *109*

9. Breast — 116

Breast Anatomy *116*; Breast Cysts *117*; Antibioma *118*; Intramammary Lymph Node *119*; Fibroadenomas *119*; Gynecomastia *120*; Phyllodes Tumor *120*; Carcinoma Breast *120*; Carcinoma Breast with Metastases *120*; Carcinoma *In Situ* *121*

10. Miscellaneous — 124

Imaging in Sickle Cell Anemia *124*; Pycnodysostosis *125*; Solitary Dense Vertebra *125*; Rib Notching *125*; Bone Infarct *125*; Fibrous Dysplasia *126*; Kienböck's Disease *127*; Avascular Necrosis Scaphoid *127*; Hyperostosis Frontalis Interna *129*; Renal Osteodystrophy *129*; Ozone Therapy *130*; Geode *131*; Magnetic Susceptibility Artifact *132*; Cloud Computing *132*; Metallic Foreign Bodies *132*

11. Ossification Centers — 134

Index — *139*

Plate 1

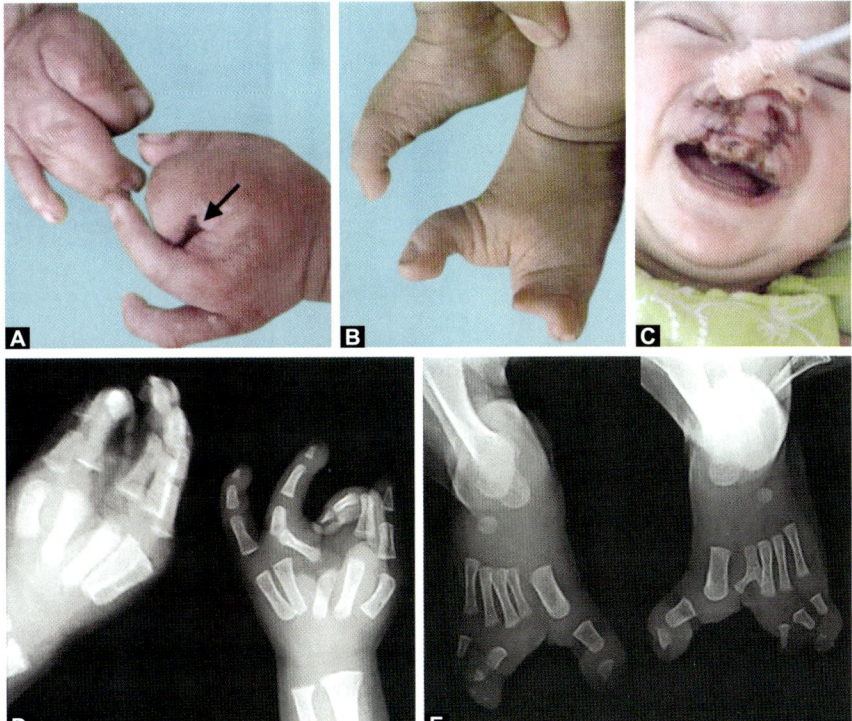

Figs 1.2A to E Both hands have claw like appearance due to cone shaped defect (arrow). Soft tissue fusion of the middle and ring finger of the right hand and index and middle finger of the left hand is seen (A). Both feet show claw like appearance due to soft tissue fusion of the 3rd, 4th and 5th toes (B). Surgery has been performed for cleft lip (C). X-ray hands (D) show a cone shaped defect. There is absence of middle and distal phalanges of middle finger on the left side. X-ray feet (E) show cone shaped defect due to absence of 2nd toe on either side. Syndactyly of the metatarsals of the left foot is seen. There is absence of middle and distal phalanges of 3rd, 4th and 5th toes on either side

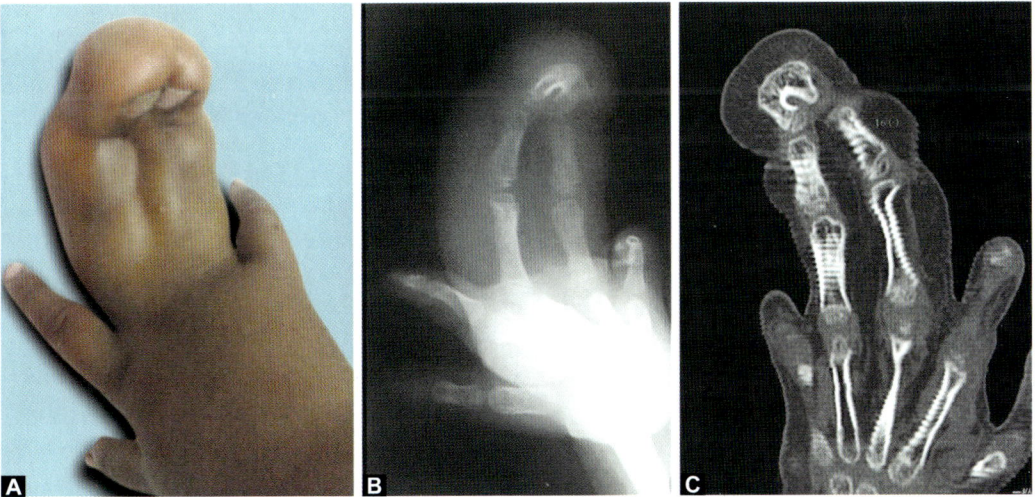

Figs 1.7A to C Clinical photograph of right hand shows enlarged, fused ring and middle finger. Plain radiograph (B) and coronal reformatted CT (C) shows soft tissue swelling and proliferation of fat on palmar aspect of the ring and middle fingers, along with dorsal angulation and syndactyly

Plate 2

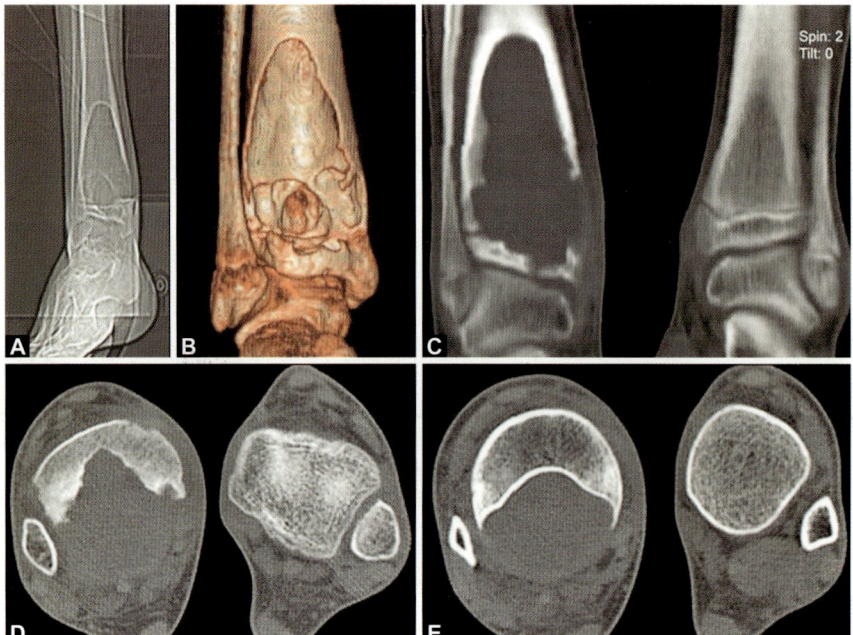

Figs 7.1A to E A 16-year-old male had history of painful swelling just above right ankle was subjected to CT, shows an eccentric expansile lytic lesion is seen in the distal diaphysis and metaphysis region of right tibia. Multiple septae are seen. The inner portion is sclerotic. No periosteal reaction is seen. The lesion does not cross the epiphyseal plate. Scanogram (A), volume-rendered image (B), coronal-reformatted image (C), axial images (D and E)

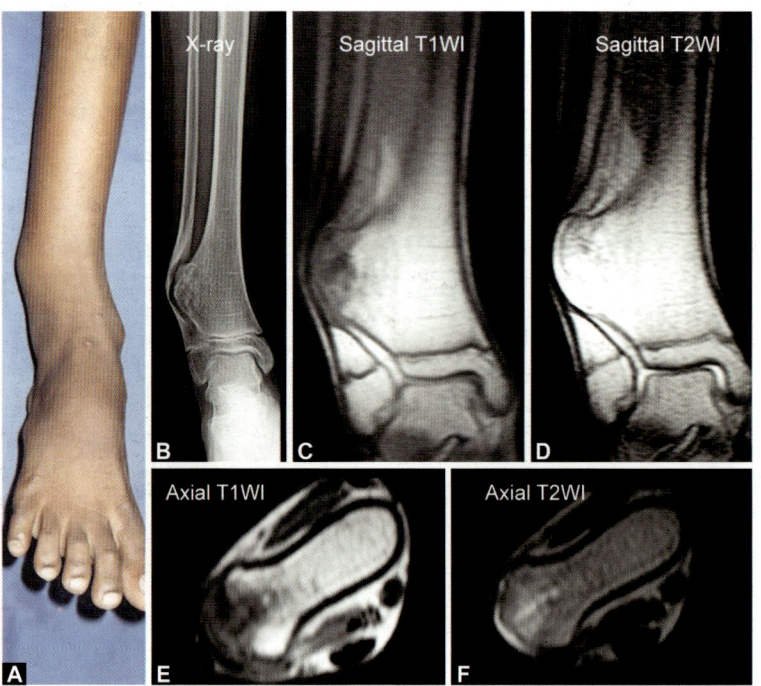

Figs 7.5A to F A 10-year-old female presented with pain and swelling in right lower leg. (A) and X-ray of both ankles anteroposterior view (B) reveals sessile bony outgrowth from right lower tibia, lateral aspect with continuity of cortex and medullary cavity with the parent bone, causing significant pressure erosion and thinning of the adjoining fibula. Mineralized areas in the cartilage cap remain low signal intensity with all MR pulse sequences. The high water content in no mineralized portions of the cartilage cap had intermediate-to-low signal intensity sagittal and axial on T1-weighted images (C and E) and very high signal intensity on sagittal and axial T2-weighted MR images (D to F)

Plate 3

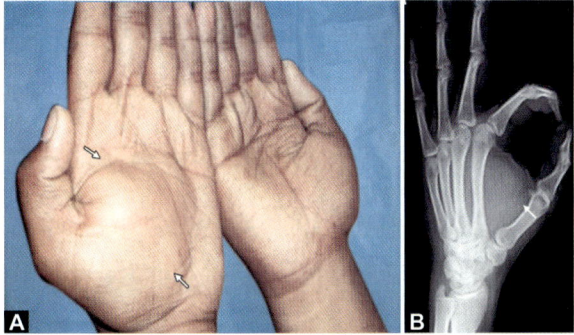

Figs 7.15A and B (A) Swelling over the thenar eminence of the left palm (arrows). (B) Oblique radiograph the left hand of patient showing soft tissue mass lesion in the thenar aspect of the left hand (arrows)

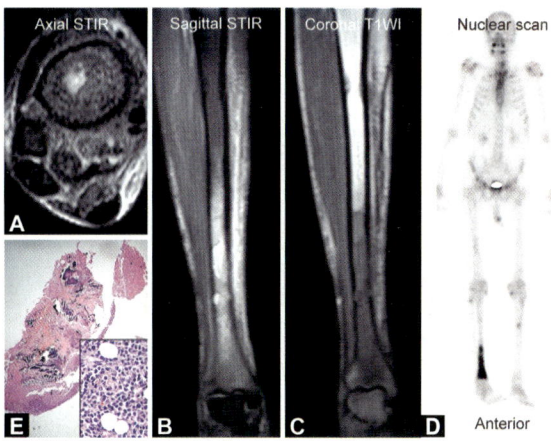

Figs 7.17A to E A 65-year-old male presented with vague pain right leg of 6 months duration on STIR axial (A) and sagittal (B) images of right leg lower third of tibia shows hyperintense signal. Coronal T1W (C) image shows the lesion to be hypointense. Whole body nuclear scan (D) shows avid uptake of tracer in right leg lower third of tibia. High power view of the sheets of plasma cells (E) shows eccentric nucleus with typical cart wheel nuclear chromatin and dense eosinophilic cytoplasm confirming the diagnosis of plasmacytoma

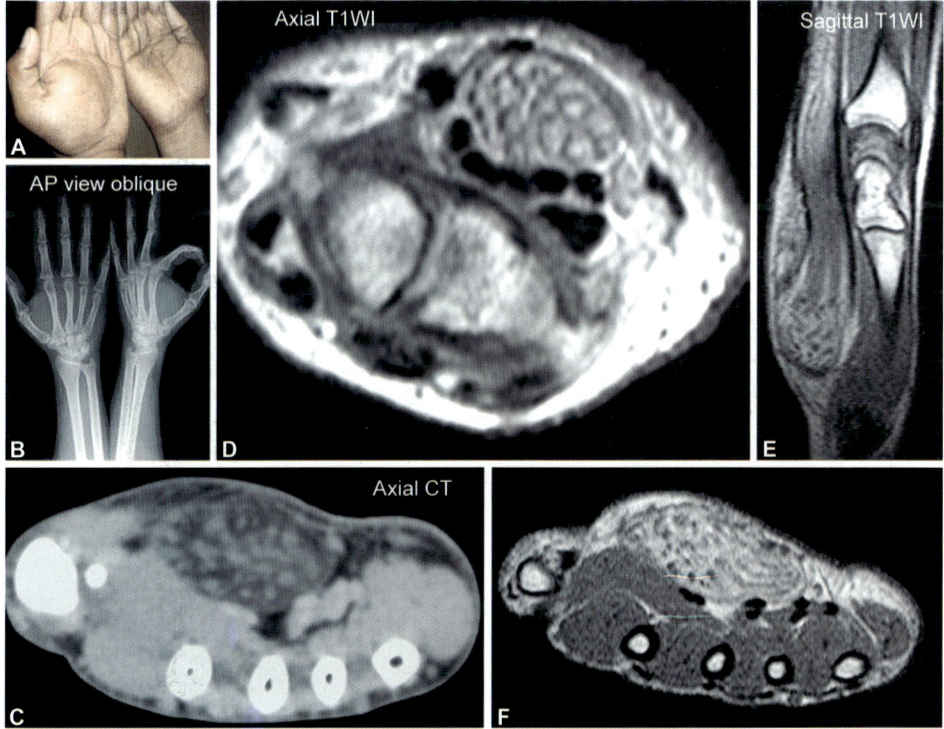

Figs 8.5A to F Photograph of hands show swelling of the left thenar eminence (A). X-ray AP and oblique views (B) of left hand show soft tissue swelling in the region of thenar eminence. Axial CT section shows a well-defined heterogeneous lesion seen in ventral aspect distal to wrist, anterior to the flexor tendons having fatty density within the lesion (C). Axial T1WI and sagittal T1WI (D and E) shows well-defined oval lesion on ventral aspect just distal to wrist appearing hyperintense with flow voids within it. In the fatty lesion, flow voids are seen abutting the flexor tendons with polka dot appearance (D to F) because of enlarged median nerve with fat infiltration in between fascicles of median nerve

Plate 4

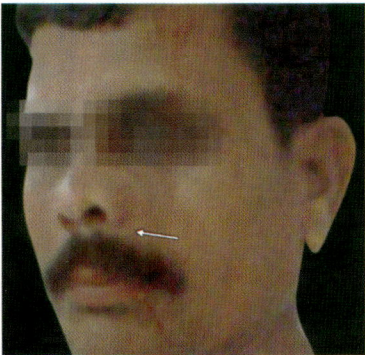

Fig. 8.9 Photograph of patient shows swelling (arrow) on left side in the nasolabial region

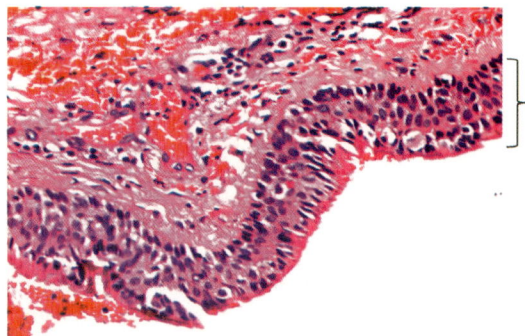

Fig. 8.12 Histopathological examination shows pseudostratified columnar epithelium (}) with fibrocollagenous tissue, the feature of a cyst wall

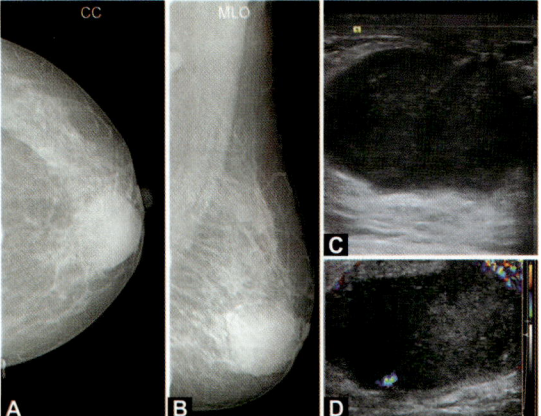

Figs 9.3A to D In patient with complaints of breast pain and antibiotic administration, mammography shows a well-defined soft tissue density mass with smooth margins in the outer lower quadrant of the left breast with no microcalcifications (A and B). No axillary lymphadenopathy seen. On ultrasound a well-defined heterogeneous mass with dense internal echoes and thick wall is seen in the outer lower quadrant of the left breast measuring 28 × 24 mm. It wider than taller (C). Color Doppler reveals peripheral vascularity (D)

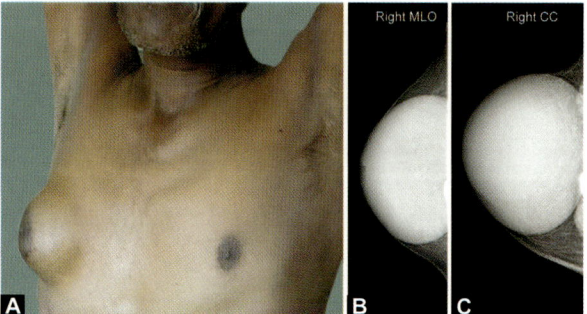

Figs 9.8A to C A 47-years-old male with history of gradually increasing painless, firm, mobile, well-circumscribed, nontender swelling of right breast (A). Mammogram show a large dense encapsulated lesion with smooth margins, typical appearance of phyllodes tumor

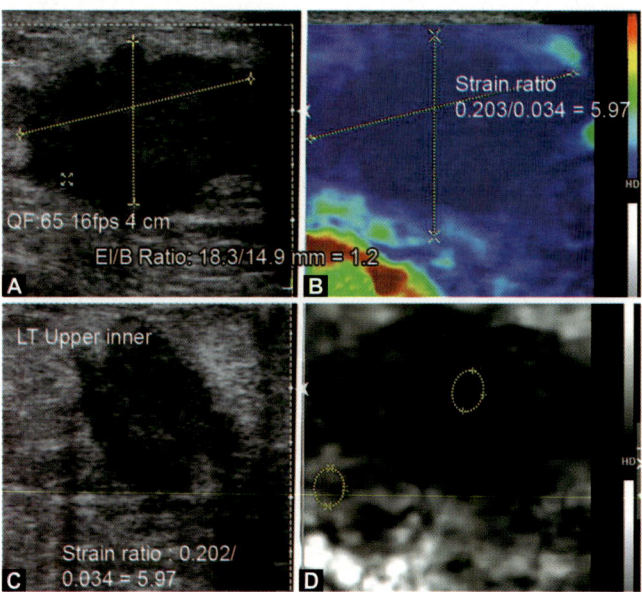

Figs 9.10A to D Breast ultrasonography shows heterogeneous, hypoechoic lesion with microlobulations or angulated margins. Elastography breast shows EI/B mode (elastography imaging B mode) ratio—1.2, strain ratio—5.97 and elasticity score—5 (not seen in figure). The lesion was categorized as BI-RADS 5

Congenital Skeletal Anomalies and Dysplasia

Preaxial and Postaxial Polydactyly

Polydactyly may be preaxial (radial) or postaxial (ulnar). It may range from an ossicle to complete duplication of fingers or toes. On occasion the hand may be duplicated. When present, should search for an associated syndrome. Syndactyly may be associated with polydactyly. Postaxial polydactyly is more frequent congenital often seen as fifth digit duplications in hands or feet **(Figs 1.1A to D)**.

Ectrodactyly Ectodermal Dysplasia Cleft Lip Syndrome

Ectrodactyly ectodermal dysplasia cleft lip (EEC) syndrome is a uncommon condition with multiple congenital anomalies with normal intelligence characterized by ectodermal dysplasia, clefting of hands, feet, lip and palate. It is an autosomal dominant syndrome. Management of the cases requires a multidisciplinary approach. Early diagnosis allows precise counseling of parents with reassurance of normal intelligence.

Examination of that baby revealed ectrodactyly (splitting of hands and feet), ectodermal dysplasia, cleft lip and palate, sparse scalp hairs and eyebrows and absence of eyelashes **(Figs 1.2A to E)**. These abnormalities constitute the EEC syndrome.

Madelung's Deformity

Madelung's deformity is commoner in girls and is generally bilateral and presents during adolescence. The defective development of the inner third of the epiphysis of the lower end the radius result in bowing of radial shaft thus increasing the interosseous space.

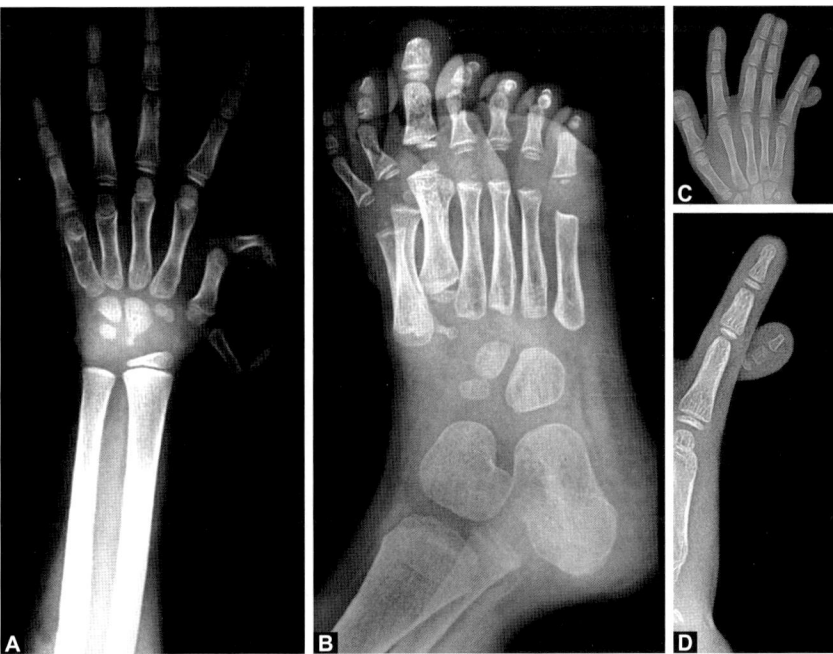

Figs 1.1A to D (A) AP radiograph of hand shows pre-axial (radial) polydactyly in a 6-year-old female; (B) Oblique radiograph of foot shows pre-axial polydactyly in 14-year-old male; (C) Shows post-axial (ulnar) polydactyly; (D) is magnified view of C

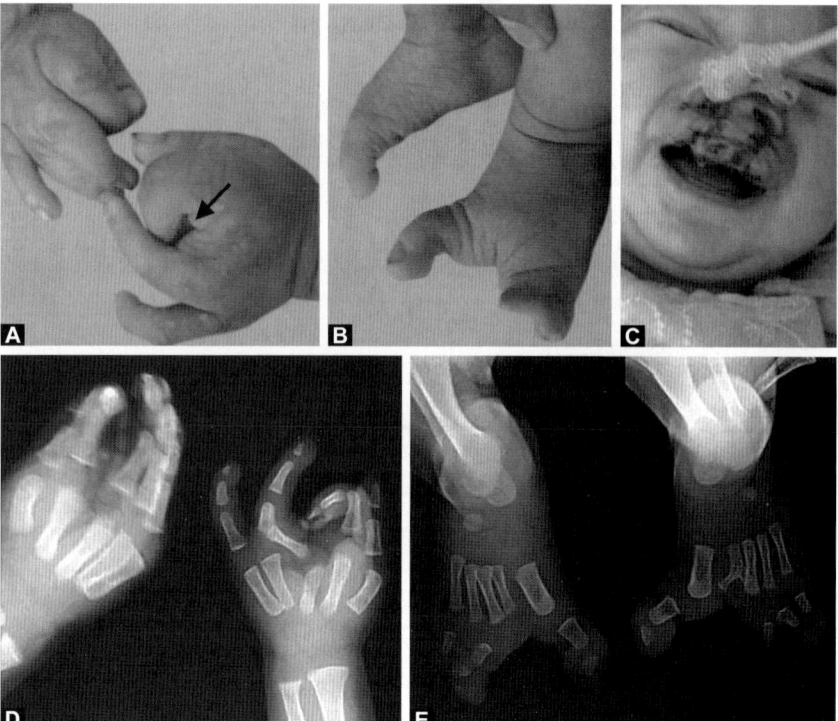

Figs 1.2A to E Both hands have claw like appearance due to cone shaped defect (arrow). Soft tissue fusion of the middle and ring finger of the right hand and index and middle finger of the left hand is seen (A). Both feet show claw like appearance due to soft tissue fusion of the 3rd, 4th and 5th toes (B). Surgery has been performed for cleft lip (C). X-ray hands (D) show a cone shaped defect. There is absence of middle and distal phalanges of middle finger on the left side. X-ray feet (E) show cone shaped defect due to absence of 2nd toe on either side. Syndactyly of the metatarsals of the left foot is seen. There is absence of middle and distal phalanges of 3rd, 4th and 5th toes on either side *(For color version, see plate 1)*

The lower end of ulna is subluxed backward. The hand project forward at the wrist joint to produce a bayonet-like appearance in a lateral projection **(Fig. 1.3)**.

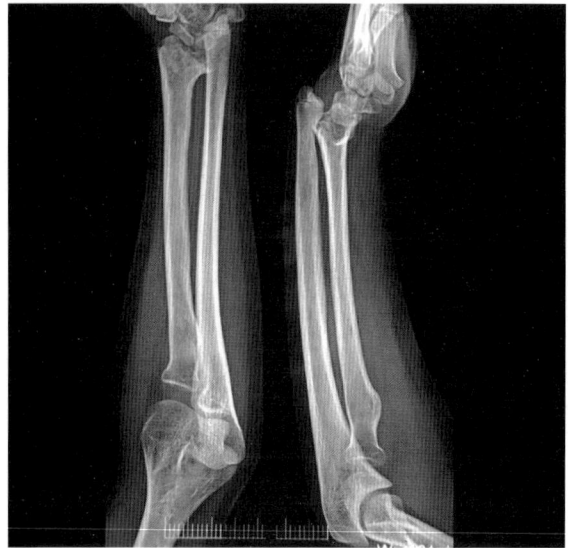

Fig. 1.3 Madelung deformity of right wrist in a 13-year-old female

Congenital Hip Dislocation

Congenital hip dislocation is a very important condition as treatment depends upon early recognition. Females are more commonly affected (F>M, 5:1). Dislocation is usually unilateral (L>R, 11:1), both hips may be involved. Ultrasound is now the accepted method of primary investigation of suspected developmental dysplasia of the hip **(Figs 1.4A and B)**.

Osteopetrosis

Osteopetrosis or Albers-Schönberg disease or marble bone disease is a rare disorder in which due to deficiency of carbonic anhydrase in osteoclasts resulting defective bone resorption by osteoclasts, when resorption fails and formation persists leads to excessive bone formation. Hence all the bones become hard dense and brittle. Radiological hallmark is generalized markedly increased bone density giving rise to a bone-in-bone appearance, Erlenmeyer flask type deformity of the tubular bones and sandwich vertebrae seen as dense bands of sclerosis parallel to the endplates **(Figs 1.5A to D)**.

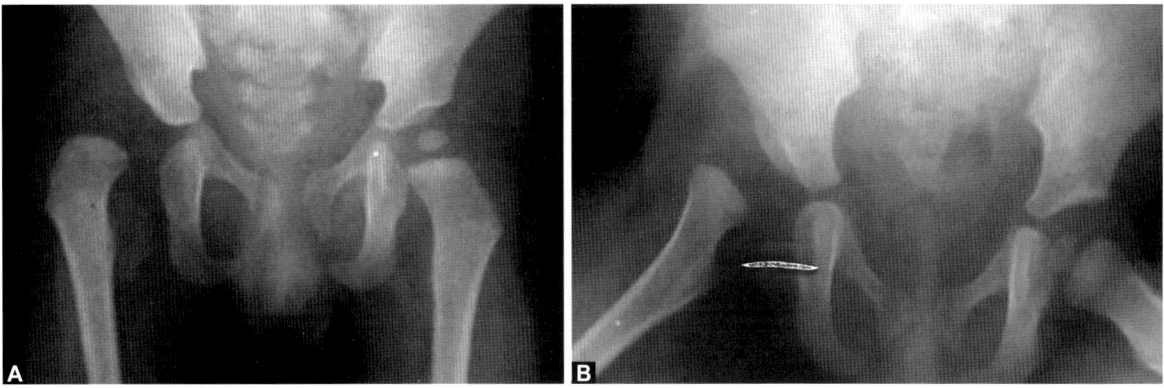

Figs 1.4A and B AP and frog pelvis radiographs shows congenital hip dislocation in a 3-year-old male

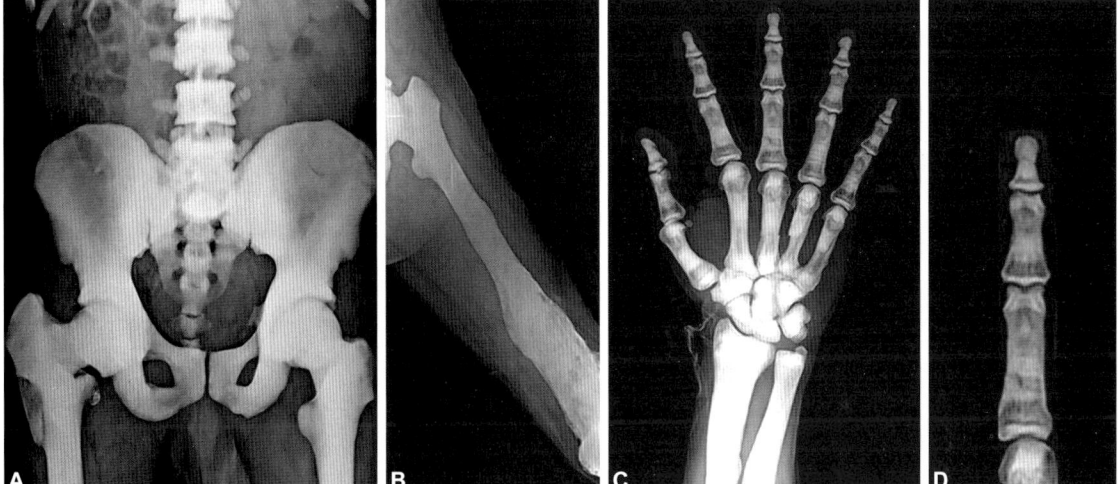

Figs 1.5A to D CT scout images of pelvis with both hips, left thigh and both hands show generalized markedly increased bone density indicative of osteopetrosis

Sprengel Deformity

Sprengel described 4 cases of upward displacement of the scapula in 1891 and named the entity as Sprengel deformity. It is also known as high scapula or congenital high scapula. It is a rare congenital skeletal abnormality where one shoulder blade sits higher on the back than the other. It is failure of descent of scapula secondary to fibrous or osseous omovertebral connection; it may be associated with Klippel-Feil syndrome, renal anomalies, and webbed neck. It results in elevation and medial rotation of scapula. It may be associated with Gorlin basal cell nevus syndrome **(Figs 1.6A and B)**.

The deformity is due to a failure in early fetal development where the shoulder fails to descend properly from the neck to its final position. Treatment includes surgery in early childhood and physiotherapy.

Macrodystrophia Lipomatosa

Macrodystrophia lipomatosa is a congenital local gigantism of the hand and foot characterized by proliferation of all mesenchymal components, particularly fibroadipose tissue. Macrodystrophia lipomatosa comes to clinical attention because of cosmetic reasons, mechanical problems secondary to degenerative joint disease or development of neurovascular compression **(Figs 1.7 and 1.8)**.

Multiple Epiphyseal Dysplasia

It is characterized by an abnormality of mucopolysaccharide and glycoprotein metabolism and develops in early childhood. Radiographs show delayed ossification and delayed mineralization of the

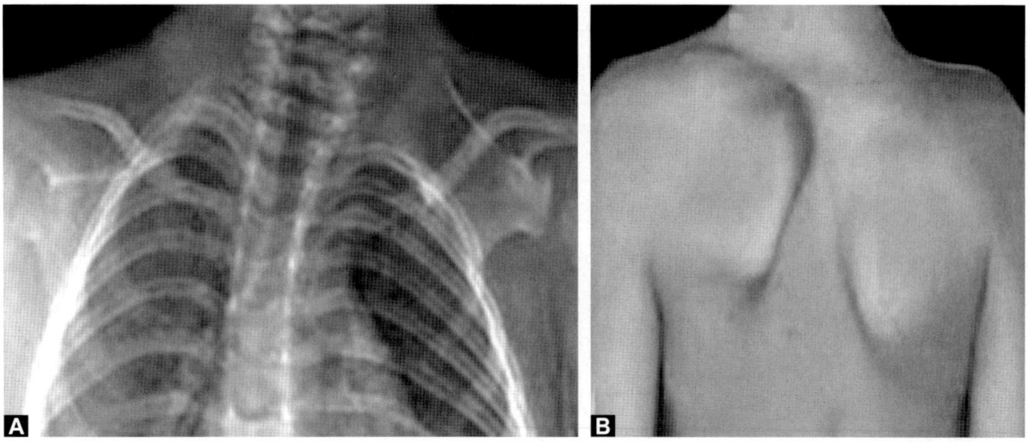

Figs 1.6A and B Chest X-ray PA view and photograph shows sprengel deformity of left scapula

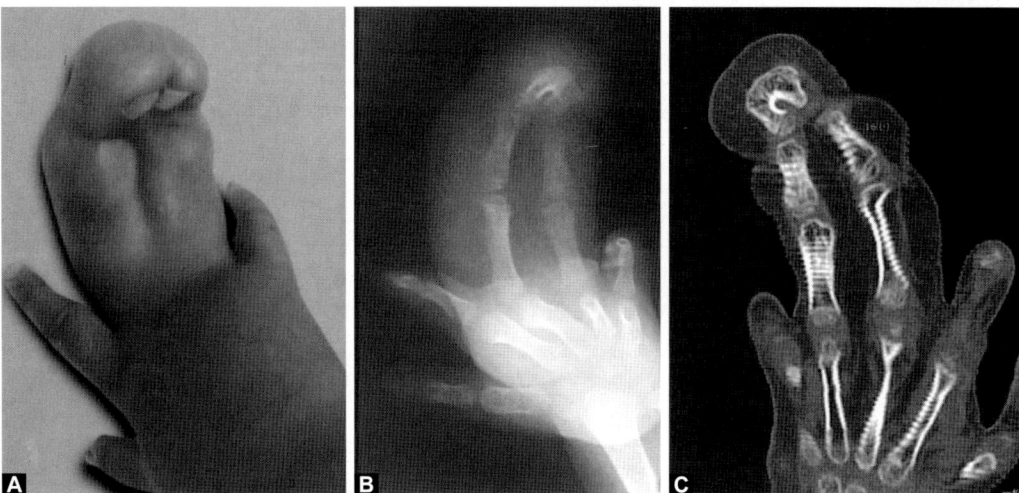

Figs 1.7A to C Clinical photograph of right hand shows enlarged, fused ring and middle finger. Plain radiograph (B) and coronal reformatted CT (C) shows soft tissue swelling and proliferation of fat on palmar aspect of the ring and middle fingers, along with dorsal angulation and syndactyly *(For color version, see plate 1)*

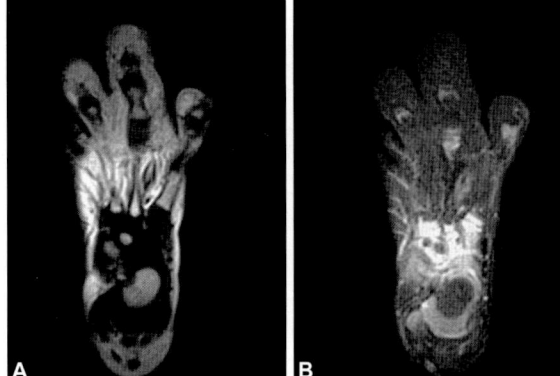

Figs 1.8A and B T1 coronal MRI (A) reveals proliferation of fatty tissue on plantar aspect of the second and third toes of right foot with signal intensity similar to that of subcutaneous fat as seen by fat suppressed STIR coronal image (B)

epiphysis of long bones which are fragmented small and flattened, loose bodies may also occur in joints. Metaphyseal irregularity is seen in tubular bones, when spine is involved there is irregularity of vertebral end plates **(Fig. 1.9)**.

Cleidocranial Dysostosis

Cleidocranial dysostosis, also called cleidocranial dysplasia is an autosomal dominant disorder resulting in delayed or failed ossification of midline bones, especially membranous bones but endochondral bones are also affected.

Patient usually present with large head, disproportionate small facial bones, narrow chest, sagging shoulders and may be with dwarfism or defective or delayed dentition.

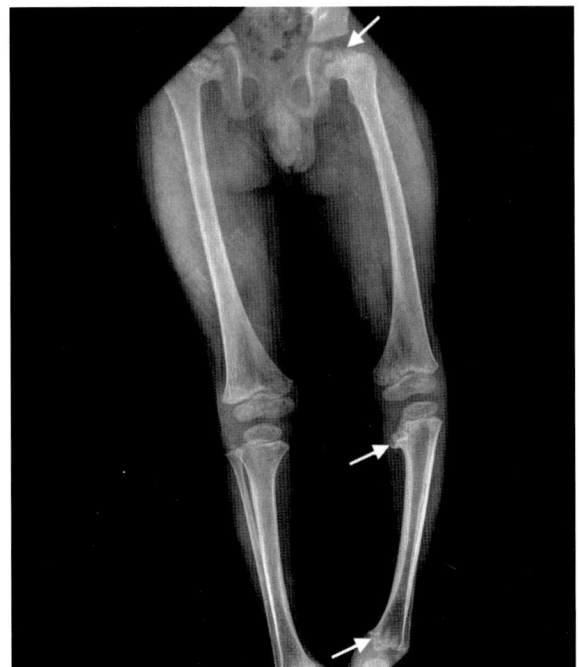

Fig. 1.9 A 5-year-old male with multiple epiphyseal dysplasia showing bilateral involvement long bones of lower limbs

Skull and Head

Radiographs of the skull show large head, large unossified areas, and failure of fusion at the fontanelles and sutures, and the presence of multiple wormian bones. Metopic suture is persistent. The bones of the base of the skull and face are small with small. Paranasal sinuses are hypoplastic. The jaws are often prognathous. Delayed eruption of the permanent teeth which may have faulty implantation and enamel defects. There may be an absence of some of the permanent teeth, or development of supernumerary teeth.

Chest

Defective formation of one or both clavicles is the most common finding from roentgen examinations. A variety of changes in the clavicles, from a simple transverse defect of the middle third, to complete absence of both clavicles. In the majority of cases the defects are found at the sternal ends. Thorax may be narrow or bell shaped. Sometimes supernumerary ribs are present.

Spine

Kyphosis, lordosis, and scoliosis may occur. Cervical ribs are common.

Pelvis

The pelvic bones frequently are abnormal in development. The pelvic canal is narrowed and the joint spaces are considerably widened, including the spaces between the ischium, ilium, and pubis at each acetabulum. The mature pelvis has broad, squat appearance associated with malformed, defective joints. Sacrum, iliac bones may be underdeveloped.

Extremities

There may be partial or complete absence of the radius. The distal phalanges are short and conical in shape. The middle phalanges are much shorter than normal and their lateral borders are concave, almost resulting in a dumb-bell shape. The metacarpal bones are expanded at their extremities and narrowed in the middle thirds, with some increase in the compact tissue at this level. Epiphyses frequently are seen at both ends of the basal phalanges and metacarpal bones. Femoral neck may be deformed, absent resulting in coxa vara.

Holt-Oram Syndrome

Holt-Oram syndrome is an inherited disorder that causes abnormalities of the hands, arms, spine and heart. Occurs approximately one in every 100,000 and affects both sexes equally **(Figs 1.10A to D)**.

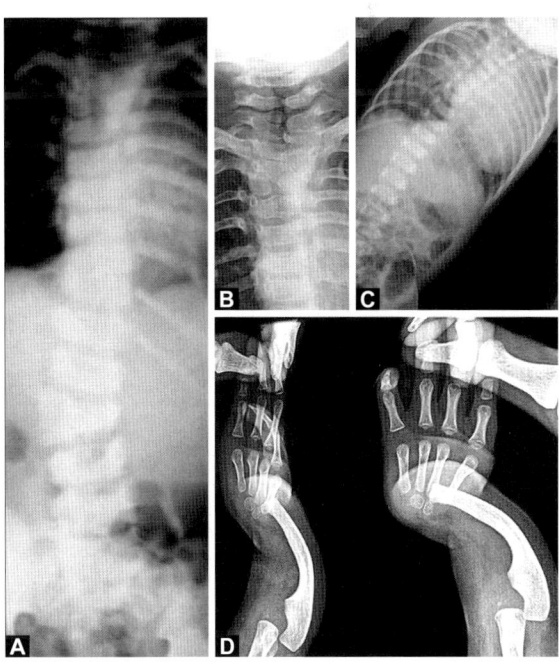

Figs 1.10A to D (A and B) X-rays spine show multiple spinal anomalies; (C) shows congenital heart disease; (D) shows absence of radius. All these are features of Holt-Oram syndrome

It falls into two groups: (A) Defects in arm and hand bones involving one or both sides of the body. Most commonly the defects are in the carpal bones and thumb. The thumb may be malformed or missing. In severe cases the arms may be very short such that the hands are attached close to the body (phocomelia). (B) Heart abnormalities—Three forth of cases with Holt-Oram syndrome heart abnormality. It may be abnormal rhythms, atrial or ventricular septal defect.

Fibrous Dysplasia

Fibrous dysplasia is a developmental anomaly of the mesenchymal precursor of bone, an idiopathic lesion of the medullary portion of bone. There is replacement and distortion of the medullary bone by fibro-osseous tissue of woven bone. Bones affected with fibrous dysplasia rarely undergo malignant degeneration. The appearance of new lesions usually terminates after skeletal maturity. Its cause is unknown and is usually found in the proximal femur, tibia, humerus, ribs, and craniofacial bones in decreasing order of incidence. These resemble tumor hence the name pseudotumoral fibrous dysplasia is used to describe rapidly growing and expanding lesions, giving rise to facial deformity and asymmetry. Fibrous dysplasia can be monostotic or polyostotic. Only one bone is involved in monostotic fibrous dysplasia. Less often, multiple bones are involved (polyostotic fibrous dysplasia). The polyostotic form is generally more severe and is discovered earlier. This form can involve as few as two bones in the same limb or multiple bones throughout the skeleton. Males and females are equally affected by the disorder. Cases are usually diagnosed within the first three decades of life. It is usually asymptomatic, though pain and swelling may accompany the lesion.

Polyostotic fibrous dysplasia is known to have multiple associations with other disorders. The combination of polyostotic fibrous dysplasia, precocious puberty, and Café au lait spots is called McCune Albright's syndrome. The association of fibrous dysplasia and soft tissue tumors has been given the name Mazabraud's syndrome. Other endocrine abnormalities including hyperthyroidism, Cushing's disease, thyromegaly, hypophosphatemia, and hyperprolactinemia have been associated with fibrous dysplasia.

Radiologic appearance in fibrous dysplasia varies according to the degree of fibrous tissue present which is seen replacing the medullary bone. Bone texture varies from a ground glass appearance to inhomogeneous mixture of bone and fibrous tissue. It appears as a well circumscribed lesion in a long bone with a ground glass or hazy appearance of the matrix. There is a narrow zone of transition and no periosteal reaction or soft tissue mass. The lesions are normally located in the metaphysis or diaphysis with occasional focal thinning of the overlying cortex due to scalloping from within. The radiological appearance can also be cystic, pagetoid, or dense and sclerotic. Repeated fractures through lesions in the proximal femur can result in the formation of a shepherd's crook deformity. MRI is helpful in delineating the extent of the lesion **(Figs 1.11 and 1.12)** and identifying possible pathological fractures and also sarcomatous

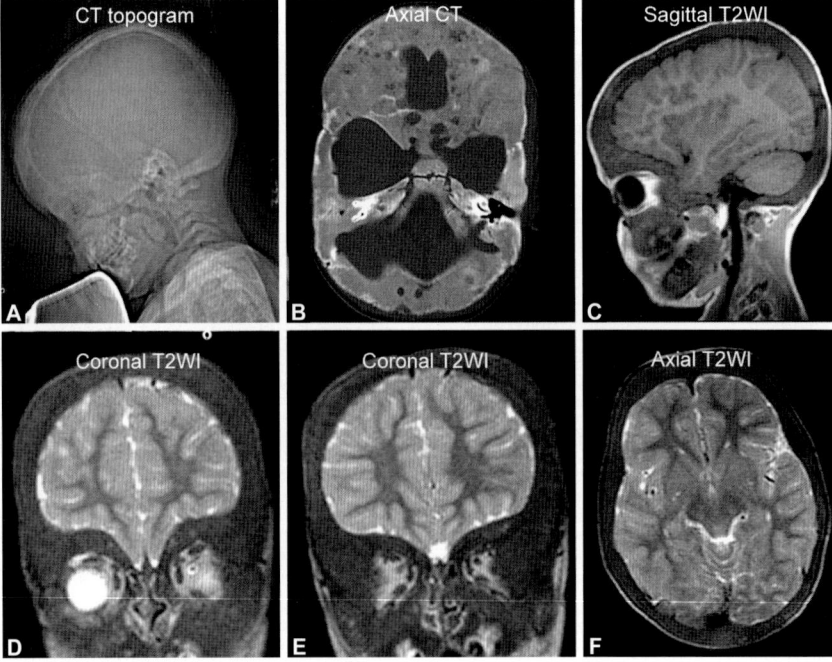

Figs 1.11A to F CT topogram (A) reveals diffuse thickening of calvarium. Axial CT (B) reveals diffuse thickening of calvarium, skull base with ground glass appearance. Sagittal, coronal and axial T2-weighted images (C to F) shows diffuse thickening of calvarium, skull base and maxillofacial bones

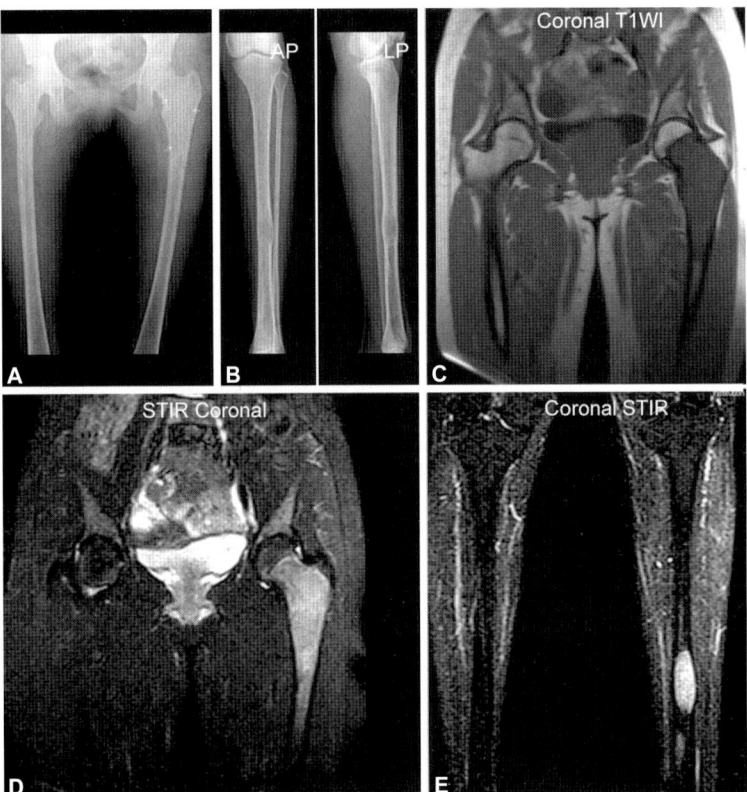

Figs 1.12A to E Fifteen-year-old female patient presented with complaint of left leg pain since seven months. X-ray of both hips and thigh AP (A) view shows expansile trabeculated lytic lesion in left femoral meta-diaphysis causing expansion of medullary cavity with thinning of cortex. X-ray left leg including knee joint, AP and lateral view (B) shows expansile lytic lesion seen in distal third shaft of tibia causing expansion of medullary cavity and thinning of cortex. T1W coronal image shows iso- to hypointense lesion in meta-diaphyseal region of left femur causing expansion of medullary cavity and thinning of cortex. Coronal STIR image (D) shows the lesion as hyperintense. STIR coronal (E) image of left thigh shows hyperintense lesion in distal third of left tibia causing expansion of medullary cavity and thinning of cortices. These findings suggest diagnosis of polyostotic fibrous dysplasia

change within the lesion. The lesions shows heterogeneous intermediate signal on T1W images and heterogeneously low signal on T2W images but may have regions of higher signal. Postcontrast T1W images show heterogeneous contrast enhancement. Bone scans demonstrate increased tracer uptake on Tc^{99} bone scans.

Fibrodysplasia Ossificans Progressiva

Fibrodysplasia ossificans progressiva (FOP) is a rare connective tissue disorder. A mutation of the body's repair mechanism causes fibrous tissue (muscle, tendon, and ligament) to be ossified when damaged. In many cases, injuries can cause joints to become permanently frozen in place.

The gene that causes ossification is normally deactivated after a fetus' bones are formed in the womb, but in patients with FOP, the gene keeps working. Aberrant bone formation in patients with FOP occurs in injured connective tissue or muscle cells at the sites of injury or growth **(Figs 1.13A and B)**.

The bone that results occurs independently of the normal skeleton, forming its own discrete skeletal elements. These elements, however, can fuse with normal skeletal bone. The symptoms are often misdiagnosed as fibrosis or malignancy. This leads to biopsies, which can actually exacerbate the growth of the lesion. The diaphragm, tongue and extra-ocular muscles cardiac and smooth muscle are spared.

Mucopolysaccharidoses

Mucopolysaccharidoses (MPSs) are a group of lysosomal storage diseases, due to an inherited deficiency of a lysosomal enzyme involved in the degradation of acid mucopolysaccharides leading to mental and motor retardation and bone changes. These diseases are autosomal recessive, except for type II, which is X-linked. The diagnosis is biochemical and based on assay of urinary excretion of the mucopolysaccharidoses. Seven distinct clinical types and numerous subtypes have been identified. Although each MPS differs clinically, most patients generally

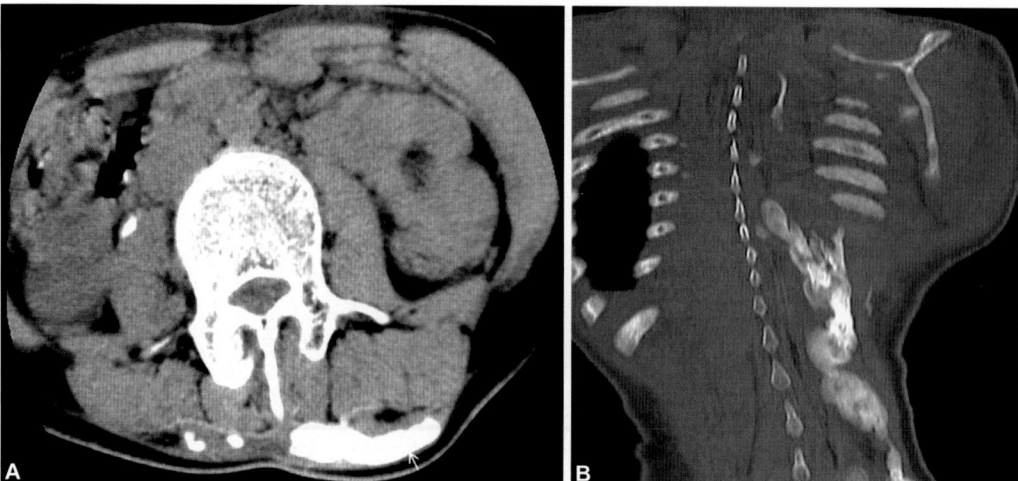

Figs 1.13A and B Plain CT scan coronal reconstructed and axial images showing abnormal extensive ossification in soft tissues

experience a period of normal development followed by a decline in physical and/or mental function.

MPS I H (Hurler Syndrome)

Hurler syndrome is caused by the enzyme deficiency alpha-L-iduronidase. There is excess urinary excretion of dermatan sulfate and heparan sulfate. Clinically, there is severe, progressive mental retardation. The children have a coarse facies, short stature, protuberant abdomen, hernias, joint contractures and a thoracolumbar gibbus **(Figs 1.14A to F)**. There is also hepatosplenomegaly, cardiomyopathy and cardiac failure. Radiologically, there is a large skull with a J-shaped sella, shallow orbits, breaking and flattening of the anterior portion of the vertebral bodies at the thoracolumbar junction, wide, thick ribs, thick clavicles, generalized symmetric damage of the epiphysis, widening of the shafts of the long bones with flaring of relatively small iliac wings with acetabular roofs. All the mucopolysaccharidoses share in common pointing of the bases of the metacarpals.

MPS I S (Scheie Syndrome)

Scheie syndrome (earlier called MPS V) is caused by deficiency of the alpha-L-iduronidase. There is abnormal urinary excretion of dermatan sulfate and heparan sulfate. Children have normal intelligence, stiff joints and corneal clouding. Radiologically, the changes are similar to Hurler's syndrome but with milder expression.

MPS II

Hunter syndrome is caused due to deficiency of alpha-iduronate sulfatase. Clinically, the physical appearances are similar to those of Hurler's syndrome but milder in expression. Intelligence has a spectrum ranging from near normal intelligence to mental retardation. Hepatosplenomegaly, hirsutism, flexion joint contractures and dorsolumbar kyphosis occur. Radiologically, the changes are similar though milder than in Hurler's syndrome.

MPS III

Sanfilippo's disease is divided into four types dependent upon alteration of a different enzyme needed to completely break down the heparan sulfate sugar chain. Clinically, there are mildly coarse facial features, corneal clouding, mild joint stiffness and severe mental and motor retardation, which is progressive. There is hepatosplenomegaly and cardiomyopathy. There is storage of heparan sulfate in the tissues. Radiologically, changes are similar to those in Hurler's syndrome.

MPS IV

Morquio's disease has two subtypes. In subtype: (a) the defect is N-acetylgalactosamine-6-sulfatase. In subtype (b) the enzyme defect is b galactosidase. Clinically it becomes evident between the age of one and three as the children present with short trunk, short stature, abnormal posture with a lumbar kyphois, pectus deformity, knock knee deformity, abnormal hands and feet, hyperextensible joints but are of normal intelligence. Corneal clouding is seen in type (b). Radiologically, the skeletal changes are different to Hurler's syndrome in that the skull shows only mild changes with underdevelopment of the mastoid air cells. There is platyspondyly, a small odontoid process of the axis with atlantoaxial subluxation, flaring of the ribs, pectus carinatum, constricted small iliac wings with steep acetabular roofs, coxa valga, secondary aseptic necrosis of the femoral head, often widening of the metaphyses and epiphyses at the knees with

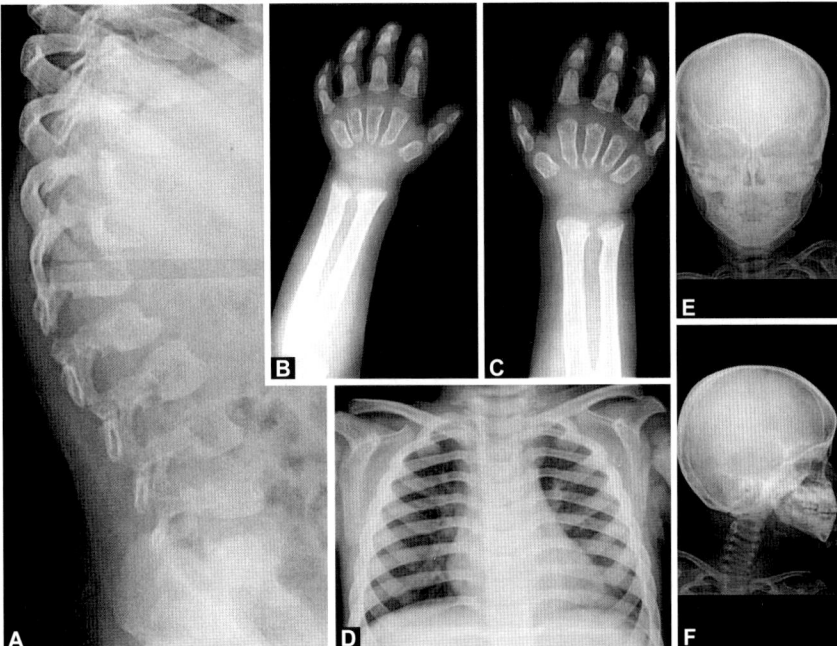

Figs 1.14A to F Spine shows thoracolumbar gibbus with breaking and flattening of the anterior portion of the vertebral bodies at the thoracolumbar junction (A), there is pointing (B and C) of the bases the metacarpals (feature shared by all the mucopolysaccharidoses), generalized symmetric damage of the epiphysis, widening of the shafts of the long bones (B and C), cardiomyopathy, thick clavicles with wide and thick ribs (D). Large skull with a J-shaped sella and shallow orbits (E and F)

secondary degenerative changes. The hands show the typical appearance of the pointed bases to the metacarpals with, in addition, irregularity of the carpal bones.

MPS VI

Maroteaux-Lamy syndrome is caused by deficiency of the enzyme arylsulfatase B. Coarse facies, corneal opacity, and small stature are the dominant clinical features. There may also be hepatosplenomegaly, aortic and mitral valve disease. Intelligence is normal. Radiologically, there is a spectrum of severity of disease. In general, the skull vault is large and is often thick with premature closure of the cranial sutures, short mandibular rami, oval vertebral bodies with a lower thoracic or upper lumbar kyphosis with wedging anteriorly, hypoplasia of the odontoid, small scapulae with hypoplastic glenoid fossae, aseptic necrosis of the femoral capital epiphyses, poorly developed acetabular roofs and diaphyseal widening of the long bones and pointed bases of the metacarpals.

MPS VII

Sly syndrome is caused by deficiency of the enzyme beta-glucuronidase. In its rarest form, Sly syndrome causes children to be born with hydrops fetalis, in which extreme amounts of fluid are retained in the body. Survival is usually a few months or less. Most children with Sly syndrome are less severely affected. Neurological symptoms may include mild to moderate mental retardation by age 3, communicating hydrocephalus, nerve entrapment, corneal clouding, and some loss of peripheral and night vision. Other symptoms include short stature, some skeletal irregularities, joint stiffness and restricted movement, and umbilical and/or inguinal hernias. Some patients may have repeated bouts of pneumonia during their first years of life. Most children with Sly syndrome live into the teenage or young adult years.

MPS IX

Natowicz syndrome results from hyaluronidase deficiency. Symptoms included nodular soft-tissue masses located around joints, with episodes of painful swelling of the masses and pain that ended spontaneously within 3 days. Pelvic radiography showed multiple soft-tissue masses and some bone erosion. Other traits included mild facial changes, acquired short stature as seen in other MPS disorders, and normal joint movement and intelligence.

MRI is the primary imaging technique to detect CNS alterations. The presence of white matter alterations is significantly correlated with mental retardation. Other possible CNS alterations are perivascular, subarachnoid and ventricular space enlargement and abnormalities of the basal ganglia, the corpus callosum, and the atlantoaxial joint.

Perthes Disease

Legg-Calvé-Perthes disease more frequently referred as Perthes disease **(Figs 1.15A to E)**. It is idiopathic avascular necrosis (AVN) of the growing femoral epiphysis seen in children; it is seen between the 4–8 years of age. The most common presenting feature is pain with or without a limp. 10% of cases show bilateral involvement.

Plain X-rays show in early stage of the disease:
- Smaller femoral epiphysis on affected side
- Apparent increased density of the femoral head epiphysis
- Widening of the medial joint space
- Blurring of the physeal plate
- Radiolucency of the proximal metaphysis

The late (stage 2) signs in the disease process include:
a. The femoral head begins to fragment with subchondral lucency (crescent) and (b) Redistribution of weight-bearing leading to thickening of few trabeculae which become more prominent.

Advanced burnt out (stage 4) of Perthes disease include:
a. Femoral head deformity with widening and flattening
b. Proximal femoral neck deformity
c. Tongues of cartilage may extend inferolaterally into the femoral neck, creating lucencies
d. The presence of metaphyseal involvement leads femoral neck deformity, and early physeal closure resulting in leg shortening.

Magnetic Resonance Imaging

Magnetic resonance imaging (MRI) provides early diagnosis **(Figs 1.15A to E)**, before the onset of X-ray findings, and in assessing extent of cartilaginous involvement, important in prognosis and assessing joint congruency in a variety of joint positions.

Both arthrography and dynamic MRI access:
- Deformity for the femoral head
- Congruency to shows batching of femoral head contour to that of the acetabulum
- *Containment:* To show the amount of lateral subluxation of the flattened femoral head out of the acetabulum.

Differential diagnosis include:
- Slipped superior femoral epiphysis
- Osteomyelitis
- Secondary causes of avascular necrosis (AVN)
- Dysplasia epiphysealis capitis femoris (Meyer dysplasia)
- Tumors
- Hemophilia
- Juvenile rheumatoid arthritis.

Prognosis depends on the degree of primary deformity of the femoral head and the secondary osteoarthritic change. The treatment aims to maintain good femoroacetabular contact and a round femoral head. Finally hip replacements may be necessary.

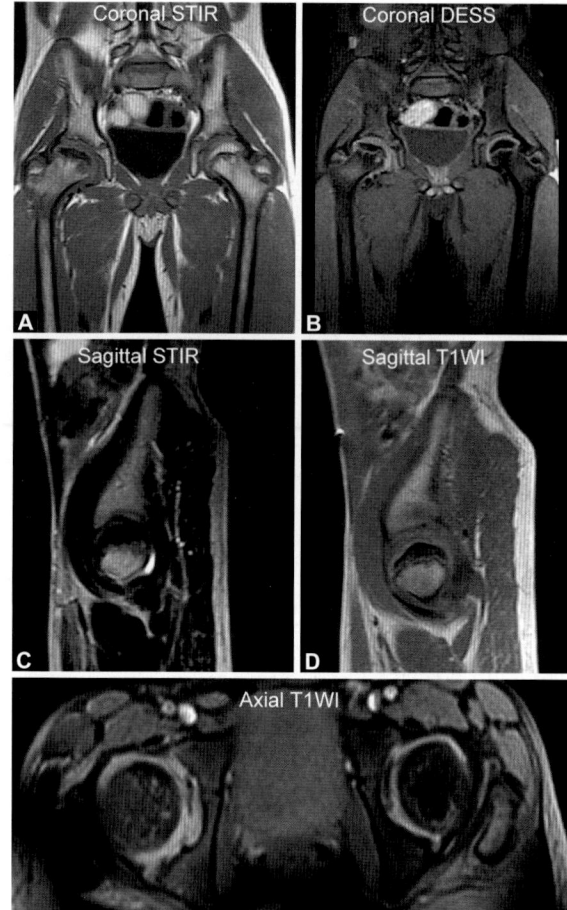

Figs 1.15A to E A 10 years male presented with pain in right hip and difficulty in cross leg sitting. MR images (A to E) show partial collapse with irregular contour of right femoral head epiphysis, predominantly hypointense signals on all pulse sequences suggestive of sclerosis. Mild effusion seen in right hip joint (E). Flattening of right femoral head is seen. Small cyst is seen in medial aspect of right femoral neck. Left femoral head, femoral neck and bilateral proximal shafts show normal appearances and signal pattern. Findings are suggestive of Perthes disease of right hip with mild joint effusion

Congenital Bifid Sternum

Congenital sternal cleft or bifid sternum is an isolated developmental defect of multifactorial etiology **(Fig. 1.16)**. It is the separation of the sternum with orthotopic normal heart and normal skin coverage. Sternal bands form in the sixth week of intrauterine life from the lateral plate mesoderm, and in the ninth week the fusion of these separate bands on either side of the anterior chest wall occurs in a craniocaudal direction. The manubrium ossification centers on each side of the mid-sternum are fused at birth and fusion of ossification centers in the sternal body is completed by the sixth year. Failure of fusion of the sternal body results in congenital sternal clefts. The treatment is the closure of primary defect in neonatal age, when flexibility of the chest wall is maximal and compression of underlying structures is minimal.

Bone Island or Enostosis

Bone island or enostosis represents a focus of mature compact (cortical) bone within the cancellous bone (spongiosa). Typically asymptomatic, this benign lesion is usually an incidental finding, with a preference for the pelvis, femur, and other long bones. On radiography it is seen as a homogeneously dense, sclerotic focus in the cancellous bone and on CT scan, a bone island appears as a high attenuation focus **(Figs 1.17A and B)**.

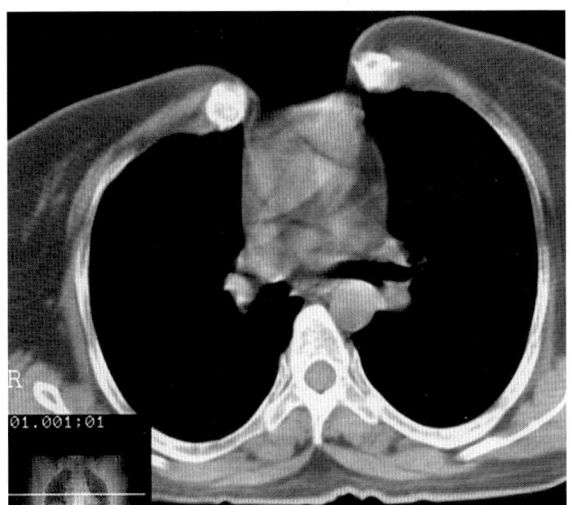

Fig. 1.16 Axial CT at mid-thorax shows broadly separated components of sternum in midline in a case of sternal cleft

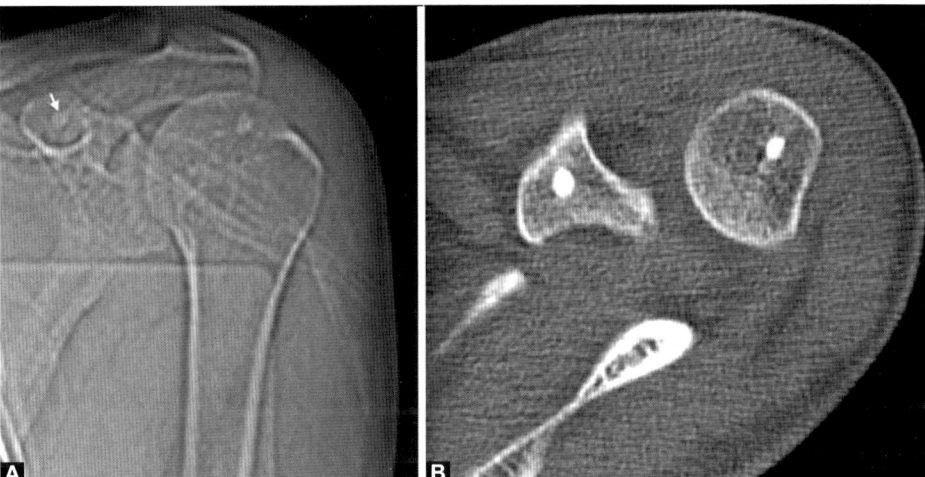

Figs 1.17A and B Scout image (A) and axial CT images (B) show two focal densely sclerotic compact bones in the spongiosa with thorny or brush borders. When the lesion is more than 20 mm it is known as giant bone island

2
Trauma

Patterns of Fracture

A fracture is a break in the continuity of a bone. It is important to assess the pattern of fracture as they can indicate the nature of causative violence.

The patterns of fracture are:
- *Incomplete fracture* involves only one cortical surface of the bone **(Fig. 2.1A)**.
- *Complete fracture* involves both the cortices with displaced or undisplaced fracture fragments **(Fig. 2.1B)**.
- *Linear fracture* could be transverse, oblique or spiral *fracture. Transverse fracture* is a fracture which forms an angle less than 30° with the horizontal line **(Fig. 2.1C)**. In oblique or spiral fractures, the angle is equal to or more than 30° with the horizontal line **(Figs 2.2A and B)**.
- *Comminuted fracture* **(Fig. 2.2C)** is characterized by three or more fracture fragments.
- *Segmental fracture* is one in which the bone breaks into segments which are at two or more levels, there may be longitudinal split or comminuted fracture **(Fig. 2.3A)**.
- *Impacted fracture* occurs when distal fragment of bone is driven into the proximal fragment.
- *Avulsion fracture* involves pulling loose of bony insertion by a muscle or ligament **(Fig. 2.3B)**.
- *Hairline fracture* is an undisplaced fracture with a fine fracture line **(Fig. 2.3C)**.
- *Occult fracture* is suspected clinically but is not visualized on initial radiographic examination.

Healing of Fracture

The pathological process of healing of a fractured bone occurs in the following stages:
- Hematoma formation
- Subperiosteal and endosteal cellular proliferation
- Callus formation **(Figs 2.4A and B)**
- Consolidation
- Remodeling

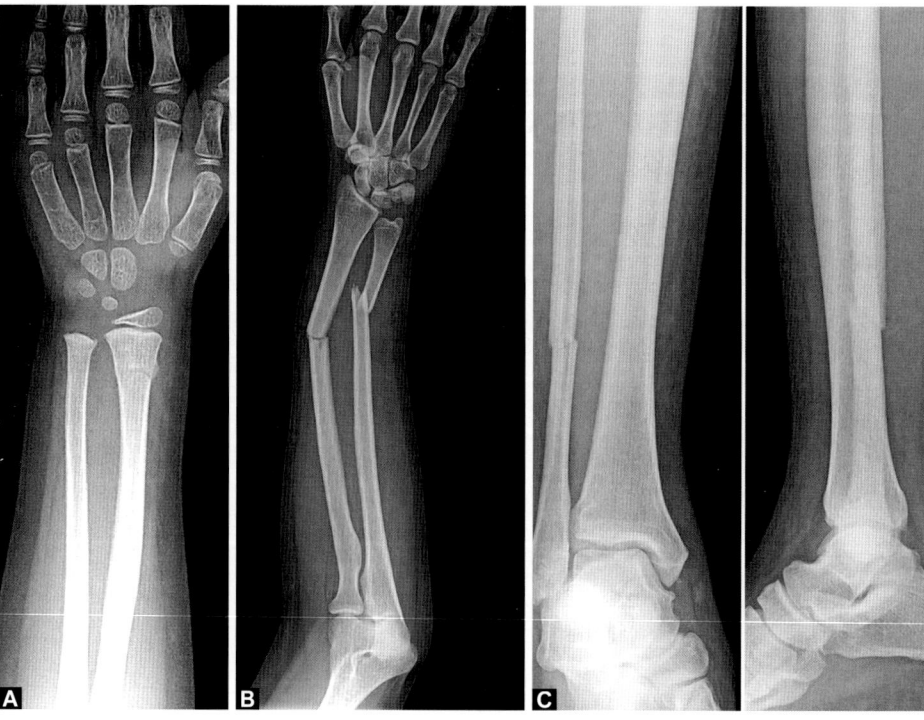

Figs 2.1A to C X-rays show: (A) Incomplete fracture; (B) Complete fracture; (C) Linear transverse fracture

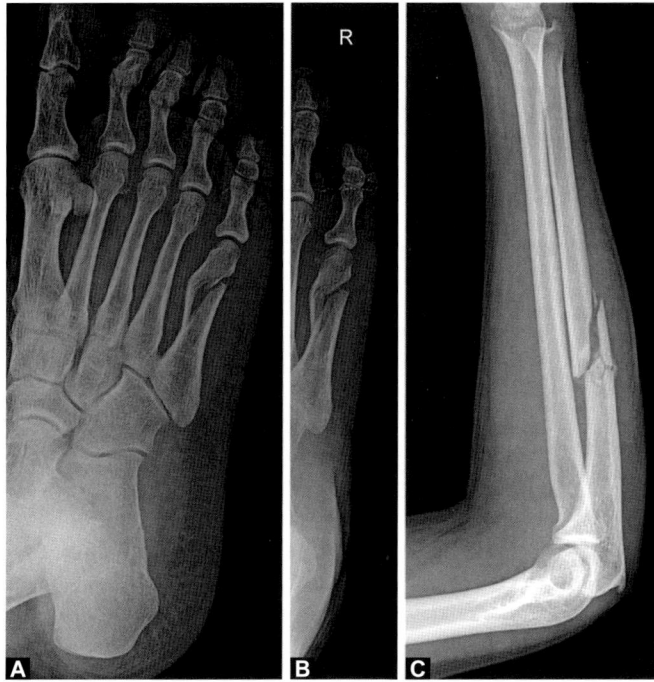

Figs 2.2A to C X-rays show: (A and B) Linear spiral oblique fracture; and (C) Comminuted fracture

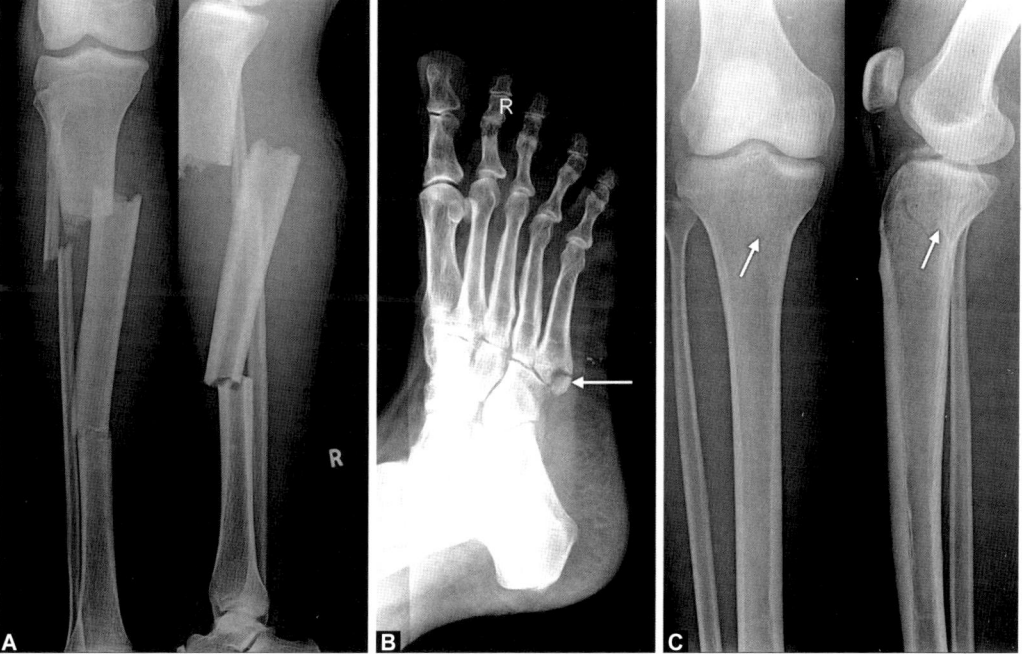

Figs 2.3A to C X-rays show: (A) Segmental fracture; (B) Avulsion fracture (arrow); (C) Hairline fracture (arrows)

Initially, there is hematoma formation which is limited by stripped periosteum. In case of torn periosteum, the hematoma is limited by the muscles, fascia and skin. This is followed by stage of cellular proliferation in the subperiosteum and endosteum in the fractured fragments, which gradually develop towards each other, with the absorption of blood clot. The cellular tissue matures to form osteoblasts, which lays down an intercellular matrix, the matrix is then impregnated with calcium, and this is callus formation, and this is the first radiological sign that indicates healing of fracture. The callus gradually transforms into more mature bone with a lamellar structure in the form of periosteal reaction, leading to union or consolidation of the fracture. After this, there is remodeling stage with gradual strengthening of the bone along the lines of stress.

Factors which influence healing process are:
- Efficacy of immobilization
- Interposition of soft tissue
- Alignment of fracture fragments vascular and neural integrity

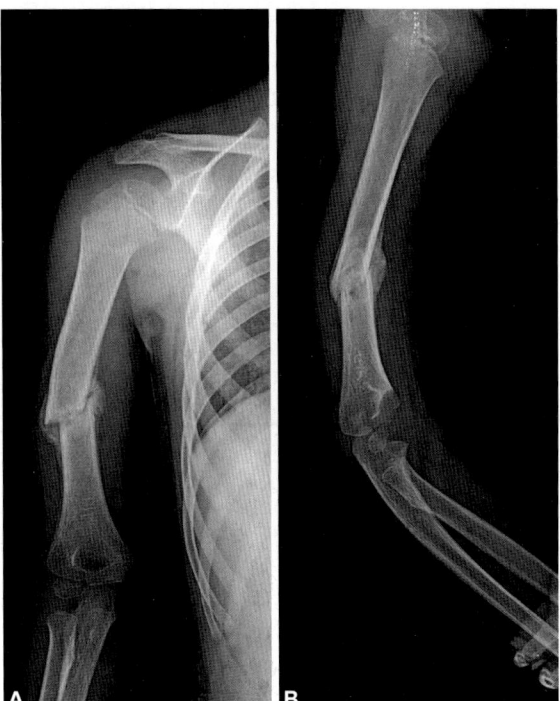

Figs 2.4A and B X-ray shows fracture of mid shaft humerus with callus formation and bridging of the fractured fragments

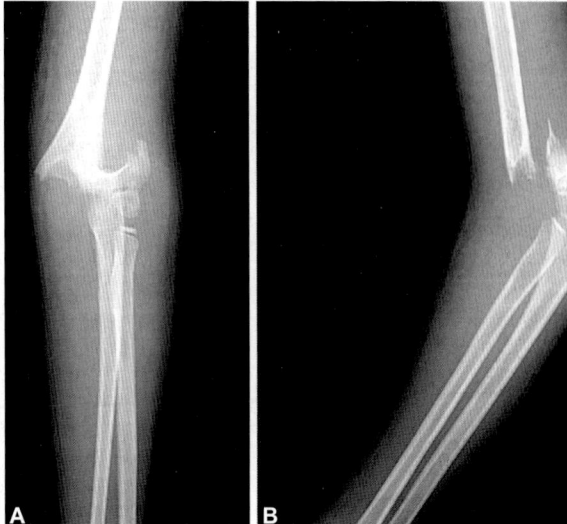

Figs 2.5A and B Supracondylar fracture of humerus takes place due to mechanism hyperextension at elbow with vertical stress. It is a transverse fracture line and the distal fragment posteriorly displaced/tilted

- Local and systemic disease
- Age of the patient.

Radiological criteria of union are demonstration of visible callus, bridging of the fracture fragments **(Figs 2.4A and B)** and blending them with continuity of bony trabeculae across the fracture.

Fall on Outstretched Hand

Fall on outstretched hand can lead to injuries at the level of arm, elbow, forearm and wrist:
- Common injuries at various levels are:
  - *Arm:*
    - Fracture proximal humerus
    - Oblique/spiral fracture of shaft of humerus
  - *Elbow:*
    - Supracondylar fracture of humerus takes place due to mechanism hyperextension at elbow with vertical stress. It is a transverse fracture line and the distal fragment posteriorly displaced/tilted **(Figs 2.5A and B)**
    - Dislocation of elbow joint
    - Radius head fracture
    - Fracture of capitellum
  - *Forearm:*
    - Colle's fracture
    - Monteggia fracture dislocation
    - Galeazzi fracture **mechanism** fall on outstretched hand with elbow-flexed radial shaft fracture with subluxation/dislocation of distal radioulnar joint **(Figs 2.6A and B)**

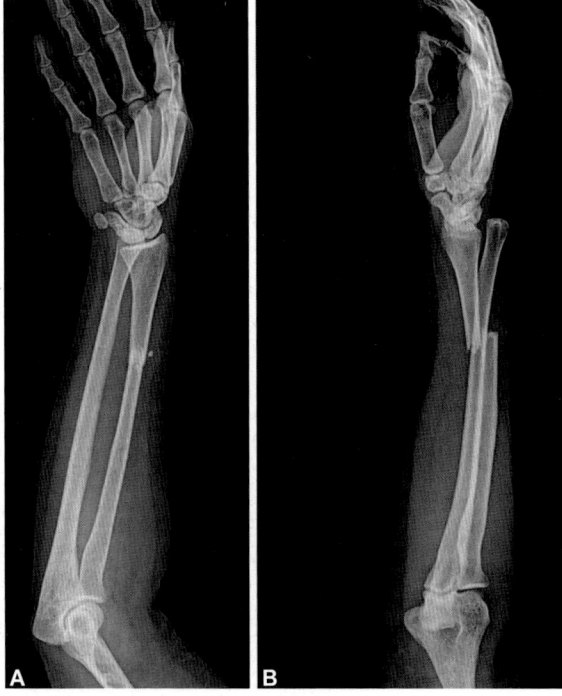

Figs 2.6A and B Galeazzi fracture mechanism fall on outstretched hand with elbow-flexed radial shaft fracture with subluxation/dislocation of distal radioulnar joint

  - *Wrist:*
    - Scaphoid fracture **(Fig. 2.7)**
    - Dorsal chip radius fracture
    - Lunate and other carpal bone fractures

Common fractures at the distal end of forearm or radius following a fall on outstretched hand are:
- Colle's fracture is the most common fracture of forearm which results from fall on outstretched hand. It is nonarticular radial fracture with dorsal

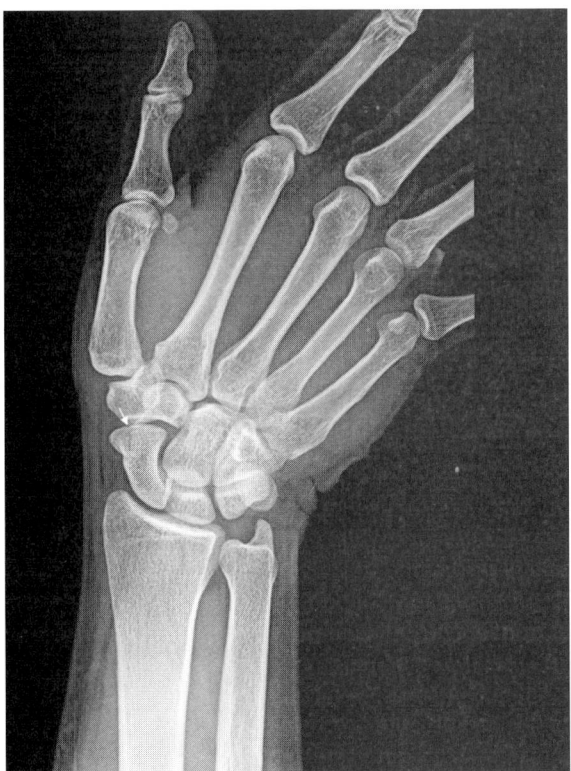

Fig. 2.7 Scaphoid fracture

displacement of distal fragment **(Fig. 2.8A)**. It is fracture of lower end of the radius, at 2.5 cm above the carpal extremity of radius with fracture dislocation of the inferior radioulnar joint. It is characterized by dorsal displacement, dorsal tilt, lateral displacement, lateral tilt, impaction and supination of the distal fragment or fragments.

Complications of Colle's fracture include:
- *Early complications:*
  - Postreduction swelling
  - Injury to proximal segment of bone
  - Median or ulnar nerve damage
  - Compartment syndrome
- *Late complications:*
  - Complications
  - Malunion
  - Rupture of the extensor pollicis longus
  - Sudeck's osteodystrophy
  - Frozen shoulder
  - Carpal tunnel syndrome
  - Nonunion

- Smith's fracture is reverse Colle's fracture; the mechanism involved is hyperflexion with fall on back of hand. It is nonarticular distal radial fracture with ventral displacement of fragment **(Fig. 2.8B)**.
- Barton's fracture is intra-articular oblique fracture of ventral or dorsal lip of distal radius **(Fig. 2.9A)**.

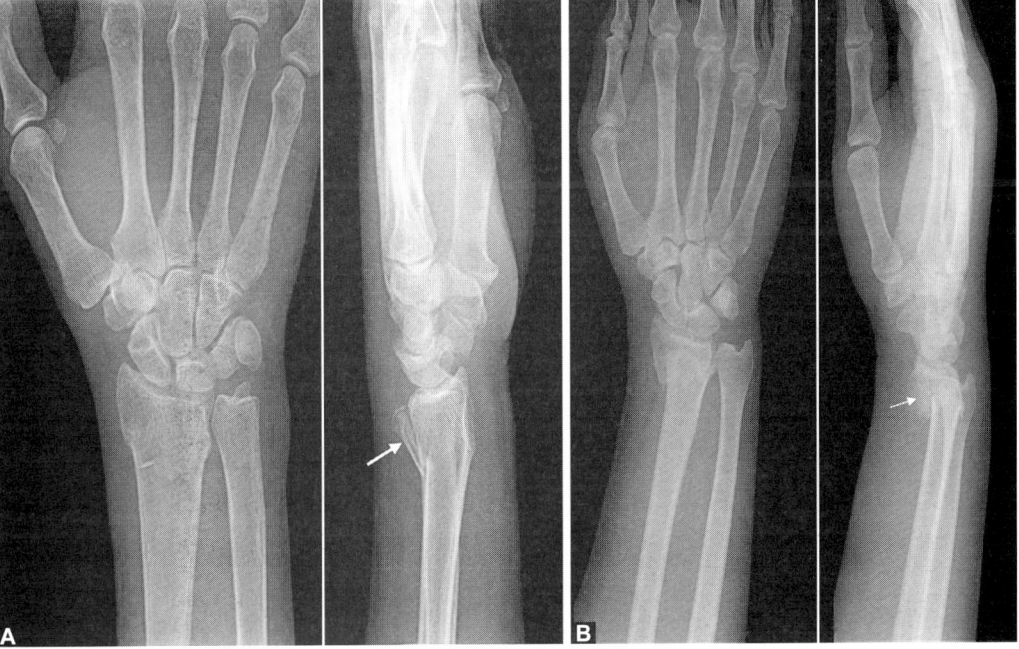

Figs 2.8A and B (A) Colle's fracture is the most common fracture of forearm which results from fall on outstretched hand. It is nonarticular radial fracture with dorsal displacement of distal fragment; (B) Smith's fracture is reverse Colle's fracture; the mechanism involved is hyperflexion with fall on back of hand. It is nonarticular distal radial fracture with ventral displacement of fragment

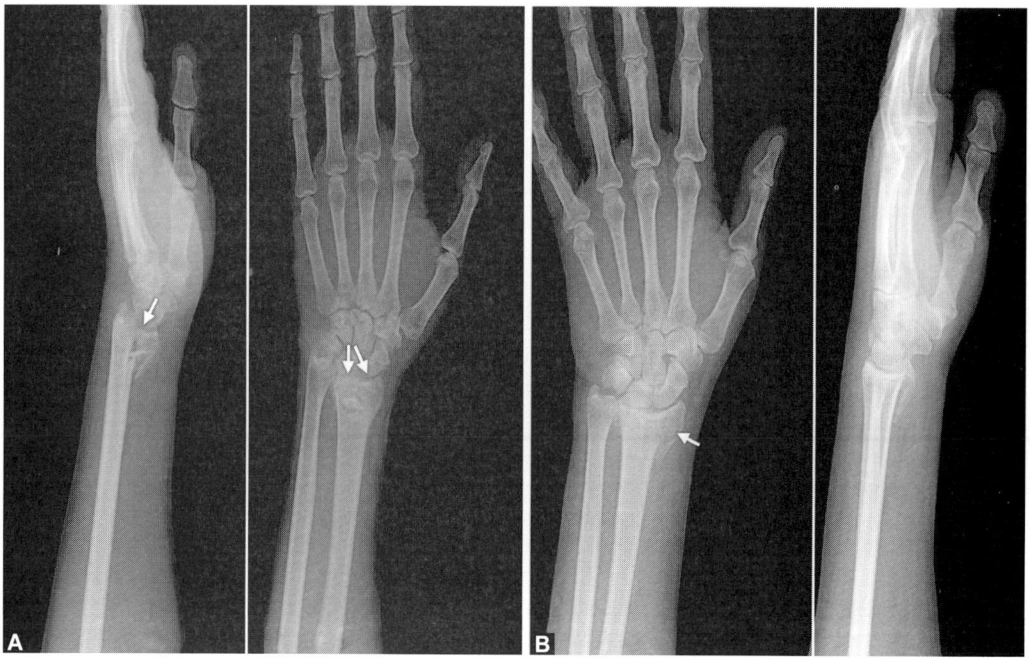

Figs 2.9A and B (A) Barton's fracture is intra-articular oblique fracture of ventral or dorsal lip of distal radius; (B) Chauffeur's fracture is also known as Hutchinson, backfire or lorry driver fracture. The mechanism involved is direct trauma to radial side of wrist sustained from recoil of crank; vintage vehicles were started with a crank resulting in acute dorsiflexion and abduction of hand. This resulted in distal radial styloid process fracture of triangular appearance

- Chauffeur's fracture also known as Hutchinson, backfire or lorry driver fracture. The mechanism involved is direct trauma to radial side of wrist sustained from recoil of crank; vintage vehicles were started with a crank resulting in acute dorsiflexion and abduction of hand. This resulted in distal radial styloid process fracture of triangular appearance **(Fig. 2.9B)**.

Fracture

Fracture is defined as complete disruption in the continuity of the bone. Types of fracture include:
- *Incomplete fracture* involves only one cortical surface of the bones, e.g. acute plastic bowing, torus, i.e. buckling of cortex and greenstick, i.e. fracture of one cortex. All these varieties are seen in children.
- *Complete fracture* involves both the cortices with displaced or undisplaced fracture fragments.
- *Linear fracture* could be transverse, oblique or spiral fracture. Transverse fracture is a fracture which forms an angle less than 30° with the horizontal line. In oblique or spiral fractures, the angle is equal to or more than 30° with the horizontal line.
- *Comminuted fracture* is characterized by three or more fracture fragments.
- *Segmental fracture* is one in which the bone breaks into segmental two or more levels, there may be longitudinal split or comminuted fracture.
- *Impacted fracture* occurs when distal fragment of bone is driven into the proximal fragment.
- *Avulsion fracture* involves pulling loose of bony insertion by a muscle or ligament.
- *Hairline fracture* is an undisplaced fracture with a fine fracture line.
- *Occult fracture* is suspected clinically but is not visualized on initial radiographic examination.

Imaging Features of Fracture

Fracture line is the direct evidence of fracture which is seen as a cortical break or cortical discontinuity. Indirect signs include:
- *Soft tissue swelling:* Skeletal trauma is always associated with soft tissue swelling. Absence of soft tissue swelling, however, virtually excludes the possibility of acute fracture.
- *Obliteration or displacement of fat stripes:* Subtle fractures, particularly in the distal radius, carpal scaphoid, trapezium and base of the metacarpal result in obliteration or displacement of fascial planes. Fracture of distal radius results in the appearance of the pronator quadrates fat stripe, which may be anteriorly displaced, blurred or obliterated. Obliteration of scaphoid fat stripe (which is usually visible as a thin radiolucent line paralleling the lateral surface of scaphoid) occurs in most fractures of scaphoid, styloid process of radius bone trapezium, base of the first metacarpal.
- *Periosteal and endosteal reaction:* Fracture line may not be visible sometimes but the periosteal or endosteal response may be the first radiographic sign visible.

- *Joint effusion:* It results in the radiographic appearance of the fat pad sign which is particularly useful in diagnosing elbow injuries. The posterior (dorsal) pad of fat lies deep in the olecranon fossa and is not visible in the lateral projection. The anterior fat pad occupies the shallower anterior coronoid and radial fossae and is usually seen as flat radiolucent strip ventral to the anterior cortex of the humerus.
- *Intracapsular fat-fluid level:* If the fracture involves a joint, then blood and bone marrow fat enter the joint (lipohemarthrosis) and produce characteristic layering of these two substances called the fat-blood interface or fat-blood interface (FBI) sign.
- *Double cortical line:* This finding indicates a subtle but depressed fracture.
- *Buckling of the cortex:* It is also known as the torus fracture which may be the only sign of a tubular bone fracture in children.
- *Irregular metaphyseal corners:* It is secondary to small avulsion fractures of the metaphysis and indicates a subtle injury to the bone caused by a rapid rotation force exerted on the ligaments.

Complications of Fractures

Early Complications

- *Local:*
  - Vascular injury causing hemorrhage, internal or external
  - Visceral injury causing damage to structures such as brain, lung or bladder
  - Damage to surrounding tissue, nerves or skin
  - Hemarthrosis
  - *Compartment syndrome (or Volkmann's ischemia):* Fractures of the limbs can cause severe ischemia by damage to a major artery or by increasing the osteofascial compartment pressure by swelling due to bleeding or edema. This causes decreased capillary flow inturn leading to muscle ischemia with more edema and more pressure and finally increased capillary flow. Thus there is rapid pressure build-up leading to muscle and nerve necrosis. Compartment syndromes can also result from crush injuries (falling debris or simple compression, if patient unconscious for length of time) or an over-tight cast.
  - Wound infection, more common for open fractures
- *Systemic:*
  - Fat embolism
  - Shock
  - Thromboembolism (pulmonary or venous)
  - Exacerbation of underlying diseases such as diabetes or CAD
  - Pneumonia

Late Complications

- *Systemic complications* include gangrene, tetanus, septicemia and osteoarthritis.
- *Local:*
  - *Delayed union* refers to a fracture that does not unite within a reasonable amount of time (16-18 weeks) depending on the patient's age and the fracture site.
  - *Nonunion* refers to a fracture that simply does not unite. A pseudoarthrosis is a variant of nonunion in which there is formation of a false joint cavity with a synovial like capsule and synovial fluid at the fracture site. Radiographically, nonunion is characterized by rounded edges, smoothness and sclerosis (eburnation of the fragments ends which are separated by a gap and motion between the fragments.

    Three types of nonunion are seen which include reactive, nonreactive and infected.
    - *Reactive (hypertrophic and oligotrophic) nonunion:* Radiographically, this type of nonunion is characterized by exuberant bone reaction and resultant flaring and sclerosis of bone ends, the elephant foot or horse hoof type.
    - *Nonreactive (Atrophic) nonunion:* Radiographically, it shows absence of reaction at the fragment ends and the blood supply is very scanty.
    - *Infected nonunion:* Radiographic presentation of infected nonunion depends on the infectious activity. Old inactive osteomyelitis shows irregular thickening of the cortex, well-organized periosteal reaction and reactive sclerosis of cancellous bone whereas active form shows soft tissue swelling, destruction of cortex and cancellous bone associated with periosteal new bone formation and sequestration
  - *Malunion:* It is characterized by union of the bony fragments in a faulty and unacceptable manner.
  - *Contractures:* It usually develops after fractures such as supracondylar fractures. For example, Volkmann contracture is caused by ischemia of the muscles followed by the fibrosis. Clinically, it is characterized by pulselessness, pain, pallor, paraesthesias and paralysis.
  - *Myositis ossificans:* Calcifications and bony masses develop within muscle and can occur as a complication of fractures, especially humeral supracondylar fractures. It presents with pain, tenderness, focal swelling, and joint/muscle contractions. Avoid excessive physiotherapy, rest the joint until pain subsides, NSAIDs may be helpful

and consider excision after the lesion has stabilized (usually 6–24 months).
- *Avascular necrosis:* It occurs after fracture or dislocation when the bone is deprived of a sufficient supply of arterial blood. It can occur even without trauma.
- *Algodystrophy (or Sudeck's atrophy):* Sudeck's atrophy is a form of reflex sympathetic dystrophy (or complex regional pain syndrome type 1), usually affecting hand or foot generally following trauma, especially fractures. Clinically, there is continuous, burning pain with initial local swelling, warmth and redness which progresses to pallor and atrophy. Movement is reduced significantly. Treatment is usually rehabilitation (physiotherapy and occupational therapy) to decrease sensitivity and gradually increase exercise tolerance along with psychological therapy. Pain management is often difficult. Approaches used are neuropathic pain medications (e.g. amitriptyline, gabapentin, opioids), steroids, calcitonin, IV bisphosphonates and regional blocks.
- *Growth disturbance or deformity:* A Salter-Harris type IV and V fractures involving the physis, growth disturbance may result from injury to the growth plate by the formation of an osseous bridge between the epiphysis and metaphysis. As a result of this tethering of the growth plate, localized cessation of the bone growth occurs.

Stress Fracture

Stress fracture is failure of the skeleton to withstand submaximal forces over time. Two forms of stress fracture have been defined:
- Fatigue fracture
- Insufficiency fracture.

Fatigue fracture is classically described in Army recruits and runners in whom normal bone is exposed to repeated abnormal stresses.

Insufficiency fracture results when normal stress is applied to abnormal bone (osteoporosis or Paget's disease).

Stress fractures are most common in the weight-bearing bones of the lower extremity, especially the leg and the foot. The most common sites include:
- Femoral neck
- Proximal tibia
- Distal fibula
- Tarsal bones
- Metatarsals.

A stress fracture is an overuse injury. Bone is constantly attempting to remodel and repair itself, especially when extraordinary stress is applied. When enough stress is placed on the bone, it causes an imbalance between osteoclastic and osteblastic activity and a stress fracture may appear. Muscle fatigue can also play a role in the occurrence of stress fractures. Mechanical factors such as bone density, skeletal alignment and body size and composition, physiological factors such as bone turnover rate, flexibility, muscular strength and endurance, as well as hormonal and nutritional factors are the important factors. Extrinsic risk factors include mechanical factors such as surface, footwear and external loading as well as physical training parameters menstrual disturbances, caloric restriction; lower bone density, muscle weakness and leg length differences are risk factors for stress fracture.

Imaging features of stress fractures include:

Radiography

On plain film radiography, stress fractures usually appear as sclerosed areas and often are oriented linearly. A focal periosteal reaction or a cortical break also may be present. A history of repetitive stress may not always be obtained. Occasionally, a stress fracture may have the appearance of aggressive periostitis without a linear sclerosis. Many a times, stress fractures are not seen on plain radiography, then comes the role of other modalities such as CT, MR or nuclear imaging.

Computed Tomography

Computed tomography (CT) scanning occasionally may be performed to diagnose stress fractures. Disruption of the bony cortex usually can be demonstrated through CT scanning, and evidence of periostitis can also be detected in this way. The sensitivity of CT scans is higher than that of plain films. However, compared with MRI or bone scanning, the sensitivity of CT scanning with regard to stress reactions and fractures is rather low, resulting in a high rate of false negatives. Thus, in the appropriate clinical setting, CT scanning can be skipped, and either MRI or a bone scan can be performed. Repeat CT scanning is not an attractive alternative, although it can result in the correct diagnosis because of the interval development of osteonecrosis.

Magnetic Resonance Imaging

Magnetic resonance imaging (MRI) has surpassed bone scintigraphy as the imaging tool for stress fractures, showing equal sensitivity (100%) but a higher specificity (85%), probably by giving better anatomical detail and more precisely depicting the tissues involved. Short tau inversion recovery (STIR), T1-weighted (T1WI) and T2-weighted images (T2WI) are used for characterization and grading.

Grading is based on signs seen at MRI:
- Mild-moderate periosteal edema on STIR, no marrow changes
- Moderate-severe periosteal edema on STIR + marrow changes on T2WI
- 2 + marrow changes on T1WI
- Fracture line visible

Low signal on T1- and T2-weighted images is the classic appearance of a stress fracture on magnetic resonance images **(Figs 2.10A to E)**. MRI is often useful in patients with severe osteoporosis, in whom skeletal scintigraphy may produce false negatives because of generalized poor uptake of the tracer. MRI is highly sensitive for the detection of bone marrow changes. Better anatomic resolution also is an advantage. This is particularly helpful in the case of small joints of the hands and feet, in which the relatively poor spatial resolution of the radionuclide bone scan can be a disadvantage. MRI also has the advantage of distinguishing between arthritis, osteomyelitis, and osteonecrosis all of which potentially can have the same appearance on a bone scan.

Nuclear Imaging

Typically, the stress fracture appears as a low signal band that arises from the cortex of the bone and extends perpendicular to the surface of the bone. Typically, stress fractures are associated with hyperemia in the first 2 phases of the 3-phase bone scan. This is manifested by increased tracer activity at the affected site. If an image of the contralateral side is available, the hyperemia is easier to detect. While detection of hyperemia is not difficult in adults, increased tracer activity around the epiphyses of pediatric patients may be difficult to detect in the absence of contralateral images. The first phase demonstrates increased blood flow in the arterial phase, and the second phase demonstrates the presence of tissue hyperemia. The third phase demonstrates increased osteoblastic activity in response to the stress fracture.

Segond Fracture

The segond fracture is an avulsion fracture of the lateral condyle of the tibia, immediately beyond the surface, which articulates with the femur. It occurs as a result of avulsion of the medial third of the lateral collateral ligament. It may be associated with tears of the anterior cruciate ligament (ACL) and injury to the medial meniscus as well as injury to the structures behind the knee. The mechanism of occurrence is abnormal varus or "bowing" stress to the knee, combined with internal rotation of the knee.

Plain X-ray knee AP film shows a small avulsion or chip fragment at the lateral tibial condyle. This chip

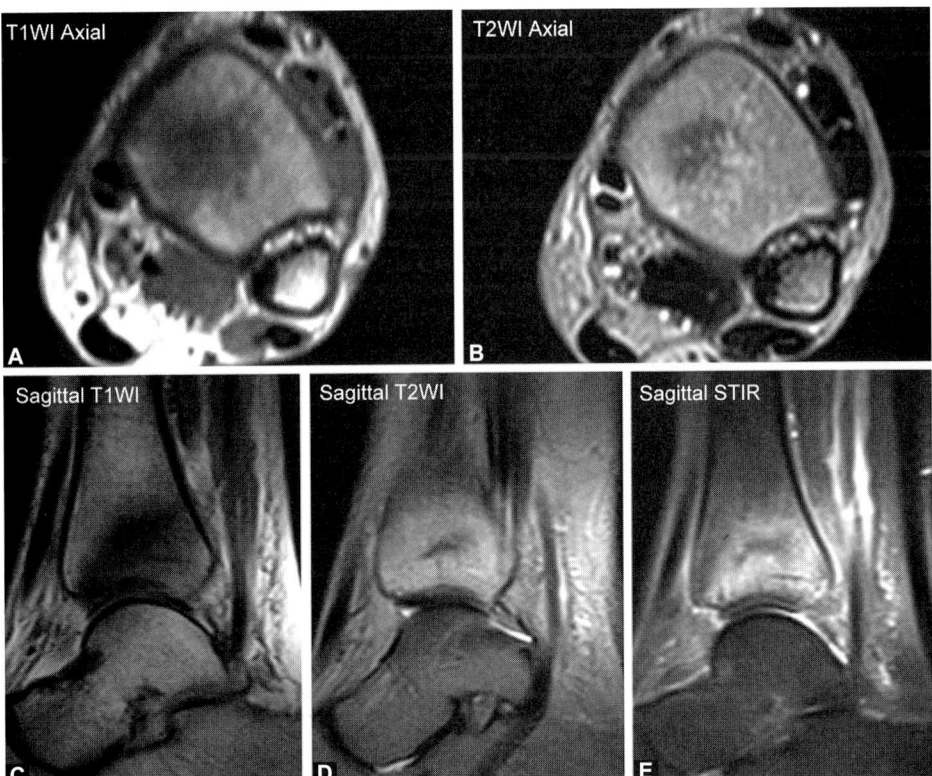

Figs 2.10A to E A 32-year male, athlete with history of ankle pain shows on MRI a linear zone of low signal intensity which indicates fracture line with surrounding boarder, poorly defined area of higher signal intensity suggestive of marrow edema on T2-weighted and STIR (B, D and E) MR images and appearing hypointense on T1W images (A and C). Similar changes are seen on axial images thus making a diagnosis stress fracture at distal metaphysis of tibia

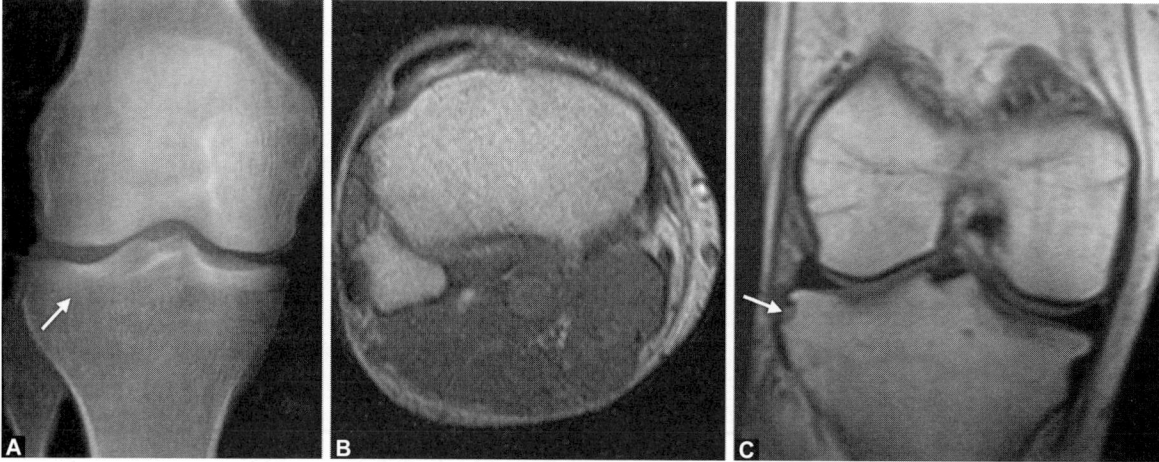

Figs 2.11A to C (A) A X-ray (anteroposterior) of knee shows a small chip of bone at the lateral condyle of the tibia immediately beyond the surface which articulates with the femur. T1W axial image (B) shows a well-defined round hypointensity at the anterolateral corner of tibial condyle, which is an avulsion fracture. Coronal T1W image (C) shows a well-defined round hypointensity at the anterolateral corner of tibial condyle similar to the avulsion fracture seen on plain X-ray

of bone is better seen on CT scan (**Fig. 2.11A**). MRI (**Figs 2.11B and C**). is useful for visualization of the associated bone marrow edema of the underlying tibial plateau on fat saturated T2W and STIR images, and to see associated findings of ligament and meniscal injury.

Avulsion Fracture

Acute avulsion injuries of greater tuberosity of humerus result from extreme, unbalanced, and often eccentric muscular contractions, and patients with such injuries present with severe pain and loss of function. In contrast, chronic avulsion injuries are the result of repetitive micro-trauma or overuse and usually occur during organized sports activities, such as athletes.

Most often the injury is abrupt and a clear history is available as in this case, which makes clinical and radiographic diagnoses easy. It is difficult to distinguish between isolated humeral avulsion fractures of the greater tuberosity and rotator cuff tears at clinical examination. The distinction is crucial, however, because treatment of the two injuries is different. At radiography, the fracture may not be readily apparent. Most of these sites, the fracture plane is through the physis of an apophysis. An apophysis acts as the insertion site for muscle and the physis represent a weak link in the immature skeleton. Radiographs generally confirm the diagnosis by demonstrating a bony fragment displaced at variable distance from the parent bone.

Magnetic resonance imaging (MRI) shows the fracture to greater advantage (**Figs 2.12A and B**).

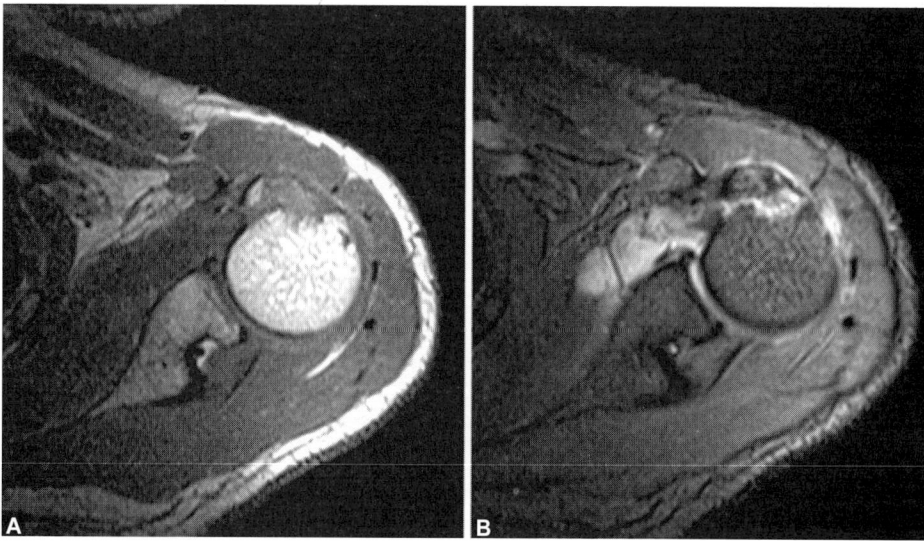

Figs 2.12A and B A 35-year-old male with history of fall from a horse onto his outstretched arm on axial T1W (A) and gradient weighted; (B) Axial images show medially displaced avulsion fracture of the greater tuberosity of humerus at the attachment of the subscapularis tendon. Joint effusion is present

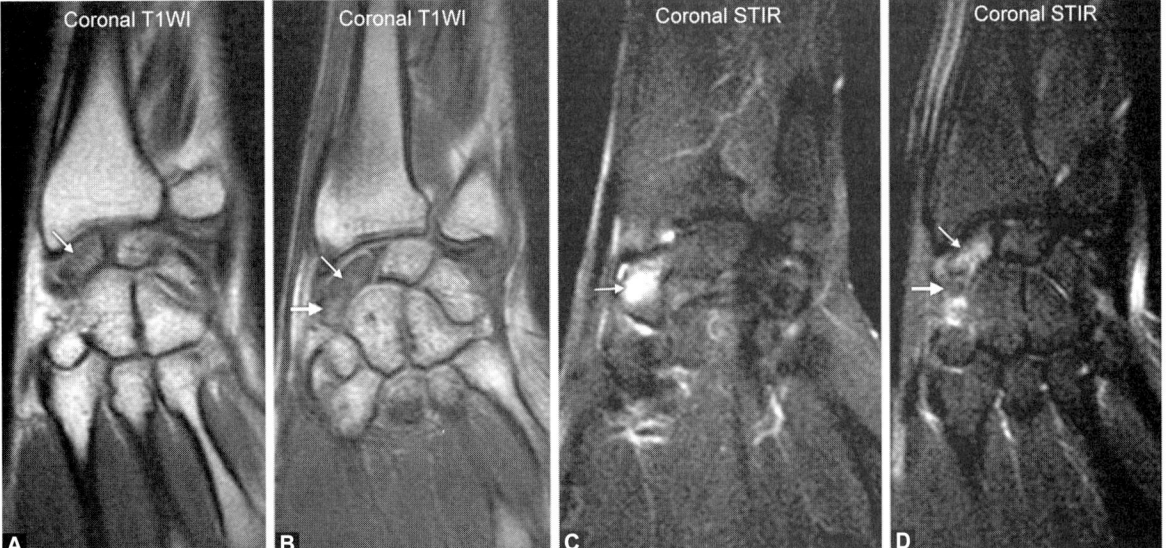

Figs 2.13A to D Complete oblique fracture is seen through the waist of scaphoid. There is hypointense signal (thin arrow) coronal on T1W images (A and B) suggestive of AVN and relatively less hypointense signal (thick arrow) represents reactive marrow edema. The signal is hyperintense in scaphoid on STIR images (C and D)

MR imaging is often requested in cases of suspected rotator cuff tear in which marrow edema is incidentally seen surrounding the greater tuberosity and denoting the margins of the occult avulsion fracture. It will demonstrate reduced signal on T1 and increased signal on T2-weighted or STIR sequences, particularly within the fatty marrow of the secondary ossification center. It is important to recognize the fracture by its characteristic site and radiographic appearance so as to avoid misdiagnosis.

Fracture Scaphoid

Trauma to the wrist may involve greater arc or lesser arc injuries to the carpal bones. In lesser arc injuries, usually only stage I (scapholunate dissociation) involves the scaphoid bone. Greater arc injuries represent fracture dislocations through the scaphoid and other bones of the carpus. Carpal fractures most frequently involve the scaphoid bone; various sites may be affected [proximal pole, waist **(Figs 2.13A to D)**, distal part of the body, tuberosity]. Often these fractures are associated with delayed union, nonunion or osteonecrosis.

In scapholunate dissociation (also known as rotary subluxation of the scaphoid), the scaphoid and lunate carpal bones are separated, sometimes after a fracture of the scaphoid or of the proximal portion of the radius. This dissociation leads to dorsiflexion instability of the wrist, or dorsal intercalary segmental carpal instability (DISI). A distance between the scaphoid and lunate bones of 2 mm or more suggests the diagnosis, and a distance of 4 mm or more is unequivocal evidence of its presence.

3
Metabolic and Endocrine Disorders

Rickets

The term rickets is said to have derived from the ancient English word *wricken*, i.e. *to bend*. It is a metabolic disease of childhood in which the osteoid, the organic matrix of bone, fails to mineralize due to interference with calcification mechanism. It manifests between six months to three years of age. Rickets is found only in children prior to the closure of the growth plates, while osteomalacia occurs at any age. Any child with rickets will have osteomalacia, while the reverse is not necessarily true.

Vitamin D deficiency causes rickets due to failure of mineralization of bone and cartilage. The normal order of maturation and mineralization of cartilage cells becomes disrupted. The cause could be:
- Vitamin D deficiency due to reduced dietary intake, pigmented skin or reduced exposure to sunlight,
- Malabsorption due to celiac disease, biliary atresia, hepatic osteodystrophy and small intestine bypass surgery,
- Anticonvulsant therapy.

The characteristic changes are seen in the growth plates prior to closure. Zone of maturation is grossly abnormal. There is overall diminished quantity of calcified osteoid and increase in uncalcified osteoid.

The radiological findings at the epiphyseal plate reveal the changed pathophysiology. The plain radiograph features show osteopenia with widening of growth plate strikingly in long bones, The metaphyseal margins are irregular due to fraying and disorganization of the spongy bone. This results in widening and cupping of the metaphysis **(Figs 3.1 and 3.2)**. Metaphyseal bands develop, they indicative of ill-defined zone of provisional calcification, bowing deformities of bones especially the lower

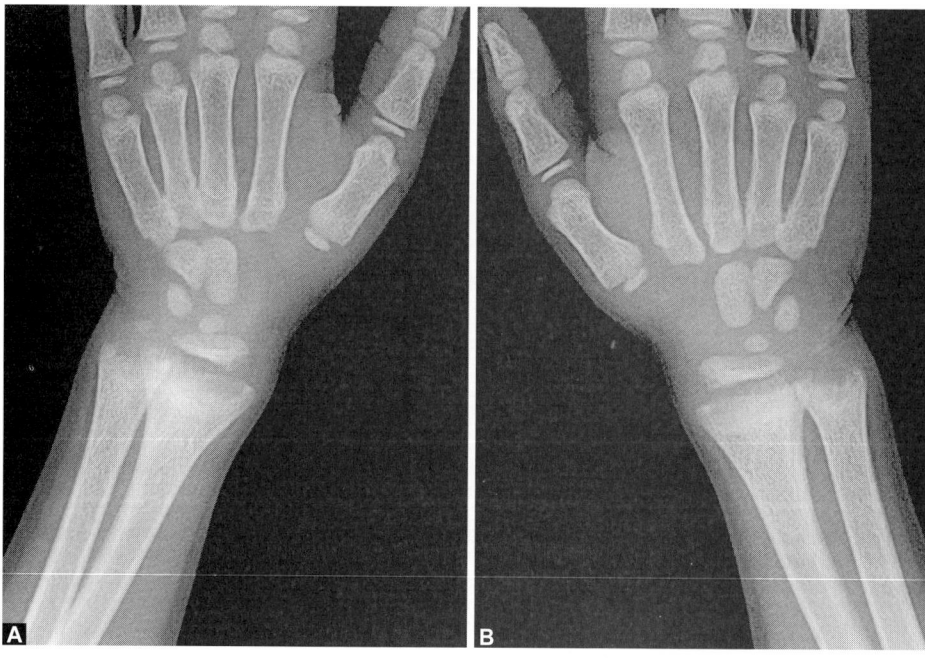

Figs 3.1A and B X-rays both wrists show widening of the growth plate, the metaphyseal margins are irregular and widened resulting in cupping of the metaphysis

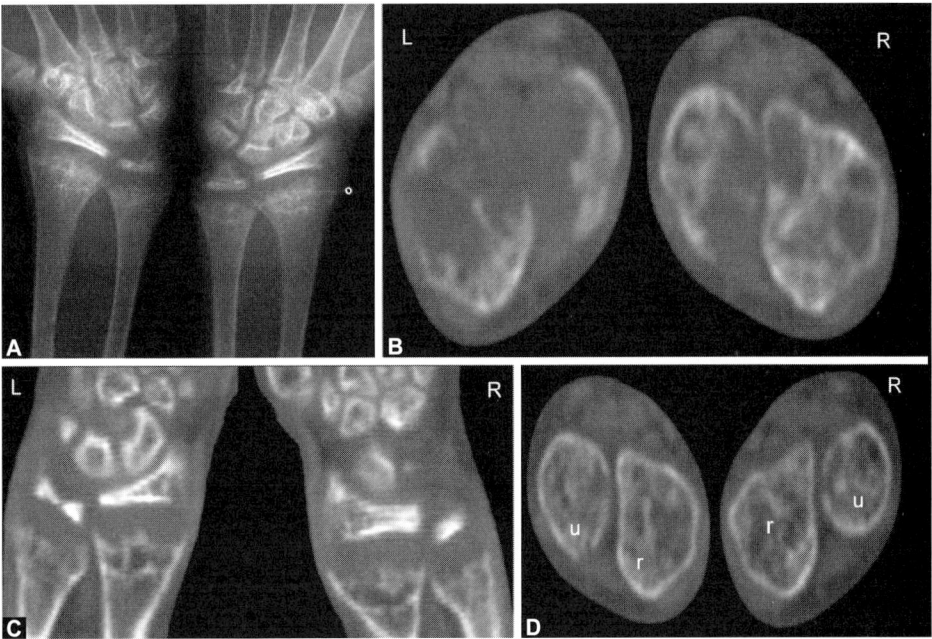

Figs 3.2A to D X-rays of both wrists and hands shows osteomalacia with widening of growth plate, splaying and cupping of distal metaphysis of radius and ulna with irregular metaphyseal margins. CT axial and coronal reconstructed images confirm the X-ray findings of defective mineralization of osteoid tissue in cortical and cancellous bone (B to D). These are features of rickets

limbs. Epiphysis is osteopenic and there is delayed appearance of the ossification center.

Skeletal deformities include broadened forehead, frontal and parietal bossing. Pigeon chest is seen due to prominent sternum, narrow chest, rickety rosary (enlargement of costochondral junction) and Harrison's sulci due to diaphragmatic pull on soft ribs. There is exaggerated curvature of spine, trefoil-shaped pelvis, coxa vara, genu valgum and bowed tibia.

Differential Diagnosis

The differential for flaring of the metaphysis includes anemia, fibrous dysplasia, storage diseases, chronic lead poisoning, bone dysplasias.

The differential for widening of the growth plate includes: scurvy, delayed maturation due to illness, endocrine disturbances, growth hormone excess, hyperparathyroidism, hypothyroidism.

The differential for leg bowing in children includes developmental or congenital bowing, Blount disease, and osteogenesis imperfecta.

Treatment is by oral vitamin D, 6 lakh IU and same dose is given again after 3–4 weeks, if no healing sign is seen on X-ray at the metaphyseal end. Followed by a maintenance dose of 4000 IU oral vitamin D, if the child is responsive.

Renal Rickets

Rickets is a disorder caused by a deficiency of vitamin D, calcium or phosphate. Rickets leads to deficient mineralization of normal osteoid and interruption of the normal orderly development and mineralization of growth plates resulting in softening and weakening of the bones. There are several subtypes of rickets, including hypophosphatemic rickets (vitamin-D-resistant rickets), renal rickets (renal osteodystrophy), and most commonly, nutritional rickets (caused by dietary deficiency of vitamin D, calcium, or phosphate).

Renal rickets is caused by a number of kidney disorders including renal tubular acidosis, chronic renal failure. Individuals suffering from kidney disease often have decreased ability to regulate the amounts of electrolytes lost in the urine. Renal insufficiency causes a decrease in vitamin D conversion into the active $1,25(OH)_2D_3$ which slows intestinal calcium absorption. Vitamin D resistance predominates and calcium levels stay low. Low-calcium levels lead to osteomalacia. Renal insufficiency with diminished filtration results in phosphate retention. This presumably leads to an elevation of the blood phosphates and lowered blood calcium. This abnormal calcium-phosphorus ratio seems to be entirely independent of the mineral and vitamin constituents of the diet, and hence renal rickets is not regarded primarily a food deficiency disease.

General retardation in body growth and osteopenia are observed radiographically. The skeletal effects are due to lack of calcification of osteoids. Widening and cupping of the metaphysis results from irregular cartilage cell growth in the zone of maturation. Poorly mineralized epiphyseal centers with delayed appearance. Epiphyseal plates appear widened and distance between end of shaft and epiphyseal center is increased. The presence of bulky growth plates at the shaft bone cartilage junctions of long bones and ribs leads to a rachitic rosary at the costochondral junctions of the middle ribs. Bowing deformity and sabre-shin deformity of the tibia also are typical manifestations of rickets. With increasing age scoliosis develops. Cortical spurs projecting at right angles to metaphysis are observed. The common deformities associated are bowing of long bones, molding of epiphysis, fractures, frontal bossing.

Osteoporosis and Osteomalacia (Table 3.1)

Osteoporosis is decreased osteoid production, a metabolic disorder characterized by decreased mass per unit volume of a normally mineralized bone due to loss of bone proteins. Whereas osteomalacia in adults and rickets in children is under mineralization of osteoid, is a metabolic disorder characterized by failure of mineralization and excess of the unmineralized osteoid due to a derangement in calcification.

Both osteoporosis and osteomalacia result in generalized decrease in bone density, known as osteopenia which means decrease in the bone mineralization quantity. Other conditions which lead to generalized osteopenia are:
- Hyperparathyroidism
- Multiple myeloma or diffuse metastases
- Drugs
- Osteogenesis imperfecta

Osteoporosis

It means reduced bone mass with normal bone composition secondary to either osteoclastic resorption of bone or osteocytic resorption. It is very commonly seen in women above 60 years of age. Various diseases can lead to osteoporosis. Those diseases are:
- *Congenital:* Osteogenesis imperfecta, homocystinuria
- *Idiopathic:* Juvenile, adult, postmenopausal, senile osteoporosis
- *Nutritional disorders:* Scurvy, calcium deficiency, protein deficiency
- *Endocrinopathies:* Cushing's syndrome, hyperparathyroidism, hyperthyroidism, acromegaly, Addison's disease, diabetes, pregnancy, paraneoplastic syndromes
- Renal osteodystrophy
- Immobilization
- Collagen disease
- Rheumatoid arthritis
- Bone marrow replacement

Table 3.1 Difference between osteoporosis and osteomalacia

Osteoporosis	Osteomalacia
Etiology	
• Primary osteoporosis-senile or postmenopausal • Immobilization due to prolonged bed rest or paralysis • Endocrine-glucocorticoid excess, thyrotoxicosis, hypogonadism, hyperprolactinemia, diabetes mellitus, hyperparathyroidism • Diet—chronic alcoholism, anorexia nervosa. • Prolonged use of drugs such as heparin, ethanol. • Chronic illness like rheumatoid arthritis, cirrhosis, renal tubular acidosis • Neoplasm-multiple myeloma, leukemia, lymphoma, mastocytosis • Genetic abnormalities-Homocystinuria, Ehler-Danlos syndrome, osteogenesis imperfect, Marfan's syndrome • Hepatic disease	• Lack of dietary intake of vitamin D • Decreased absorption of vitamin D-malabsorption syndrome, partial gastrectomy • Deficiency of vitamin D metabolism—chronic renal tubular disease, anticonvulsant therapy • Decreased deposition of calcium in the bone due to drugs like diphosphonates
Imaging	
Ground glass appearance due to generalized rarefaction	Generalized osteopenia
Loss of vertebral body height due to symmetric transverse compression	Loss of transverse trabeculae
No Looser's zones	Looser's zones at axillary margin of scapula, ramus of pubis or ischium, femur neck, ribs, Protrusio acetabuli and triradiate pelvis
Pathological fractures at wrist, hip	Pathological fractures
Anterior wedge compression and Codfish vertebrae	Codfish vertebral bodies due to biconcave vertebral bodies
Treatment	
Calcitonin, sodium fluoride, diphosphonates, estrogen replacement	Calcium, vitamin D, high-protein diet

- Drugs such as heparin, methotrexate, corticosteroids, excessive alcohol consumption, smoking, dilantin
- Radiation therapy
- Localized due to Sudeck dystrophy, transient osteoporosis of hip.

Osteoporosis can be diagnosed on X-rays and by calculating bone mineral density. X-ray features can further be evaluated with the help of CT, however, bone mineral density predicts osteoporosis quite accurately even before onset of symptoms.

X-ray features are:
- Decrease in number and thickness of trabeculae
- Cortical thinning due to endosteal and intracortical resorption
- Juxta-articular-reduced bone density predominantly affecting trabecular bone
- X-ray features in osteoporosis of spine:
  - Diminished radiographic density
  - Vertical striations due to thinning of transverse trabeculae with relative accentuation of vertical trabeculae
  - Accentuation of endplates
  - 'Picture-frame' vertebrae due to preservation of outer cortex with intracortical and endosteal resorption
  - Biconcave vertebrae
  - Schmorl's nodes
  - Wedging
  - Decreased height of vertebrae
  - Absence of osteophytes.

Osteomalacia

It is characterized by accumulation of excessive amounts of uncalcified osteoid with bone softening and insufficient mineralization of osteoid due to either high remodeling rate which is excessive osteoid formation with normal mineralization or low remodeling rate which is normal osteoid production with diminished mineralization. It occurs in adult patients due to deficiency of vitamin D. Etiology of osteomalacia:
- Dietary deficiency of vitamin D and lack of solar exposure,
- Deficient metabolism of vitamin D due to chronic renal insufficiency,
- Decreased absorption of vitamin D due to partial gastrectomy or malabsorption syndrome,
- Decreased deposition of calcium in bone.
  X-ray features of osteomalacia are:
- Uniform osteopenia
- Fuzzy indistinct trabecular details, of endosteal surface
- Coarsened frayed trabeculae which are decreases in number and size
- Cortical thinning in long bones
- Bone deformities due to softening such as hourglass thorax, bowing of long bones, acetabular protrusion, buckled or compressed pelvis, biconcave vertebral bodies
- Insufficiency fractures
- Pseudofractures also known as Looser's zones
- Mottled appearance of skull.

Osteomalacia during endochondral bone growth in childhood is termed as rickets. Radiological features are:
- Poorly mineralized irregular epiphyseal centers with delayed appearance
- Axial widening of growth plate that is increase in distance between end of shaft and epiphyseal center due to increased osteoid production
- Cupping and fraying of metaphysis with thread-like shadows into epiphyseal cartilage of weight bearing bones
- Cortical spurs projecting at right angles to metaphysis
- Coarse trabeculations
- Periosteal reaction may be present
- Deformities of long bones with bowing
- Frontal bossing of skull.

Bone densitometry helps in diagnosing osteoporosis. Bone densitometry is best performed by using dual energy X-ray absorptiometry (DEXA) scan. This examination is done on outpatient basis. DEXA examination generally measures bone density in the hip and spine, the patient lies on the table, X-ray generator is located below the patient and an imaging device, or detector, is positioned above and the detector slowly moves over the area of interest, generating images on a monitor (**Table 3.1**).

Interpretation of Results

A bone density test result shows a T-score and a Z-score. A T-score is a number derived by comparing patients BMD tests results to an average score for a healthy adult of same gender and race who has reached their peak bone mass at 25 years of age.

The T-score signifies variation from "normal." It is the difference between patients BMD and the BMD of a person at peak bone mass. T-scores can be as low as one standard deviation (SD) below normal and still be considered healthy. Patients with T-scores between −1 SD and −2.5 SD have osteopenia and are considered at high-risk for developing osteoporosis. Patients with T-scores lower than −2.5 SD have osteoporosis (**Table 3.2**).

Whereas Z-score which is patients bone density compared with a person of same age group and sex and interpreted to determine whether patient has osteoporosis or not. However, T-score is most commonly used for diagnosis.

Acromegaly

Acromegaly is the result of excessive growth hormone production, most commonly from an adenoma of the pituitary. It most commonly affects adults in middle age and can result in severe disfigurement, serious

Table 3.2 Interpretation of T-score

Bone density	T-score	Diagnosis
Normal	+1.0 to −1.0	Normal
Low	−1.0 to −2.5	Osteopenia
High-risk	−2.5 or lower	Osteoporosis

complicating conditions, and premature death. It has both an insidious onset and slow progression and may be difficult to diagnose in the early stages, only being diagnosed when the external features, especially of the face, become noticeable.

Radiological changes are seen in skull, mandible, paranasal sinuses extremities and vertebrae.

Skull and mandible show:
- Enlarged occipital protuberance
- Prognathism
- Enlarged paranasal sinuses
- Enlargement Sella and its erosion
- Calvarial hyperostosis
- Vertebral scalloping, new bone formation and loss of disc space.

Extremities show:
- Flared ends of long bones
- Cystic changes in carpals and femoral trochanters
- Osteoporosis
- Spade-like hand
- Heel pad thickness > 25 mm.

Majority of cases are the result of a pituitary macroadenoma. Expansion into the sella turcica may result in compression of surrounding structures, most importantly, the optic chiasm. The majority of pituitary tumors are incidental and do not have a genetic component. MRI detects the presence of pituitary tumors and its complications like optic chiasma compression. Pituitary macroadenomas are by definition more than 10 mm mass arising from the pituitary gland, and usually extend superiorly.

Indentation at the diaphragma sellae pituitary macroadenoma can give a *snowman* or *figure eight* configuration on CT. Contrast attenuation can vary depending on hemorrhagic, cystic and necrotic components. Adenomas which are solid, without hemorrhage, typically have attenuation similar to brain (30-50HU) and demonstrates moderate contrast enhancement. Calcification is rare.

T1W and T2W MR images show the lesion as typically isointense to grey matter and may show areas of necrosis and hemorrhage. On postcontrast images, they show moderate to bright enhancement. T2WI gradient images are sensitive in detecting hemorrhage.

The differential diagnosis includes craniopharyngioma, meningioma, pituitary carcinoma and metastases.

Fluorosis

Acute high-level exposure to fluoride is rare and causes immediate abdominal pain, excessive saliva, nausea and vomiting, seizures and muscle spasms. Acute high-level exposure to fluoride is usually due to accidental contamination of drinking-water or due to fires or explosions. Chronic fluorosis is exposure to excess of fluorine or its compounds. Sources of exposure can be from:

- Drinking of water containing concentrations of fluorine greater than 4 parts per million;
- Industrial exposure to fluorine-containing compounds over a long period of time
- Treatment of osteoporosis with sodium fluoride;
- Consumption of fluorine-containing wine.

Ingestion of excess of fluorine leads dental fluorosis in children less than 8 years of age and presents as pitting and staining of the teeth, and in severe cases, all the enamel may be damaged. Children above 8 years and adults cannot develop dental fluorosis. However, low levels of fluoride intake help to prevent dental caries. The control of drinking-water quality is therefore critical in preventing fluorosis.

Other manifestations of fluorosis include nausea, vomiting, constipation, loss of appetite, toxic nephritis, joint pain and restriction of motion, back stiffness, restriction of respiratory movements, functional dyspnea, and paraplegia.

Skeleton abnormalities include hypoplasia and irregularity of dental structures, osteosclerosis, vertebral osteophytosis, calcification of ligaments and periostitis. Increasing trabecular condensation leads to the eventual appearance of chalky areas throughout the thorax, vertebral column and pelvis. Hyperostosis and bone excrescences develop at sites of ligamentous attachment, especially in the iliac crests, ischial tuberosities and inferior margins of the ribs. In advanced stages, fluorosis can lead to contractures and deformities of extraspinal joints, kyphosis, restricted spinal and chest motion, and neurologic complications. Normally, the abnormalities are reversible after cessation of exposure, but a coarsened trabecular pattern without increased radiodensity may remain.

Resorption of Terminal Tufts

Resorption of terminal tufts commonly related to occupational conditions. It is also called as acroosteolysis, i.e. destruction of bone of the acral areas (extremities). Osteolysis may be severe in persons exposed to a number of industrial materials, such as polyvinylchloride. The radiographic hallmark of the disorder is osteolysis, which occurs predominantly in the terminal phalanges of the hands. Band-like radiolucent areas across the waist of one or more terminal phalanges may occur along with tuftal resorption. The thumb is affected more commonly than the other digits. The sacroiliac joints, the foot, and sometimes other skeletal structures may also be involved in certain types of acro-osteolysis.

Various Conditions Leading to Acro-osteolysis

- *Traumatic causes:* Amputation, burns, electric injury, frostbite, and vinyl chloride poisoning

- *Neuropathic causes:* Congenital indifference to pain, syringomyelia, diabetes mellitus, myelomeningocele and leprosy.
- *Collagen vascular disease:* Scleroderma, dermatomyositis, and Raynaud's disease.
- *Metabolic causes:* Hyperparathyroidism.
- *Inherited conditions:* Familial acro-osteolysis, pyknodysostosis, and pachydermoperiostosis.
- *Other conditions:* Sarcoidosis, psoriatic arthropathy and epidermolysis bullosa.

Frostbite

It is thermal injury to the body, usually the extremities or face. As the tissues freeze, so do the blood vessels, with vascular thrombosis interrupting circulation. Injury is followed by edema. If the circulation is not restored, there is acro-osteolysis with either auto- or surgical amputation of the fingers. The initial radiological change is soft tissue swelling at the finger tips followed by osteoporosis and periosteal new bone formation, followed by bone resorption with loss of the terminal tufts.

Vinyl Chloride Poisoning

It is a polymerizing agent used industrially that may produce cutaneous abnormalities resemble those of scleroderma. It may cause occupational acro-osteolysis in workers exposed to this substance during its manufacture. A drum-stick finger is an abnormality of the fingers occurring in patients with occupational acro-osteolysis.

Diabetes Mellitus

In this, there is pencil-and-cup appearance on X ray, where the base of the proximal phalanx broadens to form a cup with which the tapered phalangeal shaft becomes associated.

Scleroderma

It is a connective tissue disease which results in fibrosis and sclerosis of the skin and mucosa, subcutaneous tissues and submucosal tissues of internal organs. Skeletal manifestations include absorption of the distal phalanges of the hands, acro-osteolysis with periarticular soft tissue swelling, joint destruction, calcification in the soft tissue and osteopenia.

Hyperparathyroidism

In patients with primary or secondary hyperparathyroidism, bone resorption is evident radiological examination, especially in the hands in the early stages of the disease. The resorption can be categorized into various types. Subperiosteal resorption of cortical bone is virtually diagnostic of hyperparathyroid bone disease. In this form, a lace-like appearance of the phalangeal bone may progress to a spiculated contour and to complete resorption of the entire cortex. Other sites of subperiosteal resorption include the phalangeal tufts.

Pyknodysostosis

It is a dysplasia manifested clinically by dwarfism, increased bone fragility and sclerotic bones. Inheritance is autosomal recessive. Radiologically, the skull base is dense. There is a widely open persistent anterior fontanelle and multiple wormian bones. The angle of the mandible is very obtuse with severe micrognathia. The vertebral bodies and long bones are sclerotic, and there is under modeling of the bones with narrowing of the medullary canals. Fracturing is frequent. There may be acro-osteolysis.

Pachydermoperiostitis

It is an autosomal dominant condition causing large skin folds of the face and scalp that occurs predominantly in males aged 3 to 38 years old, although it usually starts at puberty. There is irregular periosteal proliferation of the phalanges and distal third of the long bones of legs and forearms beginning in the epiphyseal region at tendon or ligament insertions. The distal phalanges are rarely involved. The cortex is thickened but there is no narrowing of the medulla. Acro-osteolysis may be present. Enlargement of the paranasal sinuses and finger clubbing is seen.

Psoriatic Arthritis

It is a seronegative spondyloarthropathy occurring in some patients with psoriasis. The articular disease may be monoarticular, pauciarticular or polyarticular in its distribution, and virtually any joint can be affected. Classic radiographic features of psoriatic arthritis are involvement of synovial and cartilaginous joints and entheses, involvement of interphalangeal joints of the hands and feet, sacroiliitis and spondylitis with paravertebral ossification, bone erosion with adjacent proliferation, intra-articular bone ankylosis and destruction of phalangeal tufts.

Expansile Lesions of Metaphysis

Expansile lesions affecting the metaphyses of long bones include rickets, hypophosphatasia, metaphyseal chondroplasia, enchondroma, non-ossifying fibroma, aneurysmal bone cyst, chondromyxoid fibroma, and giant cell tumor.

Rickets

Plain radiographic and CT findings are widening and cupping of the metaphyseal regions, fraying of the metaphysis, bowing of long bones, development of knock-knees, or genu valgum.

Hypophosphatasia

Hypophosphatasia is a rare and fatal metabolic bone disease. In the perinatal period, it is the most pernicious form of hypophosphatasia. The infantile subtype presents in the first 6 months of life. In childhood, hypophosphatasia's clinical expression is extremely variable. As a result of aplasia, hypoplasia, or dysplasia of dental cementum, premature loss of deciduous teeth (i.e. before the age of 5) occurs. In adult years, hypophosphatasia can present during middle age. X-rays show hypomineralization, rachitic changes, and incomplete vertebrate ossification, lateral bony spurs on the ulnae and fibulae and tongue-like radiolucent areas protruding from the metaphyses into the bone shaft.

Metaphyseal Chondroplasia

It is a heterogeneous group of intrinsic dysplasias causing changes in the metaphyses of tubular bones. Metaphyseal chondrodysplasia is associated with neutropenia, lymphopenia, immune deficiency, pancreatic exocrine insufficiency, Hirschsprung's disease, and intestinal malabsorption. The condition is first recognized in early childhood when children present with a waddling gait, exaggerated lumbar lordosis, genu varum, and short stature. Radiographs show appearance of an enlarged metaphysis and widened-cupped physis similar to rickets, coxa vara occurs without an associated bowed femur.

Types

1. *Schmidt's type:* This disorder may arise from defective type X collagen, which is typically found in the hypertrophic zone of the physis. Patients show mild short stature, leg pains, bowed legs, increased lordosis, and waddling gait. Upper extremity shows mild wrist swelling, flexion contractures of the elbows. Lower extremities are more significantly involved than upper extremities and show varus deformities of the knees and ankles are present, with bowing visible in the thigh and the leg, severe genu varum.
2. *Jansen's type:* It is a rare autosomal dominant disorder characterized by short limb dwarfism with severe hypercalcemia and hypophosphatemia. X-rays show rachitic changes of metaphysis commonly affecting knee joints with pathological fractures. Metatarsals, metacarpals and skull base also show sclerotic lesions.

Enchondroma

It is a benign cartilaginous growth in medullary cavity, usually solitary and is seen within medullary canal and metaphysis. X-rays show oval/round area of geographic destruction with lobulated contour and fine marginal line, cortical endosteal scalloping, ground-glass appearance, dystrophic calcifications within small cartilage nodules/fragments of lamellar bone which can be pinhead, stippled, flocculent or arcs and rings pattern, bulbous expansion of bone with thinning of cortex in small tubular bones of phalanx, rib and fibula is seen with Madelung deformity = bowing deformities of limb, discrepant length. No cortical breakthrough/periosteal reaction. MRI shows low- to intermediate-signal intensity on T1WI and high-signal intensity on T2WI, low-signal intensity matrix calcifications, normal fat marrow interspersed between cartilage nodules and peripheral enhancement pattern on post-gadolinium images.

Non-ossifying Fibroma

It is a lesion resulting from proliferative activity of a fibrous cortical defect that has expanded into medullary cavity shaft of long bone which is seen in bones of lower extremity. Radiographs show eccentric metaphyseal, multilocular ovoid bubbly osteolytic area with alignment along long axis of bone, about 2 cm in length, dense sclerotic border toward medulla, V- or U-shaped at one end, endosteal scalloping with thinning and overlying bulge. Nuclear scan shows minimal/mild uptake on bone scan. MR shows hypointense lesion on T1WI and T2WI or hypointense on T1WI and hyperintense on T2WI with peripheral hypointense rim and internal intense contrast enhancement.

Aneurysmal Bone Cyst

It is an expansile pathologically benign lytic lesion of bone containing thin-walled cystic cavities filled with chronic blood products with its name derived from roentgen appearance. X-rays show purely lytic eccentric radiolucency with aggressive expansile ballooning lesion called as soap-bubble pattern with thin internal trabeculations. There is rapid progression within 6 weeks to 3 months with sclerotic inner portion, almost invisible thin cortex, no periosteal reaction. CT shows blood-filled sponge-like lesion due to fluid-fluid/hematocrit levels due to blood sedimentation. MR shows multiple cysts of different signal intensity representing different stages of blood by products like heterogeneous fluid-fluid levels within loculations reflecting hemorrhage with sedimentation and low-signal intensity rim and shows heterogeneous enhancement. Nuclear scintigraphy shows doughnut sign due to peripheral increased uptake. Angiography shows hypervascularity in lesion periphery.

Chondromyxoid Fibroma

Rare benign cartilaginous tumor which initially arises in cortex and is an eccentric, metaphyseal lesion. Radiographs show expansile ovoid lesion with radiolucent center and oval shape at each end of lesion, long axis parallel to long axis of host bone, geographic bone destruction, well-defined sclerotic margin, expanded shell with bulged and thinned overlying cortex, partial cortical erosion, scalloped margin, septations which may mimic trabeculations, stippled calcifications within tumor in advanced lesions and no periosteal reaction.

Giant Cell Tumor

It is also known as osteoclastoma. Radiographs show a well-circumscribed expansile solitary lytic bone lesion with a narrow zone of transition, soap-bubble appearance due to expansile remodeling with multiloculated appearance, no internal mineralization of tumor matrix, prominent trabeculation, no sclerosis/periosteal reaction due to aggressive rapid growth, cortical penetration, cortical thinning, soft-tissue invasion, complete/incomplete pathologic fracture, destruction of vertebral body with secondary invasion of posterior elements and vertebral collapse. Nuclear scintigraphy shows diffusely increased uptake with central photopenia on delayed bone scintigraphy. Angiography shows a hypervascular lesion. CT shows tumor of soft-tissue attenuation similar to muscle with foci of low attenuation, no matrix mineralization, and well-defined margins with thin rim of sclerosis. Soft-tissue extension at metaphyseal end of tumor with significant enhancement. MR shows well-defined lesion of heterogeneous signal intensity with low-to-intermediate intensity on T1WI and T2WI with low-signal-intensity margin significant enhancement of solid-tissue component.

Hand as an Index of Disease

Variety of disorders affects the bones and joints of the hand and thus makes it an index to diagnose associations of systemic diseases leading to arthritis. Articular disorders of hand are:

Osteoarthritis

It is also known as degenerative joint disease and occurs due to abnormal stress on the bone. Sites commonly affected are proximal and distal interphalangeal joints, 1st carpometacarpal joint, and trapezioscaphoid joint. It usually shows bilateral involvement which can be symmetric or asymmetric.

It can be classified as:
- *Primary osteoarthritis:* Most common in the older age group as the result of wear and tear on articular cartilage over time.
- *Secondary osteoarthritis:* Results from a previous process that damaged cartilage such as trauma, or inflammatory arthritis.

Diagnosis is essentially done with the help of plain X-rays. CT and MRI can be used as an adjunct to diagnose, if required. Plain X-ray features are: joint space narrowing, subchondral eburnation, radial subluxation of 1st metacarpal base, marginal osteophytes with small ossicles.

Inflammatory Arthritis

It predominantly affects postmenopausal or middle-aged women due to repeated infections or inflammations. It commonly affects proximal and distal interphalangeal joints, 1st carpometacarpal joint, and trapezioscaphoid joint. It usually shows bilateral involvement which can be symmetric or asymmetric.

Plain X-ray features are central erosions combined with osteophytes known as subchondral 'gull-wing' erosions, joint space narrowing, sclerosis, rarely ankylosis can occur.

Rheumatoid Arthritis

An inflammatory process with the target organ being the synovial membrane leading to pannus formation (inflammatory exudates in the lining of the synovial cells). Areas affected are proximal interphalangeal and middle interphalangeal joints with earlier affection of 2nd and 3rd fingers, all wrist joints, and styloid process of ulna. It affects both hands in relative symmetrical fashion.

X-ray Features

- *Osteopenia:* Demineralization of the bone is the result of increased blood flow, due to inflammation, which washes out the calcium. Early on in the inflammatory process, only the periarticular portion of the bones is affected. Over time, the inflammatory pain causes disuse of affected joints leading to generalized osteopenia of whole bones.
- *Uniform joint space narrowing:* A feature which helps differentiates rheumatoid arthritis from osteoarthritis.
- Marginal erosions at bare areas where synovium lies on bone.
- Subluxation due to ligamentous or capsular laxity.
- Fusiform soft tissue swelling and joint deformities.

Gout

It occurs due to deposition of monosodium urate crystals in synovial fluid, and usually it remains asymptomatic from months to years. It commonly targets carpo-metacarpal joints but can also affect all joints of hand.

Features on X-rays or CT are development of chronic tophaceous gout which appears as lobulated soft tissue masses, well-defined, periarticular eccentric erosions with overhanging edge and sclerotic margins, preservation of joint spaces and absence of osteoporosis. Most extensive changes are seen in the common carpometacarpal compartment which shows scalloped erosions of the bases of ulnar metacarpals.

Psoriasis

It is also known as rheumatoid variant or seronegative spondyloarthropathy. It shows peripheral manifestation in monoarthritis or asymmetric oligoarthritis or symmetric polyarthritis. Target areas are all hand and wrist joints predominantly distal.

X-ray features are 'Mouse ear' marginal erosions, intra-articular osseous excrescences, new bone formation with fusion and absence of osteoporosis.

Calcium Pyrophosphate Dehydrate: Crystal Deposition Disease

Calcium pyrophosphate dehydrate (CPPD) also known as pseudogout, is a very common entity. Radiographically, the presence of chondrocalcinosis is typical of this entity. Common locations for chondrocalcinosis include the triangular fibrocartilage at the wrist. Chondrocalcinosis in the setting of CPPD is commonly associated with calcification of fibrocartilage.

X-ray Features

Chondrocalcinosis with periarticular calcifications. Degenerative changes in unusual locations causing narrowing and obliteration of space between distal radius and scaphoid with fragmentation of surfaces and scapholunate separation. Destruction of trapezioscaphoid space, no erosions and presence of large osteophytes.

Systemic Lupus Erythematosus

It leads to myositis, polyarthritis, deforming nonerosive arthropathy and osteonecrosis. It commonly targets proximal and middle interphalangeal joints and causes reversible deformities.

Scleroderma

It is also known as progressive systemic sclerosis and commonly affects distal and proximal interphalangeal joints and 1st carpometacarpal joints.

X-rays commonly show tuft resorption and soft tissue calcifications.

Nonarticular Disorders of Bones of Hand

- *Acro-osteolysis:* It means lytic destruction. Commonly affects distal and middle phalanges. It is seen in variety of diseases like: psoriasis, porphyria, Ehlers-Danlos syndrome, thromboangiitis obliterans, Raynaud's disease, diabetes, dermatomyositis, injuries, epidermolysis bullosa, rheumatoid arthritis, Reiter's syndrome, scleroderma, sarcoidosis, pyknodysostosis, leprosy, Lesch-Nyhan syndrome, syringomyelia, hyperparathyroidism. It shows lytic lesions with absence of periosteal reaction on X-rays. Epiphyseal involvement can be seen in later stages.
- *Acro-osteosclerosis:* In this entity, sclerotic lesions are seen on X-rays in the phalanges which can be an index to diseases such as rheumatoid arthritis, sarcoidosis, scleroderma, systemic lupus erythematosus, Hodgkin's disease, hematologic disorders. On X-rays, it shows focal opaque areas with endosteal thickening.
- Resorption of terminal tufts of phalanges which can be diagnosed on X-rays help in diagnosing diseases like:
    - Trauma—due to amputations, burns, electric injuries, frostbite, and vinyl chloride poisoning.
    - Neuropathic—congenital indifference to pain, syringomyelia, myelomeningocele, diabetes, leprosy.
    - Collagen vascular disease—scleroderma, dermatomyositis, Raynaud's phenomenon.
    - Metabolic causes such as hyperparathyroidism.
    - Inherited disorders such as familial acro-osteolysis, pyknodystosis, progeria or Werner's syndrome and pachydermoperiostosis.
    - Other diseases such as sarcoidosis, psoriatic arthropathy and epidermolysis bullosa.
- *Metacarpal sign:* It is the relative shortening of 4th and 5th metacarpals. It commonly is seen associated with pseudohypoparathyroidism, basal cell nevus syndrome, multiple epiphyseal dysplasia, Beckwith-Wiedemann syndrome, sickle cell anemia, juvenile chronic arthritis, Turner's syndrome, ectodermal dysplasias, hereditary multiple exostoses, melorheostosis.

    On the other hand X-rays a tangential line drawn along the heads of 4th and 5th metacarpals intersect the 3rd metacarpal indicating relative shortening.
- *Carpal angle:* It is an angle seen on X-rays formed by tangents to proximal row of carpal bones. Normally, it should be 130°.

    A decreased carpal angle which is less than 124° is indicative of diseases such as Turner's syndrome, Hurler's syndrome, Morquio's syndrome, Madelung deformity.

    Increased carpal angle is above 139° and it is seen in Down's syndrome, arthrogryposis, bone dysplasia with epiphyseal involvement.

- *Dactylitis:* It means inflammation of the fingers. Radiologically, it is seen as the expansion of phalanges with multiple radiolucencies within due to cystic changes. It is seen in tuberculosis, pyogenic or fungal infection, syphilis, sarcoidosis, hemoglobinopathies, hyperparathyroidism, leukemia.
- *Brachydactyly:* It means shortening or broadening of metacarpals and palanges seen on X-rays. It is seen with trauma, osteomyelitis, arthritis, Turner's syndrome, osteochondrodysplasia, mucopolysaccharidoses, basal cell nevus syndrome, hereditary multiple exostoses.
- *Clinodactyly:* Abnormal curvature is seen of the fingers in mediolateral plane. It is associated with Down's syndrome, multiple dysplasia, contractures.
- *Polydactyl:* It means having multiple fingers that is more than four fingers and a thumb. It is seen associated with Carpenter syndrome, Ellis-van Creveld syndrome, Meckel-Gruber syndrome, short-rib polydactyl syndrome, Trisomy13.
- *Syndactyly:* It means osseous and cutaneous fusion of digits. It is seen in Apert syndrome, Carpenter syndrome, Down's syndrome, neurofibromatosis, Poland syndrome.
- *Fingertip calcifications:* Calcific densities can be seen in the soft tissues of fingers indicative of following diseases such as scleroderma, Raynaud's disease, systemic lupus erythematosus, dermatomyositis, hyperparathyroidism.
- *Lucent lesions in fingers:* Various lesions can lead to radiolucent lesions in the fingers which can be seen on X-rays. These lesions can be a glomus tumor, gouty arthritis, metastasis, enchondroma, simple inclusion cyst, pancreatitis, aneurysmal bone cyst, giant cell tumor, epidermoid, etc.

Thus, by routine X-ray examination of the hand can show a variety of appearances and can provide a guide to various systemic and articular disorders.

4
Infections

Periosteal Reaction (Periostitis)

Periosteum is the outer surface of bone which separates bone from surrounding soft tissues. It is firmly adherent to the underlying bone. It is normally not visible on X-rays. An underlying inflammatory or neoplastic process provokes hyperemia that activates fibroblasts to osteoblasts that produce osteoid tissue which gets mineralized and appears as layers of new bone termed as periostitis **(Fig. 4.1)**. Presence of periosteal reaction indicates the biologic underlying process. It takes 10-21 days from the intial insult for the periosteal reaction to become visible on X-rays.

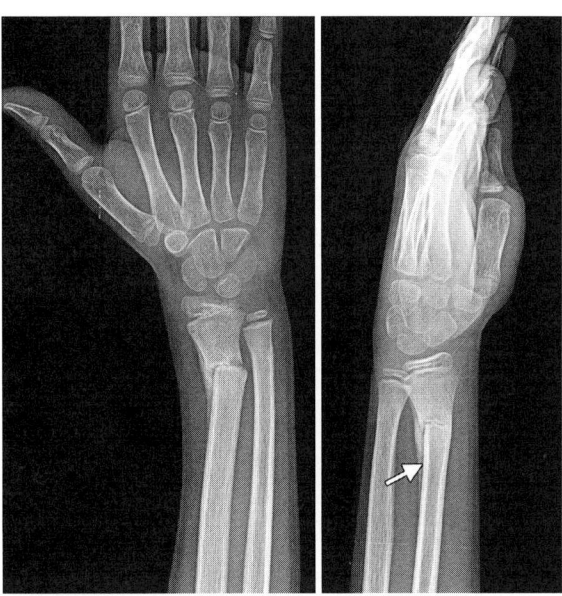

Fig. 4.1 X-ray forearm shows periosteal reaction (arrow) in the process of healing of fracture

Causes of Periosteal Reaction

- Trauma
- Infection
- Inflammatory arthritis
- Neoplasm—osteoid osteoma, osteosarcoma. Ewing's sarcoma
- Congenital—physiological in infants during first 1-6 months
- Metabolic—hypertrophic pulmonary osteoarthropathy, thyroid
- Acropachy, hypervitaminosis A, fluorosis
- Venous insufficiency.

Types of Periosteal Reaction

- Continuous—it may be solid, lamellar, multilamellar or parallel spiculated
  - Solid—seen as thickening of periosteal surface and indicates benign etiology as in osteoid osteoma, eosinophilic granuloma
  - Single lamellar—thin 1-2 mm faint radioopaque line from the cortical surface as in histiocytosis, healing fractures
  - Multilamellar or onion peel-multiple concentric layers of periosteum as in Ewing's sarcoma
  - Parallel speculated-bony spicules may appear perpendicular to the cortex, i.e. hair on end appearance as seen with thalassemia. Sunburst appearance is due to bony spicules fanning out in focal divergent manner and seen with osteosarcoma.
- Discontinuous or interrupted mineralization forms an angular configuration with underlying cortex resembling both sides of an angle (Codman angles) as in osteogenic sarcoma
- Complex reaction includes combination of lamellated, divergent spiculated reaction and Codman's angle.

Osteomyelitis

Osteomyelitis refers to bony inflammation that is almost always due to infection, typically bacterial. In most instances, osteomyelitis results from hematogenous spread, although direct extension from trauma and ulcers is also relatively common.

In the initial stages of infection, bacteria multiply setting up a localized inflammatory reaction and resulting in localized cell death. With time the infection becomes demarcated by a rim of granulation tissue and new bone deposition.

Although no organisms are recovered in up to 50% of cases, when one is isolated, *Staphylococcus aureus* is by far the most common agent. Different organisms are more common in specific clinical scenarios. *Staphylococcus aureus*: 80-90% of all infections.

- *Escherichia coli:* Intravenous drug users and genitourinary tract infection
- *Pseudomonas:* Intravenous drug users and genitourinary tract infection
- *Klebsiella:* Intravenous drug users and genitourinary tract infection
- *Salmonella:* Sickle cell disease
- *Haemophilus influenzae:* Neonates
- *Group B streptococci:* Neonates

The location of osteomyelitis within a bone varies with age, on account of changing blood supply:
- *Neonates:* Metaphysis and or epiphysis
- *Children:* Metaphysis
- *Adults:* Epiphyses and subchondral regions

In some instances, radiographic features are specific to a region or particular type of infection, for example:
- Subperiosteal abscess
- Brodie's abscess
- Pott's puffy tumor
- Sclerosing osteomyelitis of Garre.

Considering the imaging, the earliest changes are seen in adjacent soft tissues with swelling and loss of normal fat planes. An effusion may be seen in an adjacent joint. The bone itself remains normal in appearance for 10–14 days. After this time a number of changes may be noted like regional osteopenia, periosteal reaction and may appear aggressive including formation of a Codman's triangle and eventually peripheral sclerosis.

In chronic or untreated cases eventual formation of a sequestrum, involucrum or cloaca may be seen.

CT is superior to both MRI and X-rays in depicting the bony margins and identifying a sequestrum/involucrum. Appearances are otherwise similar to plain films.

MRI is most sensitive and specific and is able to identify soft-tissue/joint complications.

Although ultrasound excels as a fast and cheap examination of the soft tissues, and allows soft tissue collections to be drained it has little direct role in the assessment of osteomyelitis, as it is unable to visualize within bone.

It does however have a role to play in assessment of soft tissues and joints adjacent to infected bone, able to visualize soft tissue abscesses, cellulitis, sub periosteal collections and joint effusion.

Ultrasound also is useful in assessing the extraosseous components of orthopedic instrumentation as it is not affected by metal artifact.

In nuclear medicine a number of techniques may be employed to detect foci of osteomyelitis. These include:
- *Bone scintigraphy (Tc-99m):* Increased osteoblastic activity results in increased levels of radiotracer uptake in the surrounding bone usually both on blood pool and delayed views. It is highly sensitive but not particularly specific.
- *In^{111}-labeled WBC and Galium^{67} scintigraphy is particularly useful in:*
  - Diabetic osteomyelitis, especially combined with Tc-99m phosphonate imaging
  - Orthopedic implants
  - Vertebral osteomyelitis (Ga^{67})
  - Ulcers in bed ridden patients with potential underlying osteomyelitis (In^{111} with Tc-99m phosphonate).

Acute Osteomyelitis

Acute osteomyelitis is an inflammation of bone (cortical bone and its marrow space) caused by an infecting organism. Pyogenic osteomyelitis is the most common and Staphylococcus aureus is the most common bacteria involved. Although on the basis of the route of infection, acute osteomyelitis can be classified as hematogenous or exogenous. Hematogenous osteomyelitis is predominantly seen in children (2–16 years) and involves the highly vascular long bones, especially those of the lower limb. In adults, hematogenous spread is more common to the lumbar vertebral bodies than elsewhere. In neonatal osteomyelitis, isotopic bone scans are reportedly normal in most patients.

Before puberty, infection starts in the metaphyseal sinusoidal veins. Because bones are relatively rigid structures, focal edema accumulates under pressure and leads to local tissue necrosis, breakdown of the trabecular bone structure, and removal of bone matrix and calcium. Infection spreads along the haversian canals, through the marrow cavity, and beneath the periosteal layer of the bone. Subsequent vascular damage causes the ischemic death of osteocytes, leading to the formation of a sequestrum. Periosteal new bone formation on top of the sequestrum is known as involucrum.

Differentiating acute osteomyelitis from bone infarction in patients with sickle cell disease is a major challenge. The 2 conditions must be differentiated on the basis of clinical findings and imaging studies because both are common in patients with sickle cell disease. The 2 diseases are managed differently.

Fine-needle aspiration (FNA) or needle biopsy may be used under ultrasonographic, fluoroscopic, or CT guidance to obtain samples of pus, tissue, or both to establish a histologic diagnosis of acute osteomyelitis. The disease process involves 5 stages:
1. *Inflammation:* This stage represents initial inflammation with vascular congestion and increased intraosseous pressure; obstruction to blood flow occurs with intravascular thrombosis.
2. *Suppuration:* Pus within the bones forces its way through the haversian system and forms a subperiosteal abscess in 2–3 days.
3. *Sequestrum:* Increased pressure, vascular obstruction, and infective thrombus compromise the periosteal and endosteal blood supply, causing

bone necrosis and sequestrum formation in approximately 7 days.
4. *Involucrum:* This is new bone formation from the stripped surface of periosteum
5. *Resolution or progression to complications:* With antibiotics and surgical treatment early in the course of disease, osteomyelitis resolves without any complications.

Clinical features vary in infants, children and adults, being related to the structural and vascular differences of bone at these ages. In children older than one year the epiphyseal plate blocks extension of the infection so the infection spreads laterally into the subperiosteal space or to the joint in which synovial reflections extend beyond the epiphysis to metaphysis, such as the shoulder and hip joints. In infants, small capillaries cross the epiphyseal growth plate, and thus, permit extension of infection to the epiphysis and the joint. In adults the epiphyseal plate is fused and no longer forms a barrier to the spread of infection from metaphysis to the adjacent joint. Thus acute pyogenic arthritis is a frequent complication of osteomyelitis in infants.

Neonatal osteomyelits presents with few clinical signs despite multiple sites of involvement, and hence, a complete skeletal survey is warranted in such cases. Premature infants requiring umbilical catheterization are at higher risk for osteomyelitis. Radionuclide bone scintigraphy is advocated in all patients with suspected neonatal osteomyelitis, following initial radiographs.

Plain radiographs are the first imaging study in the work-up of osteomyelitis. Soft tissue swelling and small single or multiple osteolytic areas affecting the metaphysis is the earliest change which is seen within 7-10 days. Elevation of the periosteum or periosteal reaction which is lamellar layered new bone formation is seen after 3-6 weeks. Typically the dead bone (sequestrum) also forms at 3-8 weeks. It appears dense. Osteopenia in the surrounding bone develops due to hyperemia. Later remodeling reverts the appearance of bone to normal in infants and children but in adults the sclerosis and cortical irregularity persist.

Ultrasonography shows deep soft tissue swelling (earliest sign). Periosteal elevation seen as a hyperechoic line with subperiosteal fluid collection. Cortical breech is seen as focal defect in the cortex. Ultrasonography detects presence of fluid in the joint especially of hip and shoulder joints in an infant.

Radionuclide scintigraphy is the most sensitive investigation for diagnosing acute osteomyelitis 99m Tc-labeled methylene diphosphonate (99m Tc-MDP), hydroxymethylene diphosphonate (99m Tc-HMDP) and gallium 67 citrate are the most commonly used radionuclide agents. They shows positive findings usually within 3 days and sometimes within 24 hours of onset of infection. Triple phase bone scanning is done; osteomyelitis shows hot areas on all phases.

MRI is an important imaging tool in the evaluation of early osteomyelitis and overlying soft tissue involvement. It is superior to scintigraphy in evaluation of axial skeletal osteomyelitis because of better anatomical delineation. In addition, MRI can distinguish soft tissue infection with periostitis from osteomyelitis.

Localized Osteomyelitis (Brodie's Abscess)

Brodie's abscess is a limited osteomyelitis caused either by organisms of low virulence of high resistance in the host. It occurs most frequently at one end of the bone, but it, may also occur in the diaphysis. It is seen as a well circumscribed osteolytic focus surrounded by a sclerotic margin. Occasionally a metaphyseal serpiginous channel with sclerotic border marks the tract of infection. This is considered characteristic of nontubercular etiology like *Staphylococcus*, *Streptococcus* or *hemophilus*. In early stage when the lesion is small, it is difficult to identify on X-rays and CT or MRI is required.

Chronic Osteomyelitis

Chronic osteomyelitis results from failure to eliminate the acute or subacute osteomyelitis, or from local spread of soft tissue infection, complication of compound fractures or following surgery. Radiographs show bone destruction and focal cortical thickening due to periosteal new bone formation, cortical defects and sequestrum with modeling deformities and soft tissue irregularities can also be seen. The sequelae include:
a. Growth plate destruction leading to limb length discrepancy
b. Extensive bone destruction with modeling deformity.
c. Avascular necrosis and sequestrum formation **(Figs 4.2 and 4.3)**
d. Chronically discharging sinus **(Figs 4.4A to D)**
e. Pathological fractures and
f. Premature osteoarthritis changes.

Sequestrum is a piece of dead bone that has become separated during the process of necrosis from normal bone. It is extra dense, more radio-opaque and more heavier than surrounding bone. It does not decalcify because of avascularity. Its surface is usually irregular due to erosive process by proteolytic enzymes in granulation tissue. Types of sequestra are:
1. Tubular or diaphyseal seen in pyogenic osteomyelitis.
2. Trapezoid seen in pyogenic osteomyelitis.
3. Ring seen at end of stumps, around Steinmann pin and wires.
4. Flake or Feathery seen in tuberculous osteomyelitis in a cavity.
5. Coarse Sandy seen in tuberculous osteomyelitis out the cavity.
6. Fine Sandy seen in viral osteomyelitis.
7. Black seen in actinomycosis.

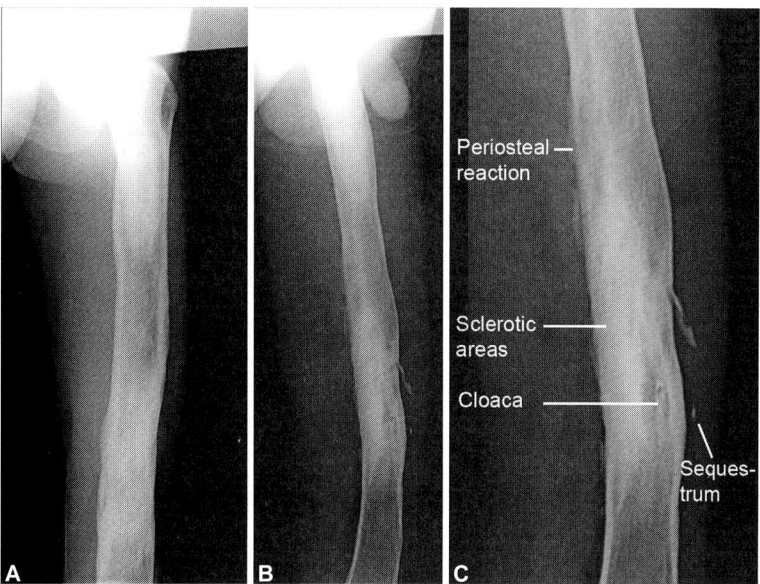

Figs 4.2A to C X-ray thigh shows chronic osteomyelitis. C is magnified view of B

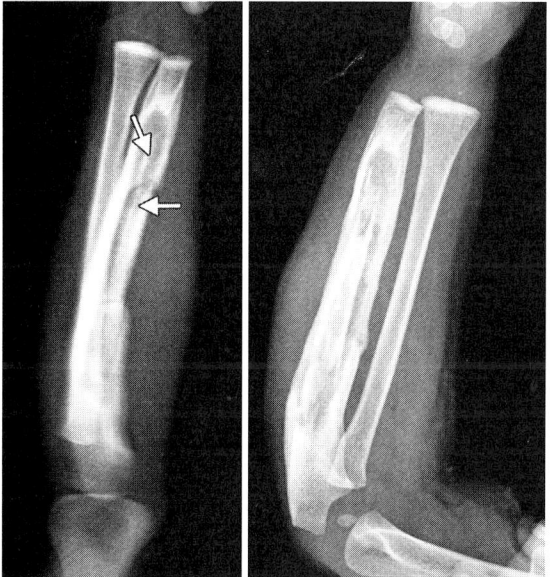

Fig. 4.3 X-ray left forearm of a 3-year-old male with chronic osteomyelitis, ulna shows cortical thickening, bone destruction and sequestrum formation (arrows)

Clinically pain, local swelling, discharge from wound, sinus formation, scars and muscle contractures, shortening of bones, deformities and decreased movements and systemic signs and symptoms may be present.

Conventional X-rays show cloacae, involucrum or sequestrum. There are sclerotic and lucent areas admixed with bony thickening and deformities. In osteomyelitis of the skull, typically no sclerosis is seen.

Scintigraphy: It is more useful in determining activity. 67Ga has been recommended as the optimal agent. Following successful treatment 67Ga uptakes should decrease to a normal level.

MRI is used to distinguish regions of active infection from uninvolved marrow or fibrotic regions.

Sclerosing Osteomyelitis of Garre

A rare type of chronic osteomyelitis occurring in children and young adults, presenting with insidious onset of local pain. There is predilection for involvement of mandible and shafts of long bones.

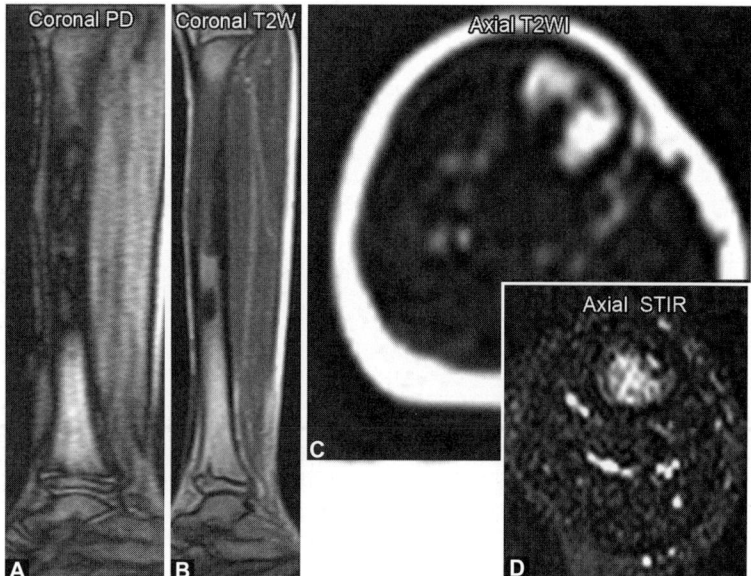

Figs 4.4A to D A 10 years old female presented with discharging sinus on right side of leg with pain and fever on MR shows altered marrow signal intensity involving the metadiaphysis of the right tibia. Patchy areas of sclerosis noted with endosteal thickening and sinus tract noted in the lower end of tibia in the anteromedial cortex. Soft tissue edema with focal collection noted in the anteromedial soft tissue of the tibia with a sinus tract in a case of osteomyelitis of right tibia

Radiological appearance is of intense sclerosis resulting in thickened bone. Areas of frank bony destruction are rare. In this the periosteal reaction and permeative bone destruction are absent.

Sequelae to Septic Arthritis

Infectious arthritis affects children and hip joint is a common site to be involved. Spread of infection may be hematogenous, local trauma, neighboring osteomyelitis or adjoining soft tissue infection. *Streptococcus* group is frequently implicated. The avascular joint cartilage gets infected through the highly vascular synovial membrane causing edema and effusion, the obliteration of cartilage leads to reduction of joint space and destroys the articular cartilage. Followed by immobilization due to pain leads to osteoporosis and destruction leading to subluxations or dislocations other sequelae are fibrous ankylosis and deformity. Initially radiographs may show joint space widening with soft tissue swelling. Later osteoporosis, loss of joint space, marginal and central erosion of articular cortex is seen (**Fig. 4.5**).

Tuberculous Arthritis

Tubercle bacilli are deposited in the synovium through a hematogenous route or direct penetration from a metaphyseal focus of osteomyelitis. A monoarticular presentation is most common involving large joints (hip, knee, and shoulder joint) are involved. Bony destruction is not usually evident on clinical presentation which, unlike acute septic arthritis, is slow and insidious with gradual onset of pain, stiffness and synovial swelling.

Initially joint effusion associated with a synovial hypertrophy is seen and is difficult to differentiate from other conditions including septic arthritis, hemophilia, Lyme disease, pigmented villonodular synovitis, and juvenile rheumatoid arthritis. Later on there is gradual proliferation of granulation tissue at the joint periphery which manifests clinically as a joint effusion with or without thickening of synovial tissue. Radiographically, there is soft tissue swelling and diffuse osteopenia, without a focal abnormality. Granulation tissue spreads across the joint, and the

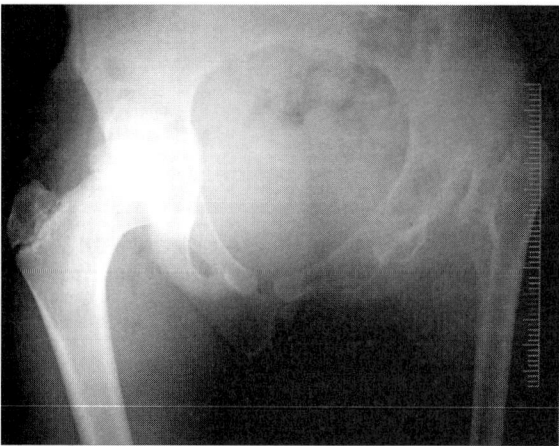

Fig. 4.5 Sequelae in septic arthritis left hip in an 8-year-old female in the form of destruction of left femoral head which is displaced superiorly with development of pseudoarthorosis

first bony changes are marginal erosions, which are evident radiographically. Over a time, there is erosion of the articular cartilage and of the underlying bone, resulting in loss of joint space on plain radiographs. Later on secondary degenerative changes in the joint are observed. The early findings on magnetic resonance imaging are nonspecific, and include a joint effusion, marrow edema, and during the stage of arthritis—abnormalities within the articular cartilage and subchondral bone **(Figs 4.6A to D)**.

Radiographic findings characteristic of tuberculous arthritis are referred as Phemister's triad which includes juxta-articular osteoporosis, peripherally located bone erosions and gradual loss of joint space. Soft tissue swelling and osteoporosis may dominate the initial radiographic findings. Marginal erosions in weight bearing joints are characteristic findings in tuberculous arthritis of hip, knee and ankle joints. These erosions produce corner defects simulating erosions of other synovial processes such as rheumatoid arthritis. The eventual outcome of tuberculous arthritis is a fibrous ankylosis of the affected joint. Bony ankylosis is seen occasionally but is more frequently observed with septic arthritis. The main differential diagnoses of tuberculous arthritis include erosive arthropathies (rheumatoid arthritis and gout), and other monoarticular processes (pigmented villonodular synovitis and osteochondromatosis).

Congenital Syphilis

In utero syphilis infection results in transmission from maternal infection of spirochete *Treponema pallidum*. The pathogen is capable of crossing the placenta any time during gestation. The following tests can be assessed on maternal blood:
- Fluorescent treponemal antibody absorbed test (FTA-ABS)
- Rapid plasma reagin (RPR)
- Venereal disease research laboratory test (VDRL)

Antenatal sonographic features are nonspecific and mimic those of the generalized in utero infection, like fetal hepatosplenomegaly placentomegaly, ascites. In severe cases there may be evidence of fetal hydrops or bowing of fetal long bones.

Skeletal lesions early in disease are osteochondritis, osteomyelitis which is diaphyseal, periostitis which occurs early in the course of disease.

Osteochondritis occurs at metaphysis in which widens the zone of provisional calcification until there is epiphyseal separation. X-ray shows, lucent metaphyseal bands which heal after six months of age. Osteomyelitis can also be seen in skull with geographic areas of destruction. Saber tibia results from growth stimulation of the tibia with forward bowing. Dactylitis, especially of proximal phalanx of index finger can be seen. Other changes seen are saddle nose, notched and narrowed incisors-Hutchinson's teeth, periosteal reaction and new bone formation more commonly seen in proximal 2/3 of tibia shaft common late manifestation.

Differential diagnosis includes birth trauma, rickets, severe malnutrition treatment is with penicillin. Fetal demise or still birth can occur in untreated cases. Fetal developing hydrops tend to have poor prognosis.

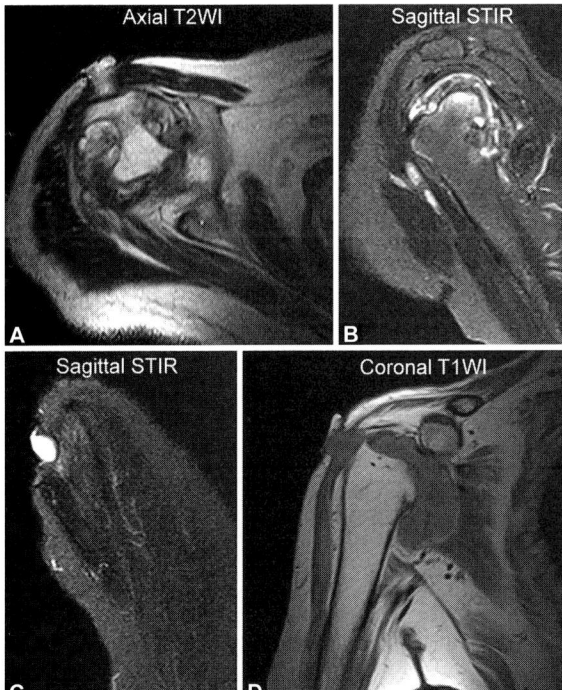

Figs 4.6A to D A 57 years old male presented with history of right shoulder discharging sinus since 5 months. No history of fever. MR shows loss of normal joint space with destruction of the articular surface involving the humerus and glenoid of right shoulder and moderate joint effusion with sinus tract extending anteriorly up to the skin surface. Atrophy of the rotator cuff muscles is seen, predominantly of the supraspinatus muscles. The effusion appears hyperintense on T2 and STIR (A to C) and hypointense on T1WI (D)

Infectious Arthritis

Infectious arthritis is classified as pyogenic (septic) or nonpyogenic. Pyogenic septic arthritis is most frequently caused by *Staphylococcus aureus*, may be caused multiple other organisms, including staphylococci, *Streptococcus pneumoniae*, group B streptococci, *Gonococcus* species, *Escherichia coli*, *Haemophilus* species, *Klebsiella* species, *Pseudomonas* species, and *Candida* species. Infection can lead to rapid and severe joint destruction.

Nonpyogenic infective arthritis tends to be less aggressive and have a more chronic course. Causative organisms include *Mycobacterium tuberculosis*, fungi, and spirochetes.

In septic arthritis the most common route of transmission is hematogenous from a distant source such as pneumonia or a remote wound infection. Direct seeding from can occur through trauma, surgery, or spread from a contiguous infection such as osteomyelitis or cellulitis.

Imaging is not the primary means of diagnosing septic arthritis. Joint fluid aspiration and evaluation is the key to the diagnosis, and samples should be obtained in all suspected cases of septic arthritis. This sampling can usually be achieved with fine-needle aspiration performed either blindly or with fluoroscopic guidance, depending on the location. Surgical exploration may be necessary in unusual cases, such as those involving sacroiliac and sternoclavicular joint infections.

Fluid should be sent for Gram staining, culturing, glucose testing, and leukocyte count and differential determination. White blood cell counts are usually 50,000–60,000/µL, with more than 80% neutrophils. Synovial fluid glucose levels are decreased. Gram-stain results are positive in 75% of patients with gram-positive cocci. Gram staining is less sensitive in cases of gonococcal infection. Only 25% of cultures of gonococcal synovial fluid are positive.

Multiple imaging modalities are available for assessing septic arthritis. Plain radiography should be used as the initial study. However, if further imaging is required, MRI is the most sensitive and specific technique. Scintigraphy, computed tomography (CT), fluorodeoxyglucose (FDG)/positron emission tomography (PET), and ultrasonography are also used, to a lesser extent.

Plain radiographs are not sensitive to early findings, such as joint effusion or soft tissue changes.

MRI is expensive and time consuming. It shows marrow edema in subchondral regions with synovial thickening **(Figs 4.7A to D)**. It is usually unnecessary if clinical suspicion is high and if the joint is easily accessible for aspiration. CT is similar to MRI, but it has the disadvantage of ionizing radiation. However, it can be useful for guiding the aspiration of certain joints. Scintigraphy is extremely sensitive but extremely nonspecific.

Ultrasonographic findings can confirm a joint effusion, but it cannot be used to assess its cause. It cannot accurately depict bony or cartilaginous abnormalities. This modality also may be useful to guide joint aspiration, and it is generally less expensive than either CT or MRI.

Sacroiliitis

Sacroiliitis is inflammation of the sacroiliac joint. The true prevalence of sacroiliac joint lesions is unknown in most population groups, either with or without low backache. Similarly, the presence of sacroiliitis on MRI has not been determined in low backache cases attributable to either mechanical or inflammatory or both these broad etiological groups. Low back pain is a common referral in routine MRI practice. Clearly, it is one of the most common symptoms evaluated and treated by practitioners. It has been observed that in any 12-month period in USA, 15–20% of the population has an episode of lumbosacral pain with back symptoms occurring in 50% of working age adults yearly. Low back pain is associated with a wide range of clinical disorders. The most common group is mechanical disorders, which occurs in more than 90% of all episodes of back pain. 10% of the remaining patients with back pain have symptoms related to systemic illness, like cancer, inflammatory back disease or infection.

Characteristic radiographic features include joint space narrowing, sclerosis, and erosions of the ilium and sacrum. Sacroiliitis is the hallmark of ankylosing spondylitis. The inflammation is evident early in the

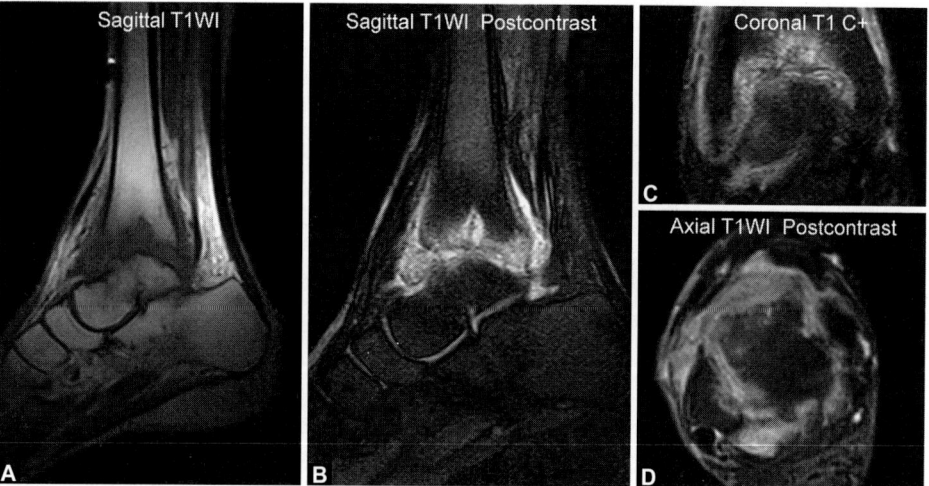

Figs 4.7A to D MR of right ankle in a 21-year-old female with history of fever and pain in ankle on T1WI sagittal image show marrow edema in subchondral regions (A). Sagittal, coronal and axial T1WI postcontrast images show synovial thickening and enhancement (B to D)

course of the disease. In later stages, the radiographic changes are almost invariably bilateral and symmetric. The alterations occur in both the synovial and the ligamentous (superior and posterior) portions of the joint and predominate in the ilium. Periarticular osteoporosis and loss of definition, superficial erosion, and focal sclerosis of subchondral bone are present initially. Sacroiliitis is evaluated by using CT to look for presence of subchondral sclerosis, osteophytosis, or cartilage loss. Sacroiliac joint is a unique joint in the human body with differences in type and thickness of articular cartilage between different regions of the sacral and iliac articular surfaces.

MRI of normal sacroiliac joint reveals an intermediate signal of the cartilage of the synovial compartment on T1 and T2 images limited by the signal void. MRI may have a role in the early diagnosis of sacroiliitis. Advantages of MRI include direct visualization of cartilage abnormalities, detection of bone marrow edema, improved detection of erosions, and the absence of ionizing radiation **(Figs 4.8A to D)**. Detection of synovial enhancement on MRI has been found to correlate with disease activity, as measured by laboratory inflammatory markers.

The marrow on T1, T2 and T1FS images has a homogeneous intermediate signal. Fat suppressed images are extremely useful in imaging of cases with sacroiliitis. Fat suppression causes rescaling of signal intensities, categorizes cartilage as the brightest structure. This additive effect along with the darkened appearance of fat in adjacent soft tissues and sacral, iliac and lumbar marrow renders improved visualization of structures and increases the conspicuity of lesion, thereby improving their pickup rate. There are two fat suppressed sequences that are available: T1-weighted with fat suppression (T1FS) and fast short tau inversion recovery (Fast STIR) sequences. These are superior to T1 and T2 images, in demonstrating the changes of sacroiliitis.

There are few normal variants, which merits consideration during MRI evaluation of sacroiliac joint. Partial volume artifact between the synovial and ligamentous compartments can be misinterpreted as erosions. There is normally a region of high signal at the immediate subchondral marrow, on Fast STIR images, which can be mistaken for early sacroiliitis. A patchy distribution of fat within the bone marrow as the sole finding should not be considered as an indicator for sacroiliitis.

The value of MRI in the diagnosis of sacroiliitis has been well established. MRI accurately delineates the cardinal features of sacroiliitis, such as changes in joint space width and symmetry, presence of erosions, subchondral edema, sclerosis, cysts and ankylosis. Furthermore, MRI plays a useful role in patients with early disease, by its superior ability to directly image changes in articular cartilage. Comparative studies between MRI and CT in the evaluation of patients with suspected sacroiliitis have further shown that the sensitivity and specificity of MR for the detection of cortical erosions and subchondral sclerosis when compared to CT images were 100 and 94.3%, respectively.

MRI offers valuable information on the lesions affecting the various structures of the sacroiliac joint

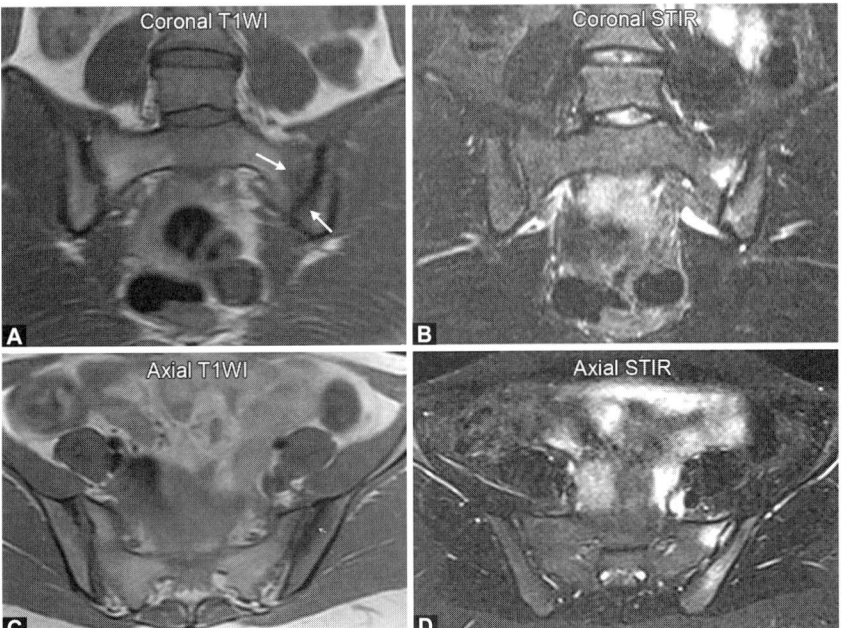

Figs 4.8A to D A 19 years female with history of low back ache since 6 months shows abnormal hypointense signal on coronal and axial T1WI (A and C) involving the articular surface of the left sacroiliac joint. Coronal and axial STIR images (B and D) show hyperintense signal involving the articular surface of the left sacroiliac joint. These imaging findings are suggestive of left sacroiliitis

in sacroiliitis. Synovial pannus tissue appears low signal intensity on T1 and high signal on T2 **(Figs 4.8A to D)**, spared cartilage exhibits persisting low-signal foci within synovial compartment, bone erosions shows high signal regions at the bone periphery and subchondral bone sclerosis displays markedly hypointense subchondral bone and infectious sacroiliitis shows diffuse high signal intensity in the bone marrow.

Seronegative and HLA B27-associated spondyloarthropathy (SpA) is a heterogeneous group of related inflammatory joint disease that share typical clinical features and a unique association with the major histocompatibility complex class I molecule HLA-B27. It comprises of five clinically defined subcategories: ankylosing spondylitis (AS), psoriatic arthritis (PsA), reactive arthritis (ReA), inflammatory bowel disease-associated arthritis and undifferentiated spondyloarthropathy (uSpA).

The value of using a 'fat suppressed' coronal sequence of the sacroiliac joint, is that it identifies sacroiliitis reliably by the presence of subchondral edema, erosions and sclerosis even when there is no joint space narrowing. Once sacroiliitis is identified on MRI, the patient is evaluated clinically, assessed for human leukocyte antigen (HLA) status, erythrocyte sedimentation rate (ESR) and C-reaction protein (CRP) for activity and subject to a periodic follow-up, wherein intravenous gadolinium is used to characterize the disease activity.

In the final analysis, the use of a 'fat suppressed' coronal sequence during the evaluation of the lumbar spine is a simple and convenient screening strategy. It reliably identifies sacroiliitis, which is a demonstrable cause of low backache, but often neglected or missed.

Cellulitis is an acute infection of the dermis and subcutaneous tissues manifesting as pain, erythema, edema, and warmth. CT scan images are used to accurately differentiate between superficial cellulitis and cellulitis associated with a deep-seated infection. In uncomplicated cellulitis, CT demonstrates skin thickening, septation of the subcutaneous fat, and thickening of the underlying superficial fascia a radiopaque foreign body associated with cellulitis may also be detected by CT scan. If the infection spreads to deeper tissues, deep cellulitis, myositis, necrotizing fasciitis, or osteomyelitis can occur, all of which can be excluded with CT. Complications like soft-tissue abscess and thrombophlebitis may also be seen on CT mages.

Necrotizing fasciitis is a progressive, rapidly spreading infection of the deep fascia, with secondary necrosis of the subcutaneous tissues, more common in immunocompromised patients with HIV infection, diabetes mellitus, cancer, alcoholism, vascular insufficiencies, and organ transplants. On CT images one can see the presence of gas in the subcutaneous tissues caused by gas-forming anaerobic organisms, thickening of the affected fascia, fluid collections along the deep fascial sheaths, and extension of edema into the inter-muscular septa and the muscles without any enhancement of the fascia, thus distinguishing non-necrotizing fasciitis from necrotizing fasciitis.

*Soft-tissue abscess is common in immuno-*compromised patients. CT shows a well-demarcated fluid collection with peripheral pseudo-capsule showing rim enhancement thus differentiating an abscess from simple cellulitis or fasciitis.

Infectious myositis is infection of skeletal muscle, seen most commonly in quadriceps muscle. On CT, there is enlargement and decreased attenuation of the affected muscle with effacement of surrounding fat planes. Involvement of a muscle group that is disproportionate to the involvement of subcutaneous tissue helps distinguish myositis from primary cellulitis. Intramuscular fluid collections may be observed, and contrast material is administered to help differentiate necrotic from viable musculature and to demonstrate a rim-enhancing abscess if present. CT guided aspiration and drainage of the muscle abscess followed by administration of appropriate antibiotics is also possible.

5
Noninfective Inflammatory Arthritis

Seronegative Spondyloarthropathy

The seronegative spondyloarthropathies are a group of conditions affecting the axial spine, presenting with back pain of an inflammatory nature. The primary feature of these disorders is sacroiliitis. The distinction between subtypes of spondyloarthritis is based on genotype (HLA-B27 positivity as in ankylosing spondylitis), peripheral manifestations of disease (psoriatic and reactive arthritis), and factors such as age, gender, and morbidity. Although radiography has long been used to diagnose the spondyloarthropathies, advanced imaging with magnetic resonance is better able to diagnose these disorders at their earliest stages and monitor disease-modifying therapies. Examples are ankylosing spondylitis, psoriatic arthritis, Reiter's syndrome and arthritis associated with chronic inflammatory bowel diseases.

Ankylosing Spondylitis

It is a chronic inflammatory disorder of unknown cause with widespread musculoskeletal involvement. The most characteristic features are sacroiliitis and spondylitis. Abnormalities occur in joints and at the sites of attachment of ligaments and tendons to bone, with an overwhelming predilection for the axial skeleton. HLA-B27 antigen is present in a very high percentage of patients with ankylosing spondylitis.

In cartilaginous joints (discovertebral junction, symphysis pubis and manubriosternal joint), the process appears to be inflammatory. Ossification produces syndesmophytes that extend from one vertebral body to another.

Enthesopathy (abnormalities in entheses or ligamentous attachments) is also a typical feature. Radiographically, erosion and eburnation of the subligamentous bone with poorly defined erosive abnormalities and surrounding sclerosis are seen.

Imaging Features

The radiographic features in synovial joints in ankylosing spondylitis are similar to those of rheumatoid arthritis. Both diseases exhibit some degree of osteoporosis, joint space narrowing and bone erosion. Proliferation about sites of erosion is more characteristic of ankylosing spondylitis.

CT scanning may possibly delineate early changes in the sacroiliac joint. Among the CT indicators of sacroiliitis are nonuniform iliac sclerosis, focal joint space narrowing and bone erosions. CT may also be used to detect spinal fractures, spinal stenosis, thecal diverticula, atlantoaxial instability and manubriosternal and costovertebral joint disease.

MR imaging can be of value in imaging certain manifestations and complications of ankylosing spondylitis. An increase in signal intensity within the vertebral body marrow, adjacent to abnormal intervertebral discs, in T2-weighted spin-echo sequences may reflect edema and indicate discovertebral inflammation.

The sacroiliac joint is among the first sites to show involvement in this disease. Changes are bilateral and symmetrical. Periarticular osteoporosis, superficial erosion and focal sclerosis of subchondral bone are observed, followed by fraying of the bone surface and widening of the interosseous space. Bone proliferation leads to the formation of irregular bone bridges that traverse the articular cavity and later result in complete ankylosis.

In the spine, the discovertebral junctions reveal osteitis, syndemophytosis, discovertebral erosions and destruction (Andersson lesions), and discal calcification. The apophyseal joints are narrowed and fused; abnormalities are observed in the lumbar, thoracic and cervical segments of the spine and are accompanied by reactive subchondral bone formation. In the cervical region, apophyseal joint ankylosis can be very striking.

Other sites that may be affected in ankylosing spondylitis are the hip joint, glenohumeral joint.

Psoriatic Arthritis

It is a seronegative spondyloarthropathy occurring in some patients with psoriasis. Five broad clinical varieties of psoriatic arthritis have been recognized; polyarthritis characterized by distal interphalangeal joint involvement, a deforming type of arthritis characterized by widespread ankylosis and occasionally arthritis mutilans, a symmetric seronegative polyarthritis simulating rheumatoid arthritis but without rheumatoid factor, monoarthritis or asymmetric oligoarthritis, and sacroiliitis and spondylitis resembling ankylosing spondylitis.

The articular disease may be monoarticular, pauciarticular or polyarticular in its distribution, and virtually any joint can be affected. In some patients, low back complaints predominate because of involvement of the spine and the sacroiliac joints. Prominent soft tissue swelling about involved joints, which may affect an entire digit (sausage digit). The histocompatibility antigen HLA-B27 is frequently present in patients with psoriasis and sacroiliitis.

Classic radiographic features of psoriatic arthritis are involvement of synovial and cartilaginous joints and entheses, asymmetric distribution more common than symmetric distribution, involvement of interphalangeal joints of the hands and feet, sacroiliitis and spondylitis with paravertebral ossification, bone erosion with adjacent proliferation, intra-articular bone ankylosis and destruction of phalangeal tufts.

Reiter's Syndrome

It is a seronegative spondyloarthropathy with skin involvement in which a classic triad of urethritis, arthritis and conjunctivitis is common. An infectious cause is suspected, as the disease often follows an infection of the bowel or lower genitourinary tract. Men are affected much more commonly than women, who tend to develop the disease after intestinal disorders, including bacillary dysentery, amoebic dysentery and shigellosis.

The characteristic skin lesion, termed keratoderma blenorrhagicum, affects the palms and soles most frequently. Superficial erythematous ulcerations may also be evident on the buccal mucosa and the tongue. The serum histocompatibility antigen HLA-B27 may be present in as many as 75% of patients.

Involvement of the lower extremity usually becomes evident initially in the knee and the ankle, followed in descending order of frequency by the metatarsophalangeal joints, the heel, the shoulder, the wrist, the hip and the lumbar spine. Heel pain and tenderness are sometimes initial manifestations of Reiter's syndrome. The arthritic attacks in this disease are usually self-limiting and of short duration but recurrences are frequent.

On radiographs, the features of joint involvement in Reiter's syndrome are similar to those in the other seronegative spondyloarthropathies and differ from the findings of rheumatoid arthritis. Soft tissue prominence, sometimes leading to a sausage digit, may be present. Regional or periarticular osteoporosis is seen. Loss of joint space, erosion of articular surfaces, and superficial bone resorption beneath inflamed bursae and tendon sheaths are additional findings.

Calcification and ossification of tendons have also been observed in patients with Reiter's syndrome. Paravertebral ossification about the lower three thoracic and upper three lumbar vertebrae is a frequent early finding in Reiter's syndrome. This is manifested as elongated vertical osseous bridges extending across the intervertebral disc but separated by a clear space from the lateral margins of both the disc and the vertebral body.

On bone scintigraphy, early findings of Reiter's syndrome include asymmetric involvement of the joints of the lower extremity, sometimes with striking increased radioactivity on the plantar and posterior aspects of the calcaneum and asymmetric sacroiliitis.

Hypertrophic Osteoarthropathy

Hypertrophic osteoarthropathy (HO) is a syndrome characterized by periostitis of the long tubular bones, clubbing of the digits, and arthritis. It this there is excessive proliferation of skin and bone at the distal parts of extremities. This condition involves symmetric periostitis involving the radius and fibula and, to a lesser extent, the femur, humerus, metacarpals, and metatarsals. Most imaging studies and histologic examinations of clubbed fingers reveal hypervascularization of the distal digits. When associated with a lung condition, it is also termed hypertrophic pulmonary osteoarthropathy. It is usually painful and associated with clubbing.

The pathologies which have clinical association with HO are shown in **Table 5.1**.

The hypertrophic osteoarthropathy is seen as a long metaphyseal and diaphyseal smooth periosteal reaction involving the long bones. With disease progression, periostitis becomes more prominent or multilayered, and extends to the epiphyses. Periosteal reaction due to venous stasis is typically solid and undulating, and initially separated from the cortex.

The etiology of HO is unknown. Several mechanisms have been proposed as contributing to the pathophysiology of hypertrophic osteoarthropathy. Paraneoplastic growth factors such as prostaglandin E, cytokines, neurologic, hormonal, immune mechanisms and vascular thrombi caused by platelets and antiphospholipid antibodies have all been proposed as possible etiologies. A popular current theory involves the interaction between activated platelets and the endothelium.

Differential Diagnosis

- *Caffey's disease:* Infantile cortical hyperostosis (Caffey disease) typically affects the young; it is usually associated with extreme proliferative periostitis of the mandible, clavicle, scapula, ribs, and tubular bones. Cranial destruction, bone

Table 5.1 Causes of hypertrophic osteoarthropathy

Cardiovascular disorders	Pulmonary disorders	Gastrointestinal disorders	Miscellaneous disorders
Bacterial endocarditis	Lung tumors (primary or metastases)	Neoplasms of liver, esophagus, or bowel	Myxedema or thyrotoxicosis
Cyanotic congenital heart disease	Pleural tumors (Mesothelioma)	Inflammatory bowel disease (e.g. Ulcerative colitis)	Hematologic malignancies
Cardiac tumors	Mediastinal tumors	Hepatic cirrhosis	Polyarteritis nodosa
Aortic aneurysm	Lung abscess or empyema	Chronic obstructive jaundice or biliary cirrhosis	Idiopathic (Primary or familial)
Infected aortic graft	Bronchiectasis	Amebiasis	
Secondary polycythemia	Pulmonary tuberculosis	Intestinal tuberculosis	
	Sarcoidosis	Subphrenic or liver abscess	
	Bronchogenic cyst	Celiac sprue (Gluten sensitive enteropathy)	
	Cystic fibrosis		
	Chronic obstructive pulmonary disease		

deformities, and soft-tissue nodules may occur in infantile cortical hyperostosis.

- *Fibrous dysplasia:* The usual appearance of fibrous dysplasia includes a lucent lesion in the diaphysis or metaphysis, with endosteal scalloping and with or without bone expansion and the absence of periosteal reaction. Usually, the matrix of the lucency is smooth and relatively homogeneous; classically, this finding is described as a ground-glass appearance. Irregular areas of sclerosis may be present with or without calcification. The lucent lesion has a thick sclerotic border and is called the rind sign. The lesion may extend into the epiphysis only after fusion. Premature fusion of the ossification centers may occur, resulting in adult dwarfism. The dysplastic bone may undergo calcification and enchondral bone formation.
- *Paget's disease:* In the long bones, osteolysis begins as a subchondral area of lucency. The advancing wedge of osteolysis often demonstrates a characteristic sharp radiolucent margin without sclerosis likened to a blade of grass or flame. In rare cases, the disease is isolated to the diaphysis, most commonly in the tibia, rather than subchondral bone, which can cause diagnostic confusion.
- *Other differential diagnoses:* The radiographic features of fluorosis, macrodystrophia lipomatosa, and *Proteus* syndrome are sufficiently distinct not to cause confusion with HPOA or HOA. When considering a diagnosis of primary hypertrophic osteoarthropathy (primary HOA, pachydermoperiostosis), also take into account congenital syphilis, diaphyseal dysplasia (Camurati-Engelmann disease), hypervitaminosis A, acromegaly, thyroid acropachy, venous stasis, endosteal hyperostosis (van Buchem disease). All these diseases have different clinical features which helps them to be differentiated from HOA.

Imaging Features of Hypertrophic Osteoarthropathy on Plain Radiograph

Plain radiography is the mainstay of radiology-aided diagnosis, although the exact sensitivity of plain radiography is unknown. Nuclear medicine studies reveal early evidence of disease. The role of magnetic resonance imaging (MRI) is currently exploratory. CT chest is useful in defining intrathoracic pathology as the cause of hypertrophic pulmonary osteoarthropathy.

Plain radiographs show 2 types of changes, **bone formation with hypertrophy** and **bone dissolution with acro-osteolysis**. The predominant radiographic feature of primary hypertrophic osteoarthropathy (HO, pachydermoperiostosis) is **periostitis**, which is depicted as symmetric osseous thickening. Periosteal changes are seen as a continuous thin line of sclerotic new bone separated from the cortex by a radiolucent space. Initially, periostitis is symmetric and involves the tibia, fibula, radius, ulna, and, less commonly, the femur, humerus, metacarpals, metatarsal, and phalanges on both sides. Periosteal proliferation is usually shaggy and is associated with irregular excrescences and diaphyseal expansion. Eventually, periosteal proliferation extends into the metaphysis. Periosteal proliferation rarely extends into the epiphysis, except in patients with congenital cyanotic heart disease, in whom the epiphysis may be affected. In rare cases, periostitis affects the ribs, clavicles, and scapula. Rarely, thickening of the calvarium and skull base is seen. Periosteal proliferation is usually single or laminated and is either regular or irregular. Laminated periostitis may have an onion-skin appearance.

Acro-osteolysis may be seen in the distal tufts in patients with long-standing hypertrophic osteoarthropathy.

Nuclear imaging bone scanning with technetium-99m (^{99m}Tc)–labeled diphosphonate shows evidence of hypertrophic pulmonary osteoarthropathy early in the course of disease. The sensitivity of isotope bone scans is greater than that of other imaging methods. Isotope uptake is symmetrically increased in the tubular bones along the cortical margins of the diaphysis and metaphysis. Uptake may be irregular, or it may create a double stripe or parallel track sign. Periarticular radionuclide uptake may be increased as a result of associated synovitis. Isotope bone scans show high rates of scapular involvement, mandibular involvement considerably higher than the involvement seen in X-rays.

Ankylosing Spondylitis

The term ankylosing is derived from the Greek word ankylos, meaning stiffening of a joint; the term spondylos means vertebra. Spondylitis refers to inflammation of one or more vertebrae. Ankylosing spondylitis, represented in the radiograph below, usually is classified as a chronic and progressive form of seronegative arthritis.

Ankylosing spondylitis (AS) is characterized by inflammation at areas where a ligament, tendon attaches to a bone. Persistent inflammation can lead to erosion of the bone. The healing takes place with formation of new bone. Eventually, the process of erosion and healing with new bone formation leads to fusion of the bones. This leads to restriction of the movement of the spine.

The majority of patients with AS exhibit the HLA-B27 antigen and high level of immunoglobulin A (IgA) in the blood. The HLA-B27 antigen is also expressed by *Klebsiella* bacteria, which are found in high levels in the feces of AS patients.

Radiograph

Sacroiliitis occurs early in the course of ankylosing spondylitis and is regarded as a hallmark of the disease. Radiographically, the earliest sign of sacroiliitis is indistinctness of the joint. The joints initially widen before they narrow. Subchondral bony erosions on the iliac side of the joint are seen; these are followed by subchondral sclerosis and bony proliferation.

CT

Computed tomography (CT) scanning may be useful in selected patients in whom ankylosing spondylitis is suggested and in whom initial sacroiliac joint radiographs findings are normal or equivocal. Features such as joint erosions, subchondral sclerosis, and bony ankylosis are visualized better on CT scans than on radiographs; however, some normal variants of the sacroiliac joint may simulate the features of sacroiliitis.

MRI

MRI has been found to be superior to CT scanning in the detection of cartilage changes, bone erosions, and subchondral bone changes. MRI is also sensitive in the assessment of activity in relatively early disease. Affected sites include the discovertebral junction and the peripheral joints. In general, areas of increased T2 signal correlate with the presence of edema or vascularized fibrous tissue.

Psoriatic Arthritis

Psoriasis is a chronic skin condition that causes red patches on the body. About 1 in 20 people with psoriasis will develop inflammatory arthritis with the skin condition. It is a seronegative spondyloarthropathy. The cause of psoriatic arthritis is considered to be a combination of environmental and hereditary factors, with as many as to 60% of patients being HLA-B27 positive. The arthritis may be mild and involve few joints, particularly, those at the end of the fingers or toes. In some people, the disease may be severe and affect many joints, including the spine. When the spine is affected, the symptoms are stiffness, burning, and pain, most often in the lower spine and sacrum. People who also have arthritis usually have the skin and nail changes of psoriasis. The inflamed joints become painful, swollen, hot, and red. Psoriatic arthritis involves the synovial and cartilaginous joints, as well as the attachment of tendons and ligaments to the bones in the appendicular and axial skeleton.

The most commonly involved sites are the interphalangeal joints of hands and feet, metacarpophalangeal and metatarsophalangeal joints, calcaneus, sacroiliac joints and spine. Findings may be bilateral or unilateral and symmetric or asymmetric. The hands and feet are frequently affected by erosive change. The distal interphalangeal joints are common site for erosions, especially the interphalangeal joint of the great toe. Erosion starts at the joint margin and proceed centrally into joint. Erosive changes are asymmetrical. Joint narrowing never occurs. Erosions are modified by proliferation of new bone giving spiculated, frayed, paintbrush appearance. Late changes include intra-articular osseous fission. The resorption of the tufts of the distal phalanx in the hands and feet is characteristic for psoriatic arthritis. The progressive osteolysis may progress to destruction of most of the phalanx. The eroded small bones are irregular in outline. The expansion of the base of the distal phalanx combined with the middle phalanx gives "pencil and cup" appearance leading to arthritis mutilans. Periostitis in psoriatic arthritis occurs along the shafts of the tubular bones on hands and feet, which become sclerotic and expanded and, in association with soft-tissue swelling, gives a 'sausage digit'.

Involvement of the larger joints is not common, but sacroiliitis may be seen in up to 50% of those with psoriatic arthritis. Often erosions, joint widening and sclerosis initially involving iliac side are noted.

Paravertebral ossification may be the only feature of osteopathy. These syndesmophytes, are vertically directed and appear fluffy and curvilinear.

Other characteristic feature is inflammation of the entheses, at the attachment sites of tendons, ligaments, fascia and joint capsule to bones.

MRI is more sensitive in detecting early bone marrow edema, bony erosion, synovitis and sacroilitis

Ultrasound can also be used in the diagnosis of early enthesitis and dactylitis. Both MRI and ultrasound are useful imaging techniques to monitor the response in treatment of psoriasis.

6
Joints

SHOULDER JOINT

Anatomy Shoulder Joint

The shoulder or glenohumeral joint is the most flexible joint in the body. It consists of bones, ligaments, muscles and their tendons, and connects the arm to the chest **(Figs 6.1 and 6.2)**. It is a ball and socket joint. The glenoid cavity forms a shallow socket and is inherently unstable. The added stability to the joint is made available by the capsule, ligaments, glenoid labrum and the rotator cuff.

The articular capsule completely encircles the joint; it is attached to the circumference of the glenoid cavity beyond the labrum. Inferiorly, it is attached to the anatomical neck of the humerus.

The ligaments of the glenohumeral joint are coracohumeral ligament and glenohumeral ligaments. Glenohumeral ligament has superior middle and inferior divisions. They are designed to stabilize the shoulder in the abducted or functional position. The labrum is a fibrocartilaginous rim attached around the margin of the glenoid cavity. It cushions and stabilizes the humeral head. It increases the superoinferior diameter of the glenoid by 75% and the anteroposterior diameter by 50%. The base of the glenoid labrum is fixed to the circumference of the cavity. It is continuous above with the tendon of the long head of the biceps, which blends with the fibrous tissue of the labrum. It deepens the articular cavity.

The tendon of the long head of biceps forms biceps labral complex with superior glenohumeral ligament and inserts on the supraglenoid tubercle. The tendon traverses laterally in the rotator cuff interval to lie in the bicipital groove. Glenohumeral joint is in connection with the sheath of biceps tendon.

The rotator interval is the portion of the joint capsule which lies between the supraspinatus and subscapularis tendons.

This lies between the superior and middle glenohumeral ligaments. The interval is reinforced by the coracohumeral ligament and underlying joint capsule. It is designed to limit flexion and external rotation.

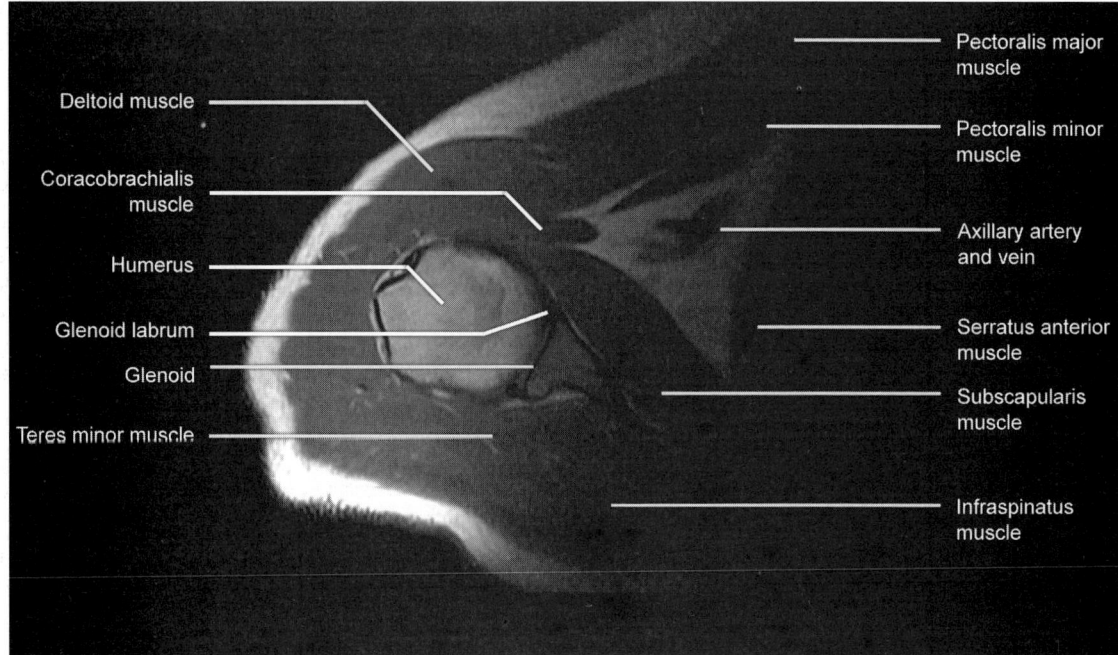

Fig. 6.1 Shoulder joint MRI: Axial T1WI

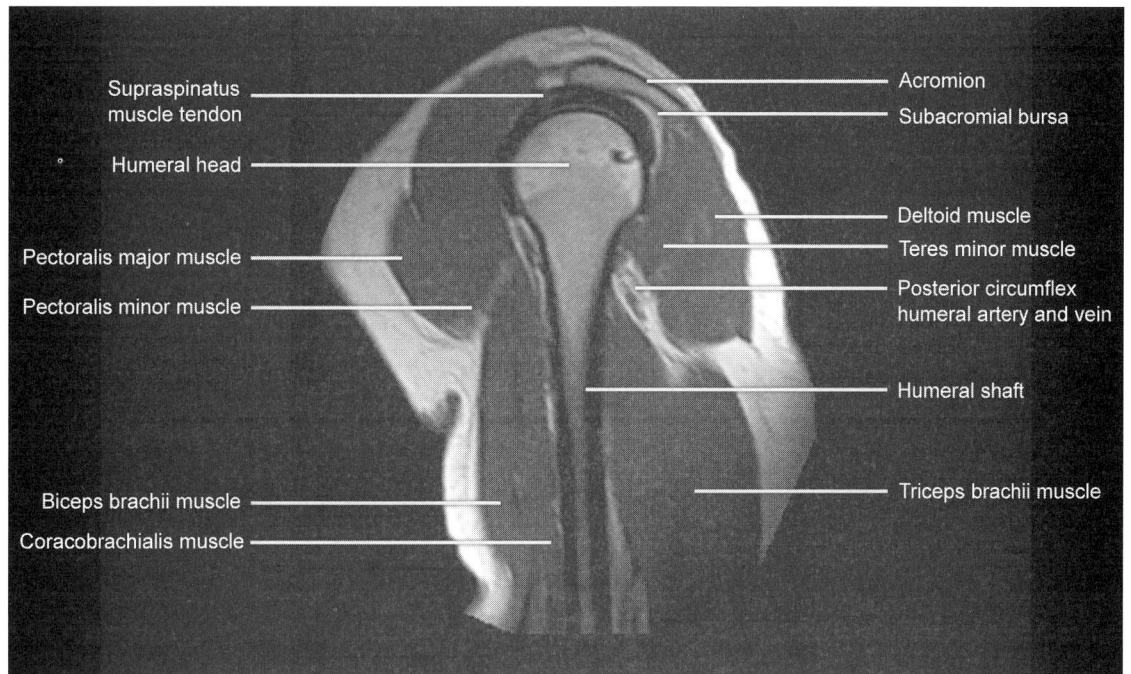

Fig. 6.2 Shoulder joint MRI: Sagittal T1WI

Rotator cuff is formed by supraspinatus, infraspinatus, teres minor and subscapularis muscles and mostly by their flat tendons **(Figs 6.1 to 6.3)**. The tendons fuse together and surround the shoulder joint. When the muscles contract, resulting in the rotator cuff tendon to rotate upward, inward, or outward. Supraspinatus tendon lies over the summit of humeral head and is an abductor. Infraspinatus and teres minor tendon cover the backside of humeral head and are external rotators. Subscapularis tendon crosses the front of the shoulder joint and is an abductor of shoulder joint.

There are two pouch-like bursae located in the shoulder which produce a lubricating fluid, which helps reduce friction between the moving parts of the joint.

Hill-Sachs Lesion

Hill-Sachs lesions are associated exclusively with anterior shoulder dislocations. It is a cortical depression in the posterolateral head of humerus. It results from forceful impaction of the humeral head against the anteroinferior glenoid rim when shoulder is dislocated anteriorly. The result is a divot or flattening in the posteromedial aspect of the humeral head, typically referred to as a 3-6 o'clock lesion for the right humeral head if seen from the bottom. The mechanism which leads to shoulder dislocation is often traumatic but may occur with history of previous dislocations. Sports, fall, seizure, assault, throwing, pulling on the arm, or just turning over in bed can be a cause of anterior shoulder dislocation. MRI shows flattening in the posterosuperior aspect of the humeral head with increased signal on T2WI **(Figs 6.4A to D)**.

Avulsion of Greater Tuberosity

Avulsion fracture is a pull-off fracture at a musculotendinous or ligamentous insertion site caused by sudden forceful muscle contraction or ligament traction. Such fractures are relatively common in athletic adolescents. The child characteristically describes acute onset of pain during muscle contraction. There is usually focal tenderness.

At most of these sites the fracture plane is through the physis of an apophysis. An apophysis acts as the insertion site for muscle and the physis represents a weak link in the immature skeleton.

Conventional radiographs generally confirm the diagnosis by demonstrating a bony fragment displaced at variable distance from the parent bone. Ultrasound can show displacement of the apophysis and dynamic examination allows confirmation that this corresponds with the site of tenderness. Ultrasound may also demonstrate associated hematoma within the adjacent muscle. MRI will demonstrate reduced signal on T1 and increased signal on T2-weighted or short tau inversion recovery (STIR) sequences, particularly within the fatty marrow of the secondary ossification center **(Figs 6.5A and B)**. It is important to recognize the fracture by its characteristic site and radiographic appearance so as to avoid misdiagnosis.

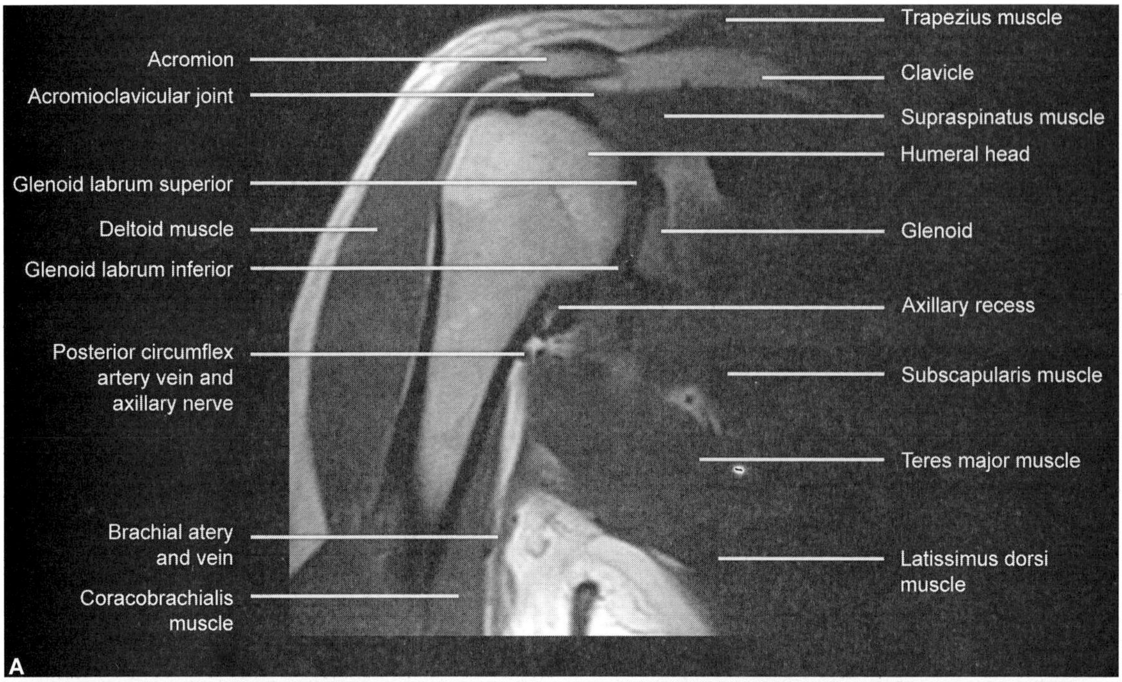

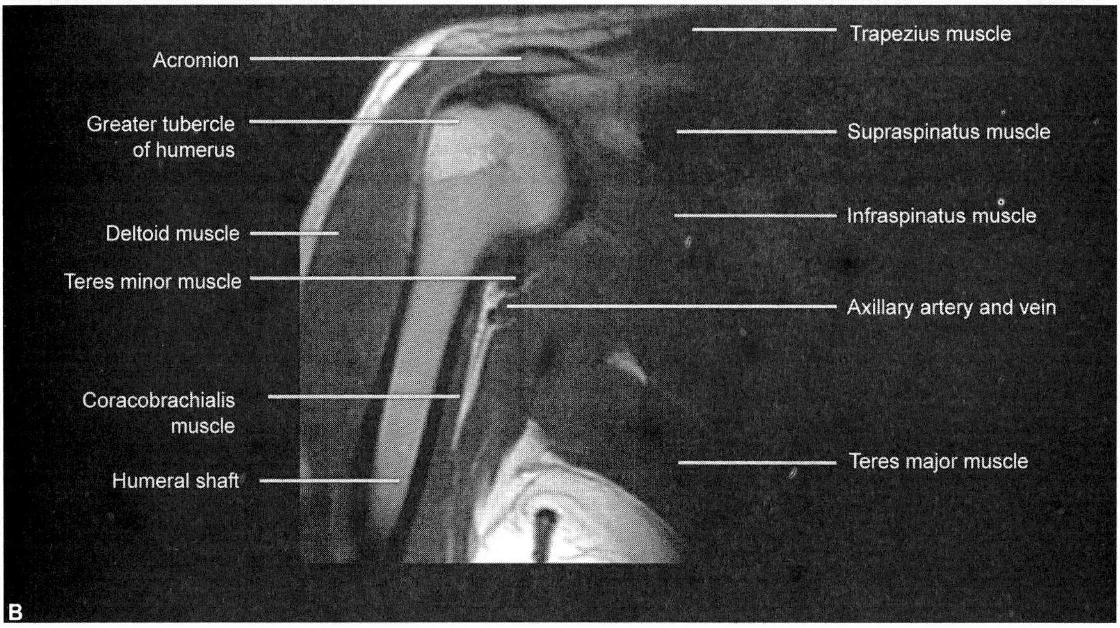

Figs 6.3A and B Shoulder joint MRI: Coronal T1WI

Acromioclavicular Degeneration

The acromioclavicular (AC) joint is the synovial articulation between the acromion process of the scapula and the acromial facet of the clavicle in the shoulder; it is a common spot for osteoarthritis to develop in middle age.

Degeneration of the AC joint can be painful and can cause difficulty in using the shoulder for routine activities. The AC joint is under constant stress as the arm is used overhead. Weightlifters and others who repeatedly lift heavy weight overhead tend to have an increased incidence, and often at a younger age.

Acromioclavicular joint osteoarthritis may also develop following an injury to the joint, such as an AC joint separation. This injury is fairly common. A separation usually results from falling on the shoulder. The shoulder does heal, but many years later degeneration causes the AC joint to become painful. Degenerative changes or osteoarthritis occur almost universally in elderly persons. Joint space loss, sclerosis and marginal osteophytes are common radiographic features. MRI shoulder generally reveals hyperintense signal along the articular surfaces of the acromioclavicular joint with loss of joint space and degenerative osteophytes **(Fig. 6.6)**.

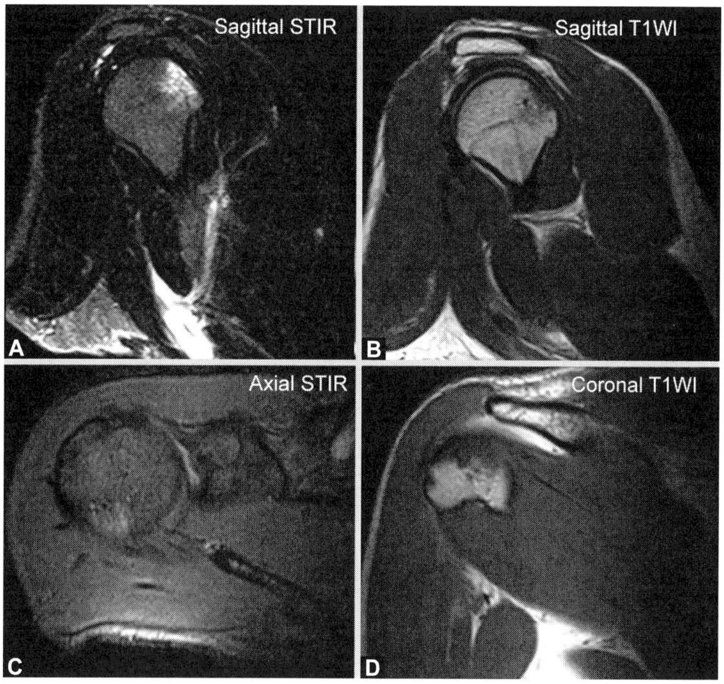

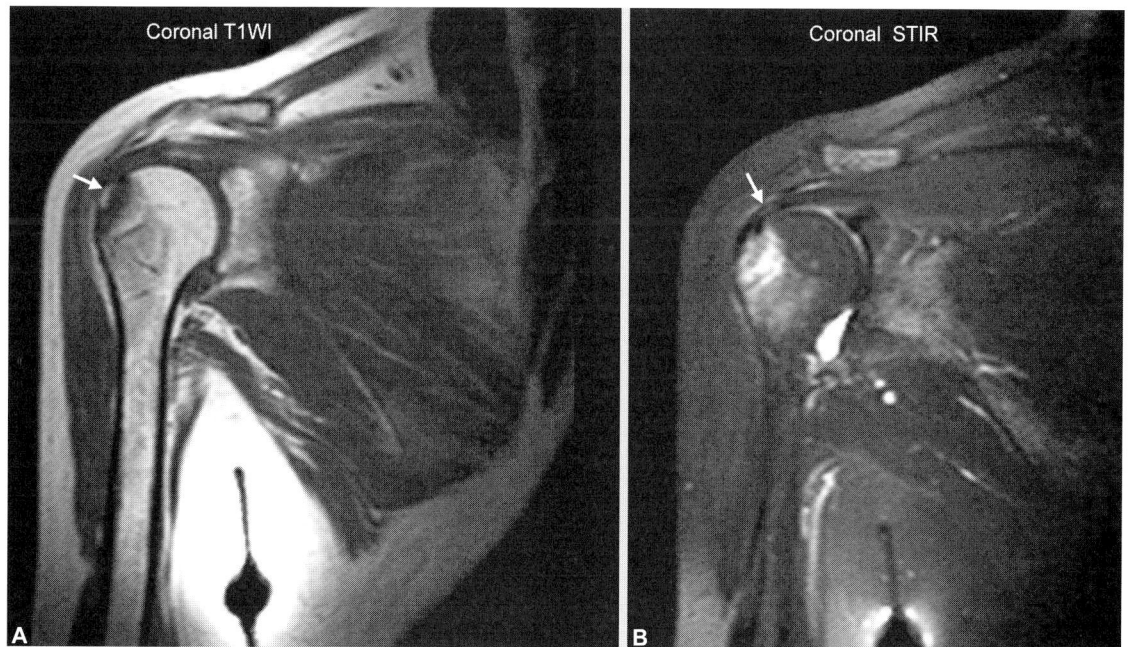

Figs 6.4A to D A 27-year-old male presented with history of shoulder dislocation. MR shows hyperintense signal along the posterosuperior aspect of the humeral head on sagittal STIR and axial STIR images (A and C) appearing hypointense on sagittal T1W and coronal T1W images (B and D), findings are suggestive of Hill-Sach's lesion

Figs 6.5A and B Coronal T1W image (A) showing avulsion fracture (arrow) of the greater tuberosity and coronal STIR images; (B) show partial tear of supraspinatus tendon (arrow)

Spinoglenoid Cyst

Paralabral cysts are common incidental findings on shoulder MR examinations. They arise from a torn glenoid labrum. The tear of the capsulolabral complex leads to extravasation of synovial fluid, which accumulates as either a unilocular or multilocular cystic structure. Paralabral cysts are classified as

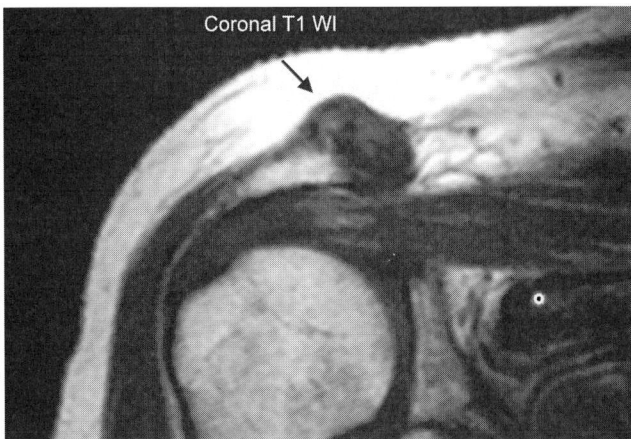

Fig. 6.6 A 42-year-old male patient with shoulder pain on T1W coronal image shows osteophyte formation at the acromio-clavicular joint (arrow) suggestive of degeneration

synovial cysts, ganglion cysts or pseudocysts. Synovial cysts occur through evagination of the joint capsule and contain a thin synovial cell lining. Ganglion cysts can arise from ligament, tendon, bone, joint capsule, or bursa. Pseudocysts are fluid-filled structures within the soft tissues that lack the cellular lining of a true cyst. Paralabral in spinoglenoid region are called spinoglenoid cyst **(Figs 6.7A and B)**. Paralabral cysts in the suprascapular notch cause entrapment neuropathies of the suprascapular nerve alone or both the suprascapular and infrascapular nerves. MR imaging findings include a thin-walled, rounded; sometimes multiloculated hyperintense structure on T2-weighted imaging and hypointense on T1-weighted imaging. Electromyographic assessment and nerve conduction studies are helpful in determining the degree and site of nerve compression.

Glenoid Labrum Tear

Glenoid labrum is a rim of fibrocartilaginous tissue attached to the edge of the glenoid cavity, which functions to add depth and greater stability to the glenohumeral joint.

Assessment of this structure is important in patients with shoulder instability. Arthroscopy provides accurate results but is invasive; consequently, conventional and computed arthrotomography are preferred. Using the latter methods, the Bankart lesion, Hill Sachs lesion, intra-articular osteocartilaginous bodies, and subluxation or dislocation of the bicipital tendon can be identified.

Magnetic resonance imaging, however, is the current imaging method of choice in assessing the glenoid labrum in patients with instability. MR arthrography may also be employed. MRI shows hypointense signal on T1WI hyperintense signal on T2WI **(Figs 6.8A to F)**, with erosions in the glenoid on CT images.

Other lesions involving the labrum are tears, anterior labroligamentous periosteal sleeve avulsion (ALPSA) lesion, glenoid labrum ovoid mass, humeral avulsion of the glenohumeral ligament (HAGL) lesion, bony humeral avulsion of the glenohumeral ligament (BHAGL) lesion, and superior labrum anterior and posterior (SLAP) lesion.

In recurrent shoulder dislocations, disruption of the integrity of the glenoid labrum is the most frequent abnormality. In addition, with age the superior portion may become partially detached from the glenoid process.

Tuberculous Arthritis Right Shoulder

Tubercle bacilli are deposited in the synovium via a hematogenous route or through direct penetration from a metaphyseal focus of osteomyelitis. A monoarticular presentation is most common and mainly large joints (hip, knee, shoulder or sacroiliac joint) are involved. Overt bony destruction is not usually evident on clinical presentation which, unlike acute septic arthritis, is characteristically slow and insidious with gradual onset of pain, stiffness and synovial swelling.

Initially joint effusion associated with a synovial hypertrophy is seen and is difficult to differentiate from other conditions including septic arthritis, Lyme disease, hemophilia, pigmented villonodular synovitis, and juvenile rheumatoid arthritis. Later on there is gradual proliferation of granulation tissue at the joint periphery which manifests clinically as a

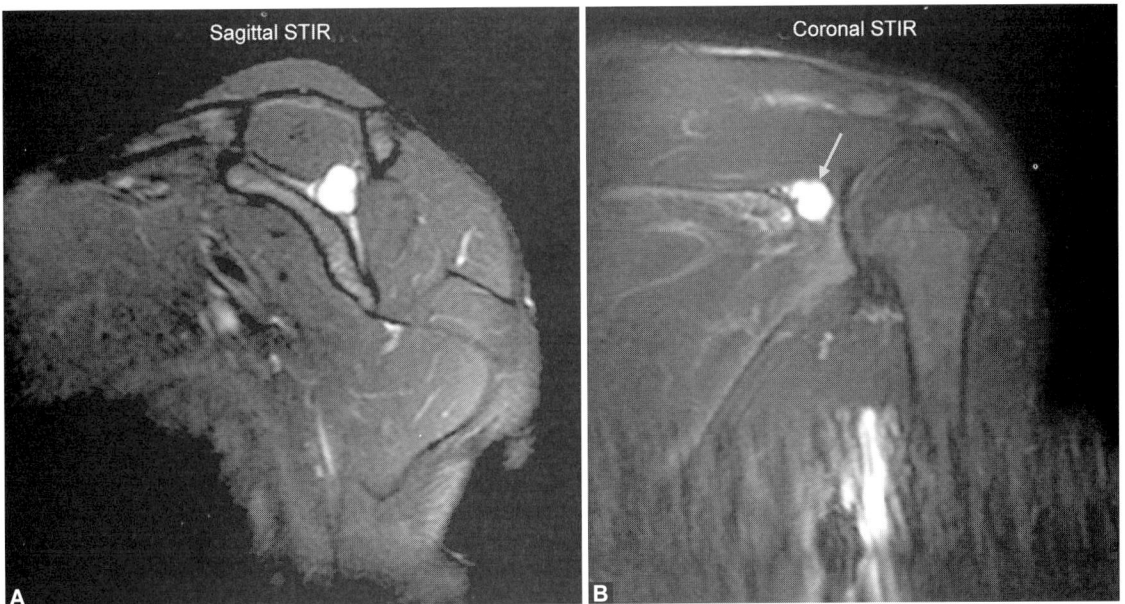

Figs 6.7A and B Sagittal and coronal STIR images show a hyperintense cystic lesion in the spinoglenoid notch, a spinoglenoid cyst

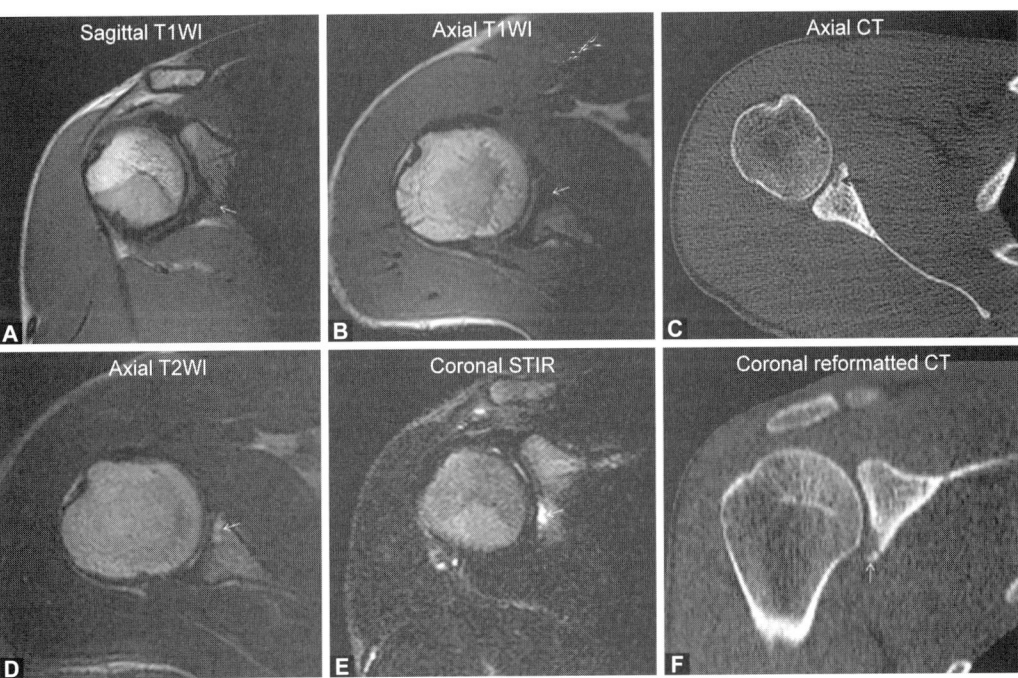

Figs 6.8A to F (A and B) Sagittal and axial T1WI reveal abnormal hypointense signal in anteroinferior aspect of bony labrum. The signal is hyperintense on axial T2WI; (D) and coronal STIR (E) images. Axial; (C) and coronal reformatted CT; (F) images show small subarticular erosive lesion in glenoid

joint effusion with or without thickening of synovial tissue. Radiographically, there is soft tissue swelling and diffuse osteopenia, without a focal abnormality. Granulation tissue spreads across the joint, and the first bony changes are marginal erosions, which are evident radiographically. Over time, there is erosion of the articular cartilage and of the underlying bone, resulting in loss of joint space on plain radiographs. Later on secondary degenerative changes in the joint are observed. The early findings on magnetic resonance imaging are nonspecific, and include joint effusion, marrow edema, and during the stage of arthritis—abnormalities within the articular cartilage and subchondral bone **(Figs 6.9A to D)**.

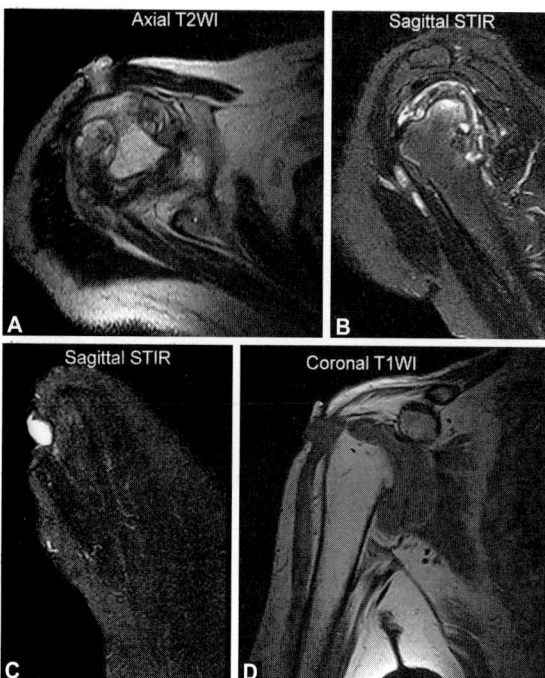

Figs 6.9A to D A 57-year-old male presented with history of right shoulder discharging sinus since 5 months. No history of fever. MR shows loss of normal joint space with destruction of the articular surface involving the humerus and glenoid of right shoulder and moderate joint effusion with sinus tract extending anteriorly up to the skin surface. Atrophy of the rotator cuff muscles is seen, predominantly of the supraspinatus muscles. The effusion appears hyperintense on T2 and STIR (A to C) and hypointense on T1WI (D)

Rotator Cuff Tears

The rotator cuff comprises four muscles that stabilize the shoulder joint: the supraspinatus, infraspinatus, teres minor and subscapularis. Tendons are fibrous tissue that connects muscle to bone. Tears in the rotator cuff can be within the muscle or at the site where the tendon attaches to the bone. Rotator cuff tears may be partial tears or full thickness tears. Complete tear of supraspinatus tendon may or may not be associated with mild joint effusion **(Figs 6.10 and 6.11)**. Precipitating factors include trauma, attrition, ischemia, and impingement.

Magnetic resonance imaging (MRI) is the investigation of choice for rotator cuff injuries, where the high signal intensity of tendons on some sequences, is indicative of tear. Full-thickness tears of the rotator cuff are characterized by presence of a tendinous defect that is filled with fluid or granulation tissue and retraction of the musculotendinous junction.

Partial-thickness tears often appear on MRI as only an intermediate signal, isointense to muscle, which disrupts the normal low-signal surface of the rotator cuff. Magnetic resonance arthrography can improve the differentiation of rotator cuff degeneration from partial or complete rotator cuff tears. In complete

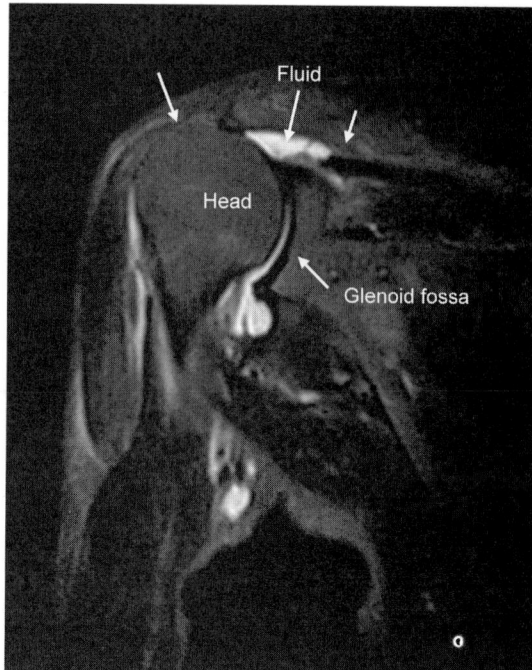

Fig. 6.10 STIR coronal image shows complete supraspinatus tendon tear with medial retraction of the tendon (short arrow) and superior displacement of the head of humerus (long arrow). Hyperintense signal due to effusion is seen in the subacromial space and glenohumeral joint cavity

tears an abnormal communication between the glenohumeral joint and bursa allows contrast material to collect within the subacromial bursa.

HIP JOINT

Anatomy Hip Joint

The hip joint is a multiaxial synovial joint (ball and socket joint). It engages the bony surface of the head of femur in the acetabulum of the hip bone. The stability of the joint is provided by the muscles and ligaments **(Figs 6.12 to 6.15)**. The three parts of the hip bone (ilium, ischium and pubis) congregate at the acetabulum to form the triradiate synchondrosis.

The acetabular labrum is attached to the acetabular rim and the transverse acetabular ligament. It forms a complete ring encircling the head of femur which fits into the acetabular cavity. The transverse acetabular ligament bridges the acetabular notch.

At the site of the subtendinous bursa of psoas, where the capsule is partially deficient and weak, the joint is only supported by the psoas tendon. The inverted Y shaped iliofemoral ligament is attached superiorly deep to the rectus femoris muscle and becomes stiffer during medial rotation of femur at the hip joint.

The ligament of head of femur connects the head of femur to the acetabular cavity. Its fibers are also

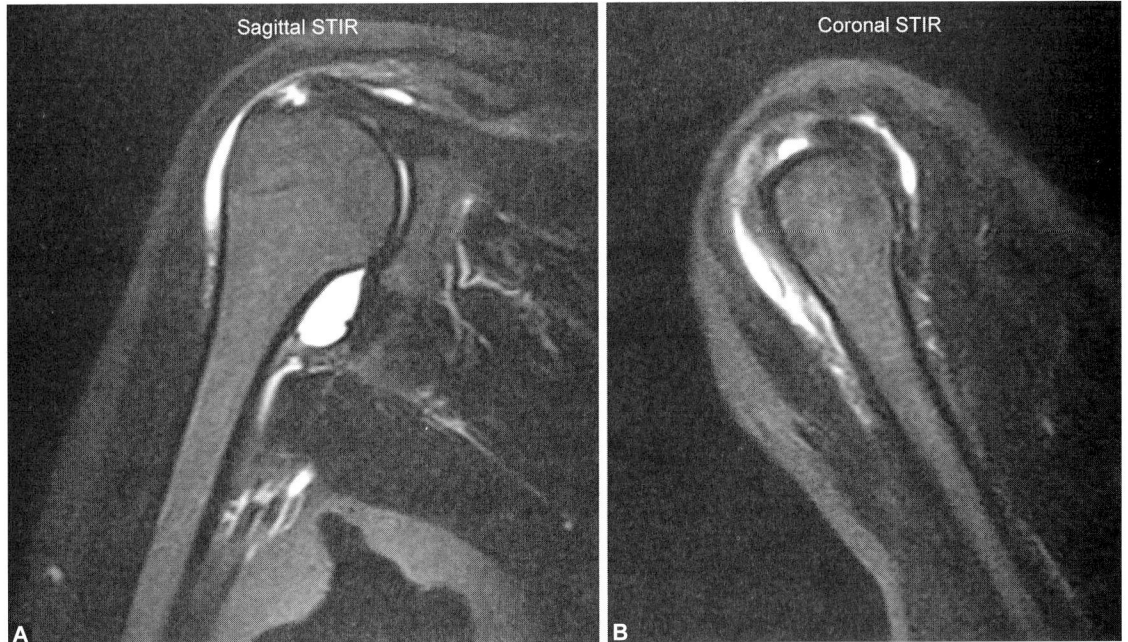

Figs 6.11A and B Another case shows complete tear in the supraspinatus tendon with mild joint effusion

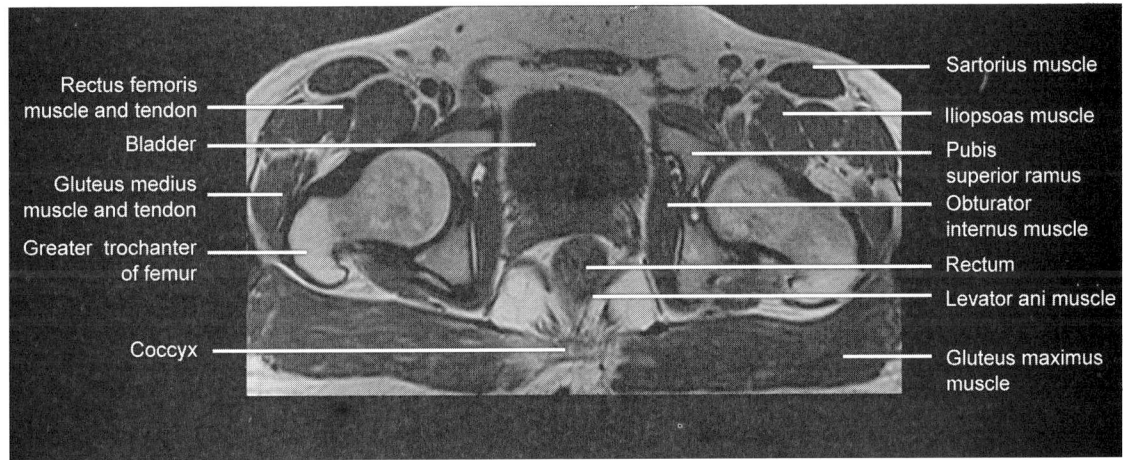

Fig. 6.12 Hip joint MRI: Axial T1WI

attached to the margins of acetabular notch. The ligament of the head of femur becomes stiffer during adduction movement of the hip joint, more so when the legs are crossed in front.

The fibrous capsule of the joint is strengthened by three ligaments—the iliofemoral ligament, the pubofemoral ligament and the ischiofemoral ligament. The fibrous capsule is thick where it forms the iliofemoral ligament and it is thinner posteriorly. The femoral sheath enclosing the femoral artery, femoral vein, lymph nodes and fat is loosely bound except posteriorly between the psoas and pectineus muscles, and is attached to the capsule of hip joint. The femoral nerve lies between the iliacus muscle and the fascia. The fibers of the capsule spiral to become stiffer during movements like extension and medial rotation of the femur.

The synovial membrane inferiorly forms a bursa for the tendon of obturator externus muscle. The subtendinous bursa of the obturator internus is seen at the lesser sciatic notch, where the tendon makes an angle of 90° to attach to the greater trochanter.

The obturator artery divides into anterior and posterior branches. The acetabular artery is a branch of the posterior branch of obturator artery. The acetabular branches pass through the acetabular foramen and enter the acetabular fossa where they diverge in the fatty tissue. The nutrient branches radiate

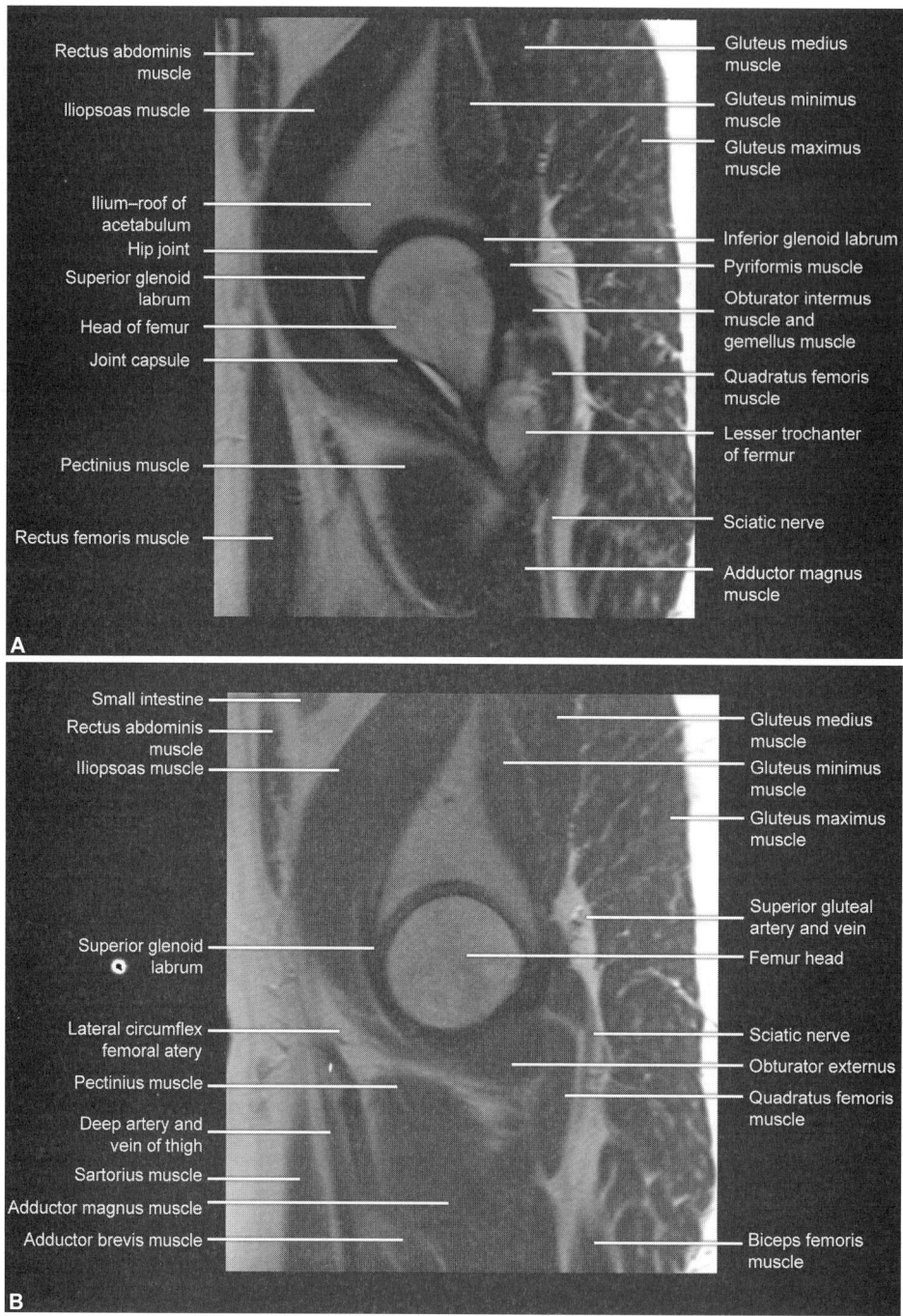

Figs 6.13A and B Hip joint MRI: Sagittal T1WI

to the margins of the acetabular fossa to enter the nutrient foramina. Major anastomosis occurs around the femoral neck involving branches from the femoral arteries (medial and lateral circumflex branches) and obturator artery branches. As the medial circumflex artery supplies a major portion of blood to the head and neck of femur, in fracture of femoral neck this blood supply is disrupted and the avascular necrosis femoral head is seen in many of these patients.

Osteoid Osteoma

Osteoid osteoma is a benign lesion frequently found in the appendicular skeleton. The tumors produce excess bone and secrete pain-causing prostaglandins, resulting in intense pain especially at night. Osteoid osteoma is more commonly see in children and adolescents. Radiograph shows sclerosis and cortical thickening due to subperiosteal bone formation. The radiolucent

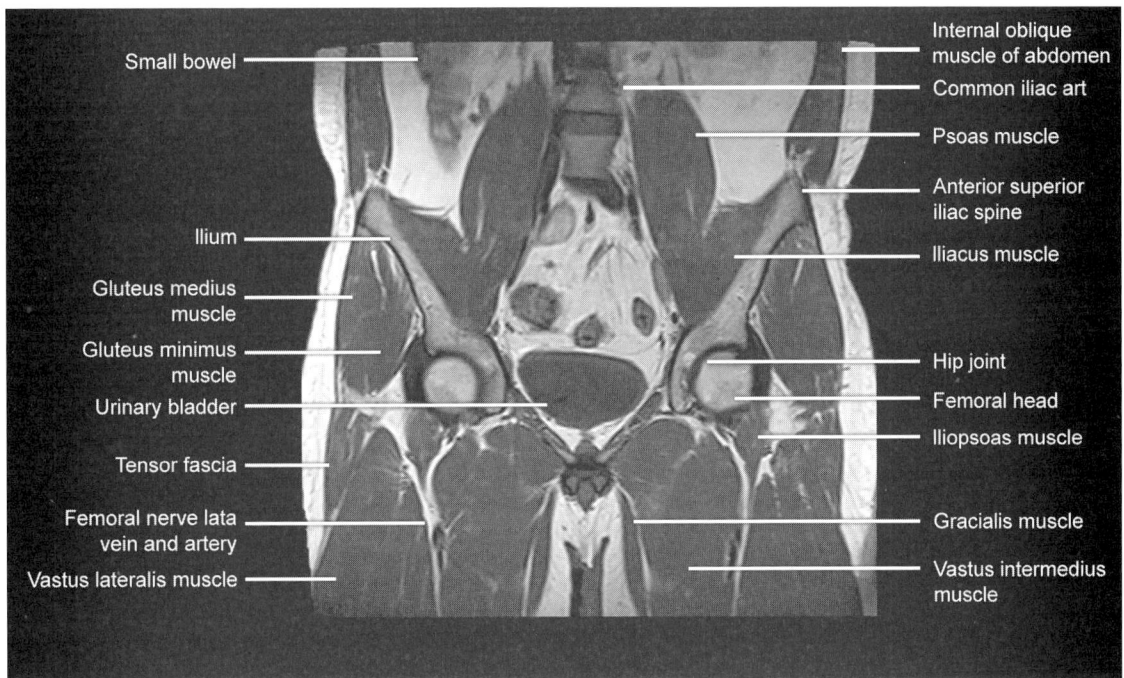

Fig. 6.14 Hip joint MRI: Coronal T1WI

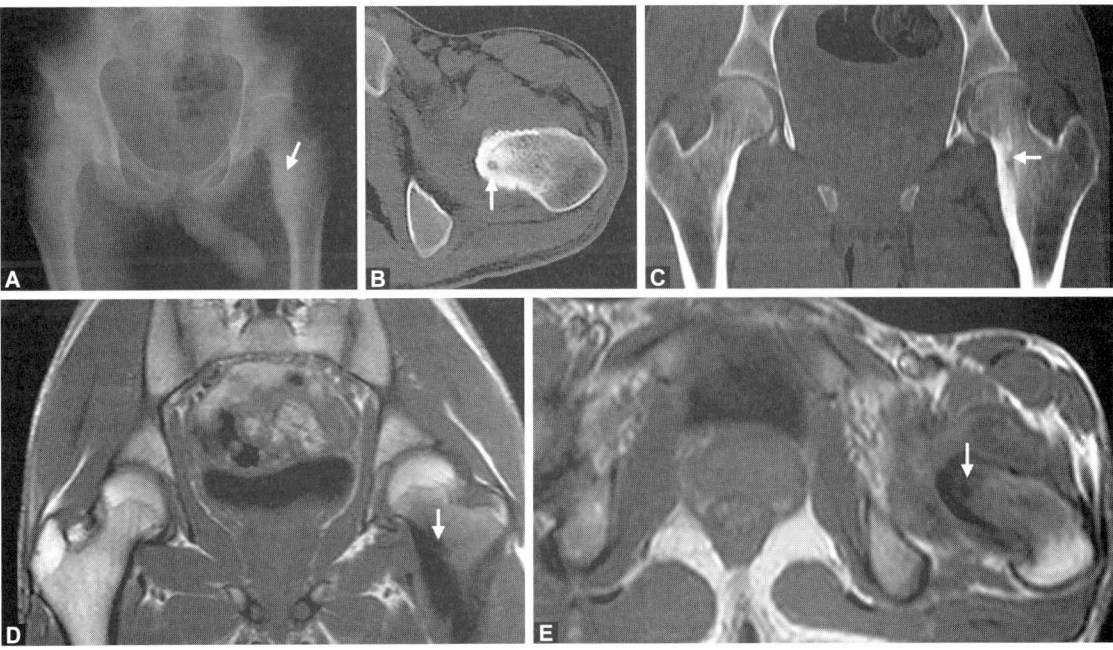

Figs 6.15A to E Plain radiograph (A) reveals an ill-defined region of increased cortical thickness (arrow) and CT axial (B) and coronal reformatted (C) reveals the presence small well-defined calcified nidus and dense cortical thickening near lesser trochanter. MRI coronal (D) and axial (E) reveals hypointense cortical thickening along lesser trochanter with well-defined small hypointense lesion adjacent to it (arrow)

nidus may be visualized on plain X-ray. The location of the nidus, intranidal calcification, sclerosis, periosteal bone formation and location of original cortex are usually precisely demonstrated on CT. MRI will show the partially calcified nidus and associated cortical thickening. In addition, MR images can also reveal marrow and soft tissue edema in the vicinity of the nidus, which is not demonstrated by CT **(Figs 6.15A to E)**.

Avascular Necrosis

Avascular necrosis (AVN) is a self-limiting osteonecrosis of the femoral head epiphysis, more common in males. AVN or osteonecrosis is the death of bone tissue due to a lack of blood supply and leads to tiny breaks in the bone trabeculae and the bone eventually collapses. It is result of interruption of blood flow to the part of bone. It is seen if the bone is fractured or the joint becomes dislocated or long-term use of steroids and excessive alcohol intake. Hip is the most common joint affected by avascular necrosis and worsens with time. Prognostic evaluation by MRI indices depends on the extent of necrosis, lateral extrusion, epiphyseal involvement and metaphyseal changes.

Ficat and Arlet classification is used for AVN of the hip. It uses a combination of clinical features, plain film and MRI.

Grade 0

- *Clinical symptoms:* Nil
- *X-ray:* Normal
- *MRI:* Double line sign on the MR image in the asymptomatic hip in this stage.

Grade I (Figs 6.16A and B)

- *Clinical symptoms:* Pain typically in the groin
- *X-ray:* Trabeculae appear normal or minor osteopenia in femoral head.
- MR imaging may show a single line on T1-weighted images and the double line sign on T2 weighted images. The double-line sign is specific and pathognomonic for AVN. The hyperintensity at the periphery of the necrotic focus is probably caused by hypervascular granulation tissue, a hyperemic response adjacent to thickened trabeculae.
- *Bone scan:* Central photon void area is noted in the femur head with peripherally increase in tracer uptake in the femoral head (arrow).

Grade II (Figs 6.17A to C)

- *Clinical symptoms:* Pain and stiffness
- *X-ray:* Mixed osteopenia and/or sclerosis in the femoral head
- *MRI:* Geographic defect in femoral head is seen in stage II with associated marrow edema from the nonischemic region of the femoral head into the femoral neck
- *Bone scan:* Increased uptake in femoral head.

Grade III (Figs 6.18A and B)

- *Clinical symptoms:* Pain and stiffness +/– radiation to knee and limp
- *X-ray:* Stage III disease is marked by the loss of the spherical shape of the femoral head. The AP radiograph may appear normal, but the lateral view often reveals a crescent sign, or radiolucency, under the subchondral bone. This represents

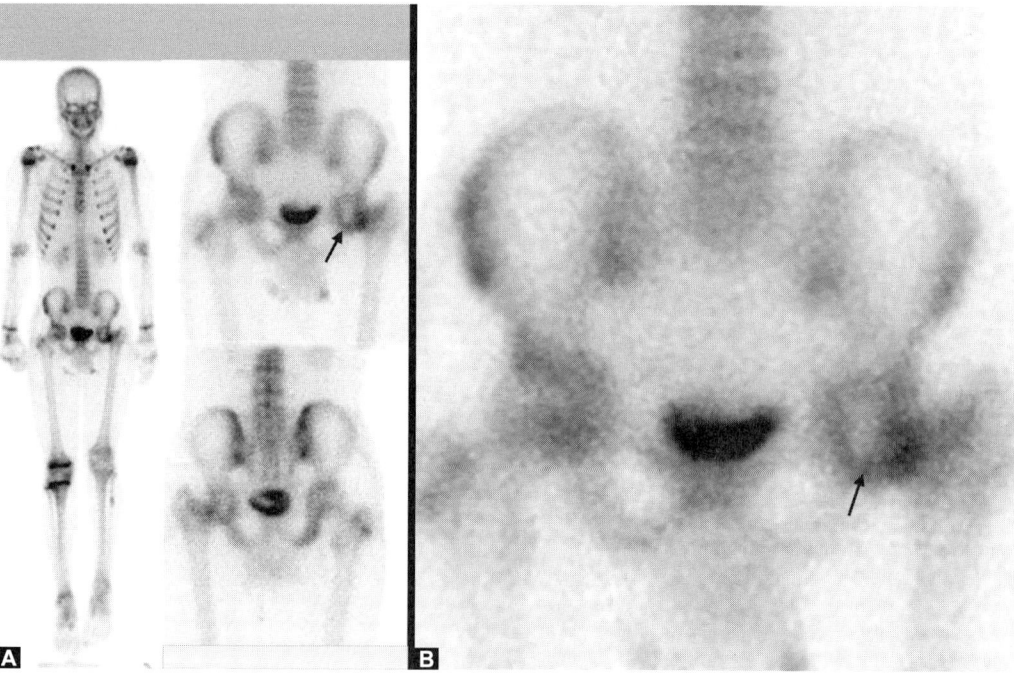

Figs 6.16A and B Tc-99m methylene diphosphonate (MDP) three phase bone scan shows central photon void area in the femoral head with peripherally increased (arrow) tracer uptake

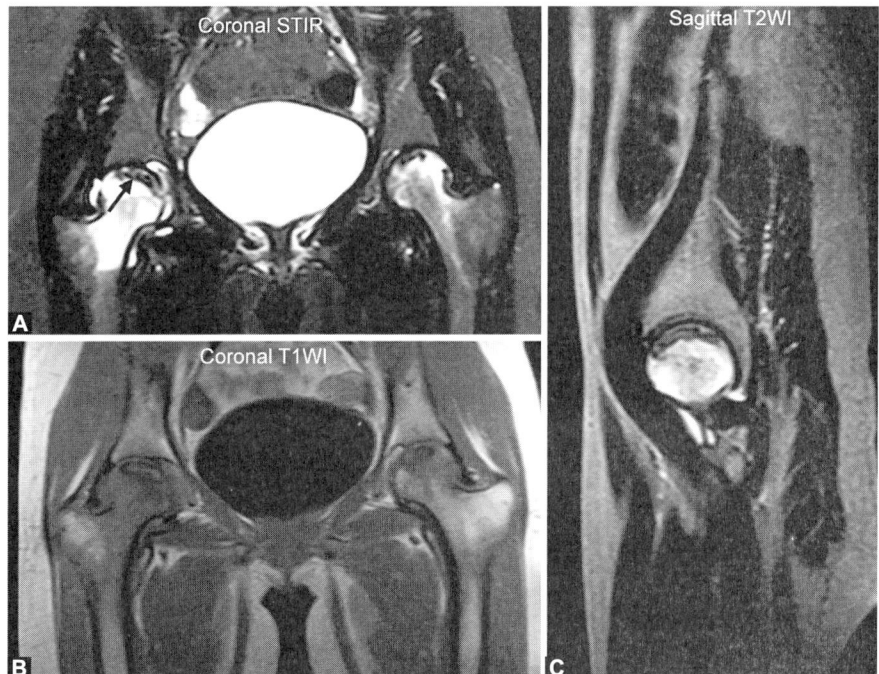

Figs 6.17A to C Coronal STIR (A), coronal T1W (B) and sagittal T2W (C) images reveal well-defined crescents (arrow) of altered marrow signal in both femoral heads. The marrow within the crescent is predominantly hypointense on T1W, T2W and STIR images, suggestive of sclerosis. Normal contour of femoral head is maintained. These findings are suggestive of Grade II avascular necrosis

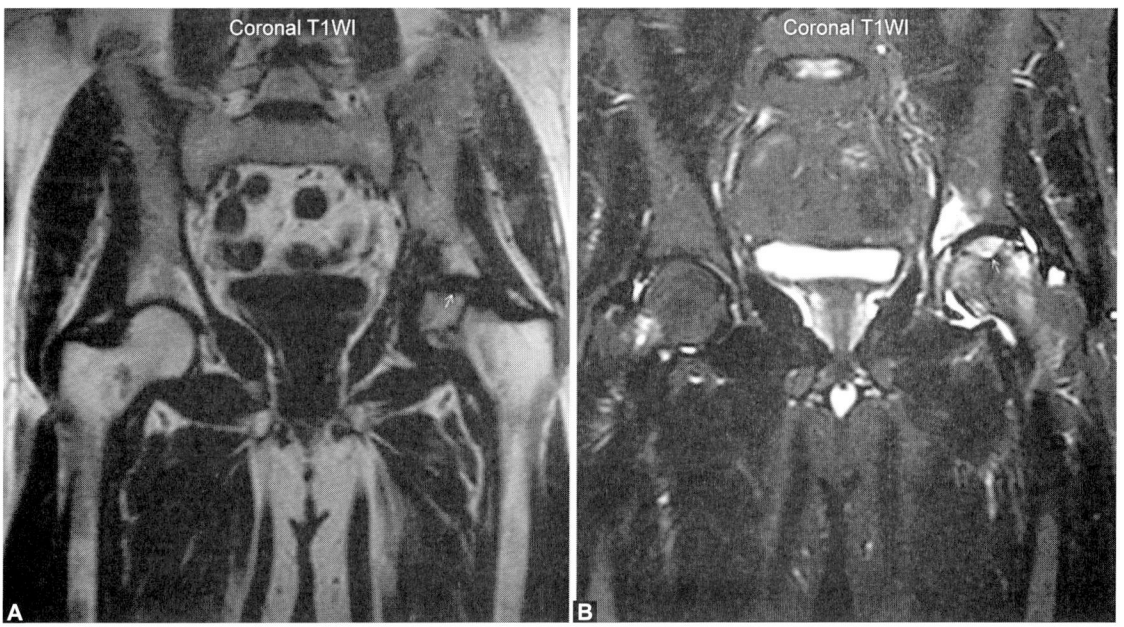

Figs 6.18A and B Coronal T1WI (A) and STIR (B) shows evidence of altered signal changes seen in left femoral head withsclerosis and subchondral collapse (arrow). These findings are of Grade III AVN

a fracture between the subchondral bone and the underlying femoral head. The crescent sign is the earliest indication of mechanical failure from accumulated stress fractures of nonrepaired necrotic trabeculae. The necrotic area becomes radio dense. The joint space remains preserved or may actually increase in height

- *MRI:* MRI findings as seen in stage II with loss of the spherical shape of the femoral head. Subchondral collapse with crescent sign.

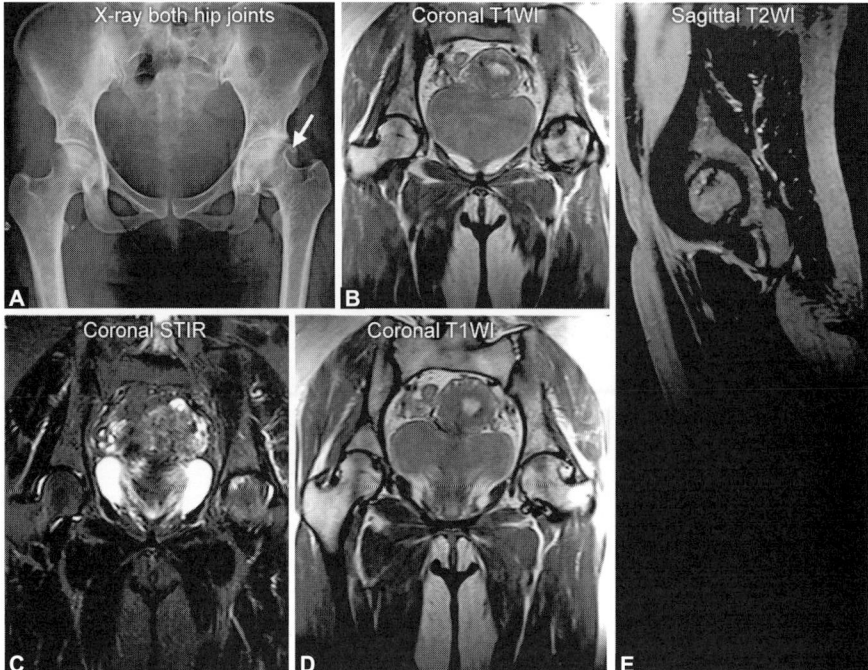

Figs 6.19A to E X-ray pelvis AP view (A) shows a well-defined crescent of hypodensity with loss of normal contour of left femoral head with degenerative changes in the form of osteophytes. Coronal T1WI (B) and STIR (C) images show a well-defined crescents of altered marrow signal in the subchondral region of left femoral head. Coronal T1WI (D) and sagittal T2WI (E) show loss of normal contour of left femoral head with secondary degenerative changes in the form of osteophytes (arrows)

Grade IV (Figs 6.19A to E)

- *Clinical symptoms:* Pain and limp
- *X-ray:* The femoral head undergoes further collapse, leading to articular cartilage destruction and joint space narrowing with evidence of secondary degenerative change in hip joint
- *MRI:* Finding as seen in stage III with further collapse of femoral head and secondary degenerative change in hip joint.

Septic Arthritis

Septic arthritis is an infectious (usually bacterial) inflammation of joints. Septic arthritis of the hip in infancy and childhood is a common entity leading to displacement of the femoral head or metaphysis.

Infection occurs by:
- Hematogenous spread of infection
- Spread from a contiguous source of infection
- Direct implantation of infectious organisms
- Postoperative infection.

Plain radiography is of limited value in evaluating a joint for infection; periarticular soft-tissue swelling is the most common finding. MR is imaging modality of choice and is most useful in ruling out underlying osteomyelitis or periarticular osteomyelitis caused by the joint infection itself. Ultrasound is sensitive for the detection of hip joint effusion.

Magnetic resonance imaging is more sensitive for distinguishing osteomyelitis, periarticular abscesses, and joint effusions. MRI is preferred because of its greater ability to image soft tissue. MRI findings include: synovial enhancement, perisynovial edema and joint effusion **(Figs 6.20A to D)**. Signal abnormalities in the bone marrow can indicate a concomitant osteomyelitis.

KNEE JOINT

Anatomy Knee Joint

The knee joint is a modified pivotal hinge joint. It is the largest synovial joint in the body. It consists of two condylar joints between the femur and the tibia and a saddle joint between the patella and the femur. The intercondylar eminence of the tibia prevents sideway slipping of femur on tibia. The ligaments and muscles make knee a very stable joint.

The medial and lateral articular surfaces of the femur and tibia are asymmetrical. The distal surface of the medial condyle of the femur is narrower and more curved than the lateral condyle. The articular surface of lateral tibia is almost circular whereas the medial surface is oval in shape. The articular surface of patella has a larger lateral and a smaller medial surface.

Inferiorly, the capsule is attached to the margins of the tibial condyles posteriorly except where the popliteus tendon crosses the bone. On either sides

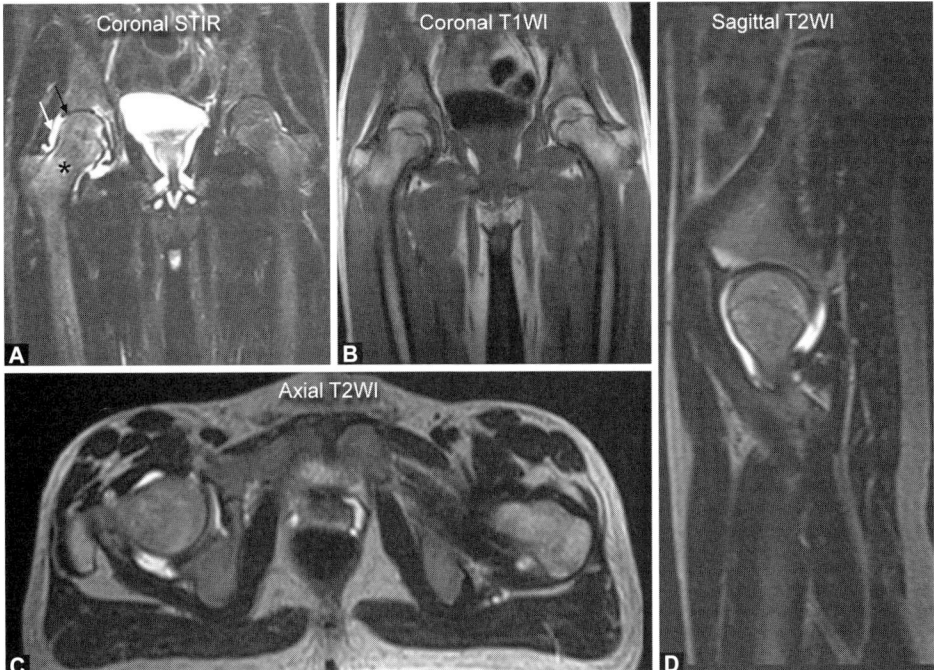

Figs 6.20A to D A 14-year-old male with history of pain in the right hip joint on coronal STIR (A) and T1W (B) images show marrow edema (*) and mild effusion (white arrow in A). Axial T2W (C) and sagittal T1W (D) image shows marrow edema involving the head of right femur and the acetabulum with mild effusion

the capsule is attached to the margins of the tibial condyles, and laterally to the head of the fibula. On its deeper aspect the coronary ligaments connect the capsule to the rims of menisci. The capsule is attached to the tibial tuberosity anteriorly on the tibia.

The ligaments of knee joint include the cruciate ligaments, arcuate popliteal ligament, the oblique popliteal ligament, fibular collateral ligament and the tibial collateral ligament **(Figs 6.21 to 6.23)**.

The cruciate ligaments are a pair of ligaments (anterior and posterior). They cross each other connecting the tibia to the femur and lie within the capsule of knee joint but outside the synovial membrane **(Figs 6.21 and 6.22)**. The anterior cruciate ligament is attached to the anterior part of the tibial plateau between the attachments of anterior horns of medial and lateral menisci. Posteriorly, the anterior cruciate ligament is attached to the posteromedial aspect of lateral femoral condyle. The anterior cruciate ligament appears as a fan shaped structure, it is 11 mm wide and 31 to 38 mm long. The posterior cruciate ligament is attached posteriorly to the intercondylar area on tibia and anteriorly it is attached to the anterolateral aspect of the medial femoral condyle. The posterior cruciate ligament is about 13 mm wide and 38 mm long. Both these ligaments stabilize the knee in a rotational fashion. Thus, if one of these ligaments is significantly damaged, the knee will be unstable when planting the foot of the injured extremity and pivoting, causes the knee to buckle and give way.

The arcuate popliteal ligament is a Y-shaped thickening of posterior capsular fibers; the stem of the Y is attached to the head of fibula. The medial limb of Y is attached to the posterior edge of the intercondylar area, while the lateral limb is attached to the lateral femoral condyle.

The oblique popliteal ligament is an expansion of the tendon of semimembranosus muscle that blends with the capsule posteriorly and ascends laterally. The tibial collateral ligament is a triangular band 8 to 9 cm in length, attached above to the medial femoral epicondyle and below to the medial surface of tibia. Its anterior margin forms the vertical base of the triangle and is free except at its attached extremities. The posterior apex of the triangular ligament blends with the capsule and is also attached to the medial meniscus.

The fibular collateral ligament is 'cord-like' and is attached superiorly to the lateral epicondyle and inferiorly to the head of the fibula. The patellar ligament **(Figs 6.21 and 6.22)** is a central band of the tendon of quadriceps femoris muscles; it is about 8 cm long. Proximally, it attaches to the anterior and posterior surfaces of patella including the apex. Distally it attaches to the smooth area of tibial tuberosity. The patellar ligament blends with the medial and lateral patellar retinaculum, which are aponeurotic expansions of vastus medialis and lateralis. The retinaculum supports the articular capsule of the knee laterally.

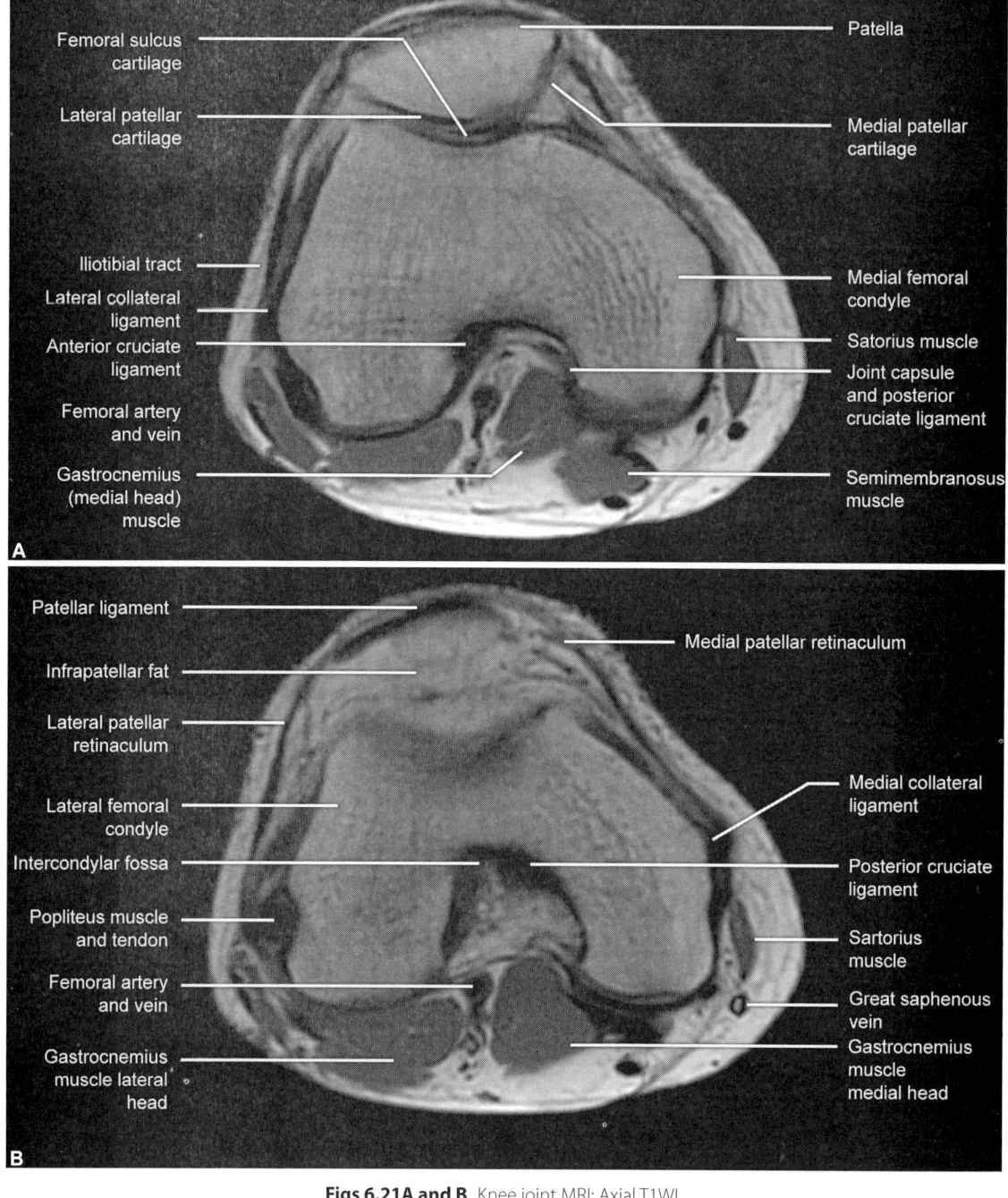

Figs 6.21A and B Knee joint MRI: Axial T1WI

The menisci are called semilunar cartilages (**Figs 6.22 and 6.23**). These are crescentic discs of fibrocartilage that act as shock absorbers. The menisci are avascular structures comprising mainly of collagenous fibrous tissue attached to the tibial plateau. There are two menisci, the lateral and the medial meniscus. They are triangular in cross-section, being thicker at their convex periphery (5 mm in height). Their distal surfaces are flat while their proximal surfaces are concave and articulate with the convex femoral condyles. The menisci demonstrate diffusely low signal on all MRI pulse sequences because of their fibrocartilaginous nature.

The medial meniscus is almost a semicircle in appearance and is broader posteriorly. Its anterior horn is attached to the intercondylar area in front of the anterior cruciate ligament; the posterior horn is attached in front of the posterior cruciate ligament in intercondylar area. The lateral meniscus is of uniform width and almost forms a complete circle. Its anterior horn is attached in front of the intercondylar eminence of the tibia behind the anterior cruciate ligament, while

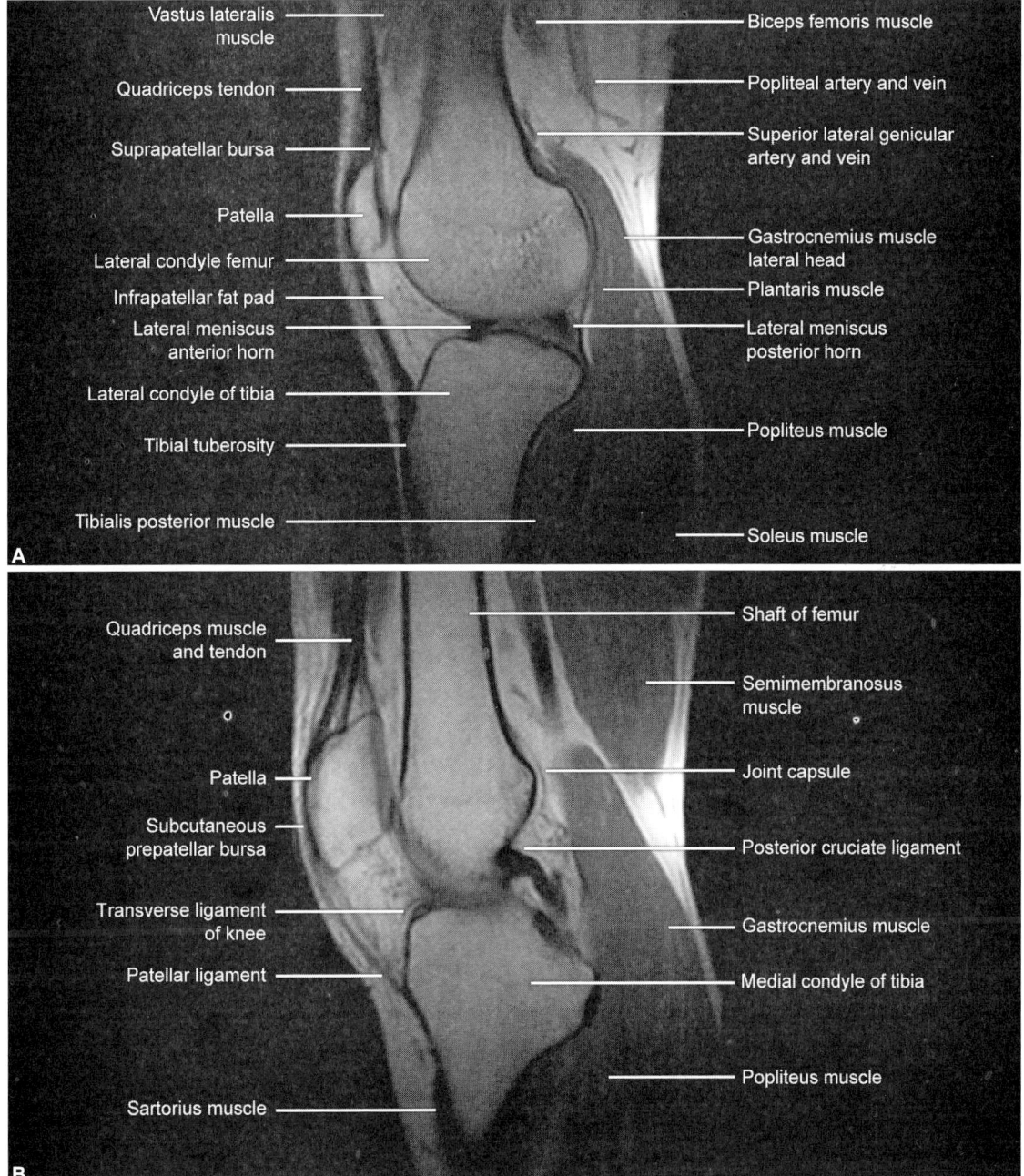

Figs 6.22A and B Knee joint MRI: Sagittal T1WI

the posterior horn is attached in front of the posterior horn of the medial meniscus.

The synovial membrane lines the internal surface of the fibrous capsule and attaches to the periphery of the patella and the edges of the menisci. The synovial membrane is continuous with the lining of the suprapatellar bursa. Normal amount of synovial fluid is 0.5 mL.

Bursae of knee joint reduce the friction between tendon and bones. The suprapatellar bursa lies between the femur and the quadriceps femoris. The prepatellar bursa lies between the skin and the patella.

The infrapatellar bursa lies between the skin and the tibial tuberosity. The deep infrapatellar bursa lies between the patellar ligament and the upper part of the tibia. The semimembranosus bursa lies between that muscle and the medial head of gastrocnemius.

Blood supply to knee joint is by anastomosis of the genicular branches of the popliteal artery. The middle genicular branches supply the cruciate ligaments.

Movements at the knee joint are the flexion, extension and rotation. Flexion is limited to about 150° due to soft tissue parts behind the knee. Flexion movements are primarily performed by the hamstring

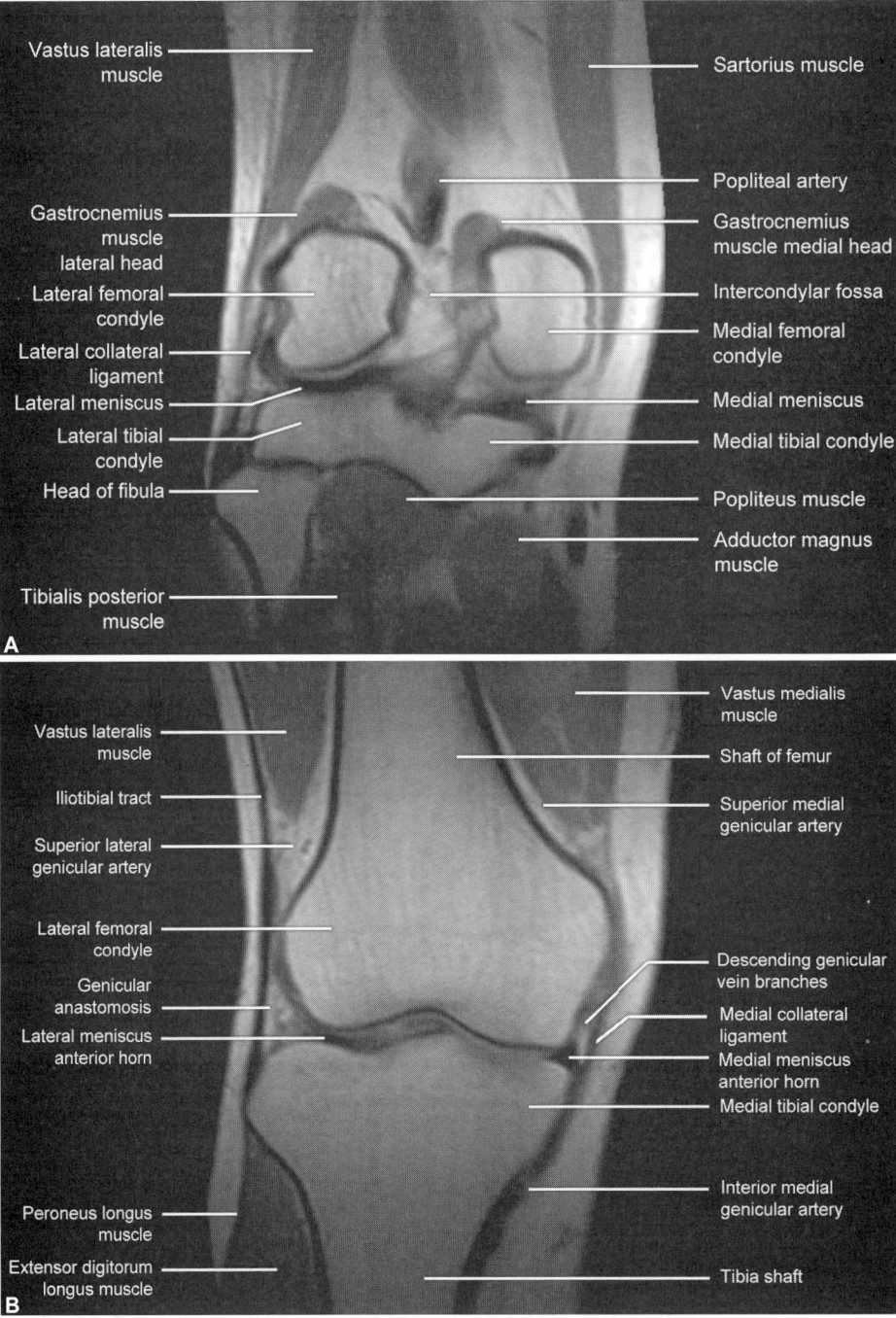

Figs 6.23A and B Knee joint MRI: Coronal T1WI

muscles. Extension is performed by the quadriceps femoris muscles assisted by tensor fascia lata. As the knee extends the shorter and rounded lateral femoral condyle completes its extension to about 30° short of full extension. The rotation movement occurs during extension with the foot on ground. Passive medial rotation of the femur is a part of a 'locking' mechanism which secures the joint in 5–10° of hyperextension when the cruciate ligaments, the collateral ligaments and the oblique popliteal ligament are all taut. Lateral rotation is produced by the popliteus muscle when flexion occurs with the foot free.

The knee joint is stabilized by the surrounding muscles and their tendons. Anteriorly, it is the quadriceps tendon. This broad tendon attaches to and surrounds the patella and continues as the patellar ligament, which is attached to the tuberosity of the tibia. Posteriorly are the popliteus, plantaris and medial and lateral heads of gastrocnemius. Laterally are the tendons of the biceps femoris and popliteus.

Medially by the sartorius, gracilis, semitendinosus and semimembranosus muscles are present.

Cruciate Ligaments

The anterior and posterior cruciate ligaments are two major ligaments of the knee. Their job is to maintain the anteroposterior relationship of the distal femur and proximal tibia to each other. This job is trickier by the fact that it needs to be done at all times during flexion or extension of the knee.

The anterior cruciate ligament (ACL) is a fan shaped linear band; **(Figs 6.24A to F)**. It attaches proximally at the internal aspect of the lateral femoral condyle, and runs distally to its broad attachment to the anterior tibia and the anterior aspect of the tibial spine. The anterior cruciate lies lateral to the posterior cruciate. The recognition of ACL is comparable to putting your hand inside the pocket of your trousers. This position represents ACL, i.e. the hand is positioned from posterior to anterior and from lateral to medial, so is ACL positioned. The reverse is true for PCL.

The posterior cruciate ligament (PCL) is a relatively simple band of tissue and attaches proximally on the internal aspect of the medial femoral condyle and runs distally to where it attaches to the posterior eminence of the tibia. It generally lies in the sagittal plane, and can usually be seen in its entirety on a single sagittal MR slice **(Figs 6.25A to G)**.

Collateral Ligaments

The collateral ligaments of the knees are found on the medial and lateral aspect of the knee joint. The medial collateral ligament and the lateral collateral ligaments are actually a series of much smaller ligaments that create a web of ligaments that go in many different directions and are comprized of different layers. The medial collateral ligament is found on the interior facing side of the knee and connects the tibia to the femur **(Figs 6.26A to C)**. The lateral collateral ligament is located on the exterior facing side and connects the femur to the fibula in the lower leg **(Figs 6.27A to C)**.

In function these ligaments regulate the side to side movement of the knee and restrict it from making abnormal motions. Also, they prevent abnormal movement of the tibia backwards towards the femur. In some injury situations, the medial ligament also assumes responsibility of limiting the knee's rotation. In coordination with both the anterior cruciate ligament and the posterior cruciate ligament, proper knee motion and limitations is achieved.

In injuries involving these ligaments, the medial ligament is more susceptible to damage. Due to the complex nature of the knee's anatomy, most problems involving the lateral or medial ligaments also involve other parts of the knee. Most frequently, the injuries are caused by traumatic contact that forces the knee

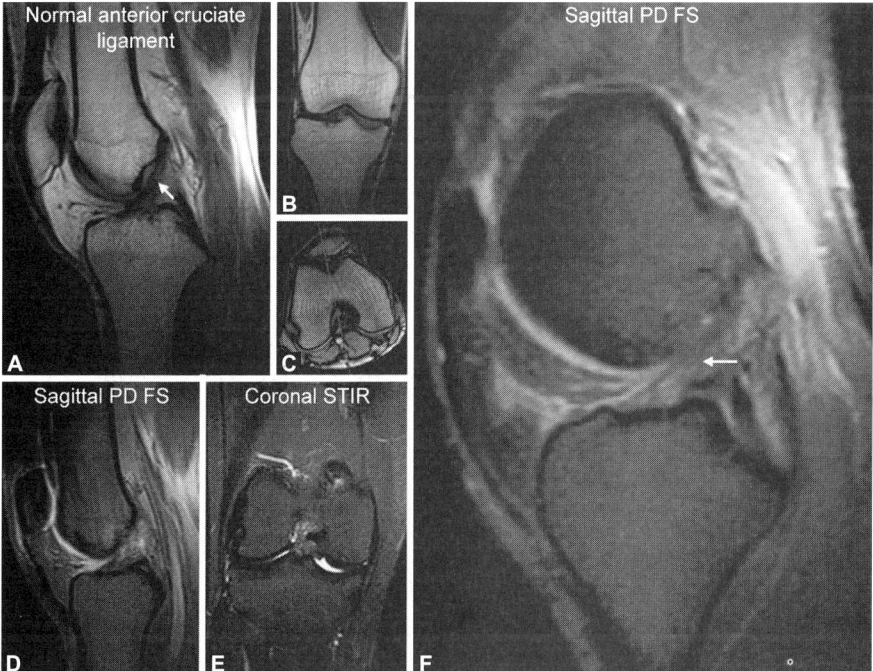

Figs 6.24A to F Normal anterior cruciate ligament (A to C). Sagittal fat-suppressed proton-density (PD FS) (D) and coronal STIR (E) image shows nonvisualization of the fibers of ACL suggestive of complete ACL tear. Sagittal PD FS (F) shows edematous (arrow) appearance of ACL with thinning of the fibers suggesting strain

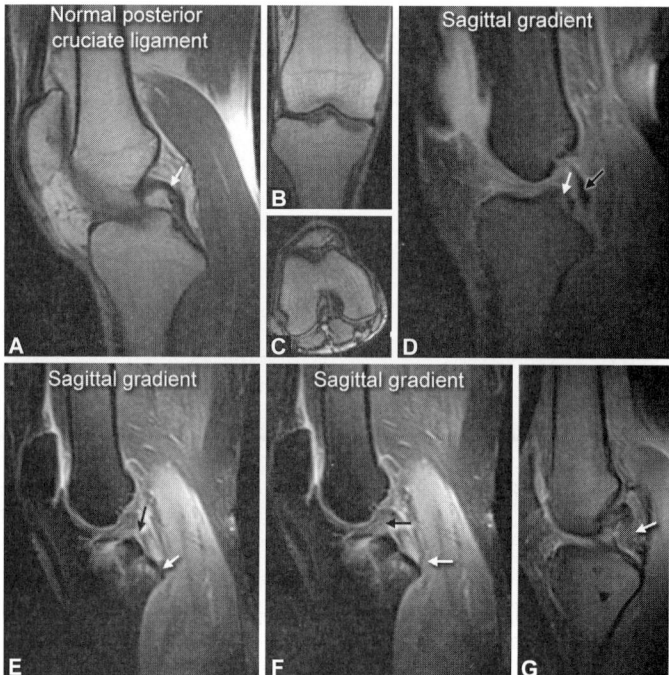

Figs 6.25A to G Normal posterior cruciate ligament (A to C). Sagittal gradient image (D) shows double PCL sign suggestive of ACL tear (white arrow), normal PCL is shown by black arrow. Sagittal gradient sequence (E) shows hyperintense signal in PCL at its tibial attachment with avulsion injury (white arrow) and also at ACL attachment with avulsion injury (black arrow). Sagittal gradient sequence (F) shows hyperintense signal in PCL at its tibial attachment with avulsion injury (white arrow) and also at ACL attachment with avulsion injury (black arrow). Sagittal PD FS image (G) shows interstitial tear of the fibers of PCL

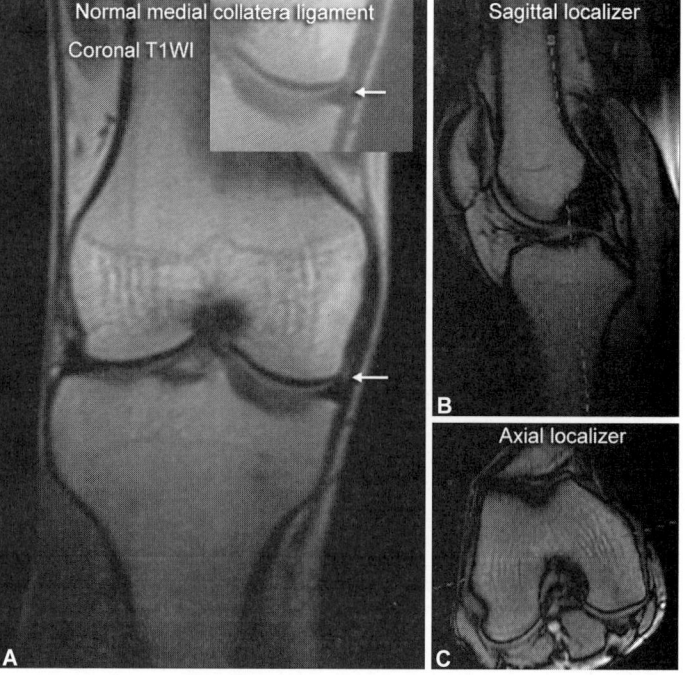

Figs 6.26A to C Normal medial collateral ligament (arrow). Localizers in sagittal and axial planes (B and C) give the exact planes in which the coronal section (A) shown has been taken

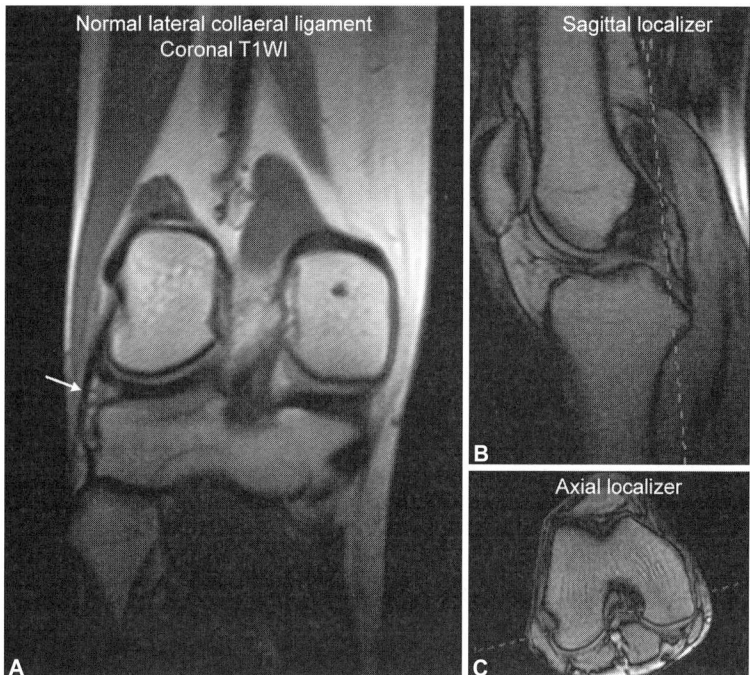

Figs 6.27A to C Normal lateral collateral ligament (arrow). Localizers in sagittal and axial planes (B and C) give the exact planes in which the coronal section (A) shown has been taken

inwards and stretches or tears the ligament. MRI shows three grades of tear in collateral ligaments:
a. *Grade I:* Microscopic tear
b. *Grade II:* Partial tear
c. *Grade III:* Complete tear **(Figs 6.28A and B)**.

Menisci

The function of meniscus is to cushion the joint from any injury. ON MRI, the medial meniscus **(Fig. 6.31A)** has sharp, triangular horns. The posterior horns are always larger than the anterior horns. The lateral meniscus has equal sized horns, the posterior horn being higher in position **(Figs 6.29A to C)**.

Meniscal degeneration on MRI is divided into 3 grades.

Grade I is a nonaritcular focal or diffuse region of increased signal intensity within the substance of meniscus and it correlates with early meniscal degeneration.

Grade II is a horizontal linear area of increased signal intensity within the substance of the meniscus that extends but does not involve the inferior surface **(Fig. 6.31B)**. Grade II is progressive degeneration from grade I.

Grade III is a region of abnormal signal intensity within the meniscus extending to and communicating with at least one articular surface of the meniscus **(Figs 6.30A to C, 6.31C and D)**.

Bucket Handle Tear

It is a longitudinal, peripheral tear of the meniscus with displacement of fragment toward the intercondylar notch of the knee. The displaced inner fragment resembles the handle of a bucket. The remaining larger peripheral portion of the meniscus resembles the bucket **(Figs 6.32A to C)**.

These tears account for about 10% of all meniscal tears.

They are either longitudinal, vertical, or oblique in direction with an attached tear fragment displaced from the meniscus. Magnetic resonance imaging (MRI) signs are widely used in the diagnosis of these tears, including the 'fragment within the intercondylar notch sign', 'flipped meniscus sign', 'double anterior horn sign', 'absence of the bow tie sign', 'double posterior cruciate ligament (PCL) sign', 'posterior double PCL sign', and 'triple PCL sign'.

Intercondylar notch sign: A meniscal fragment within the intercondylar notch was defined as a band like area of low signal intensity within the notch but not appearing on the same slice as the PCL.

Flipped meniscus sign: An abnormally tall anterior horn (greater than 6 mm) diagnoses a flipped meniscus. It is also considered to be present if an ill defined meniscus shape was seen immediately posterior to the anterior horn with a shortened posterior horn.

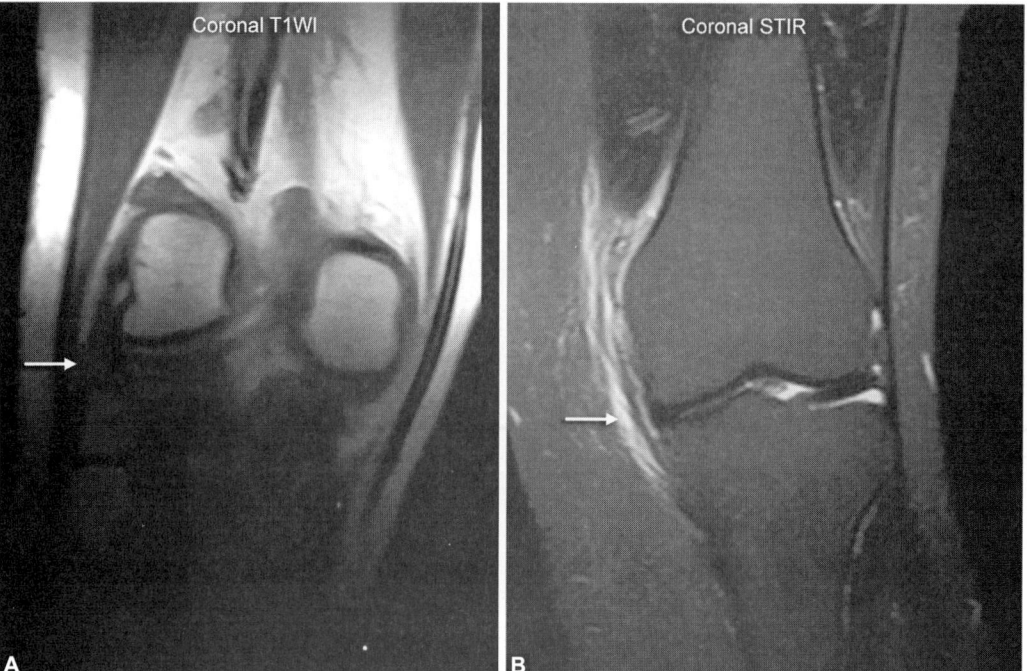

Figs 6.28A and B T1-weighted coronal image (A) shows Grade III, i.e. complete tear of the lateral collateral ligament (arrow) and STIR coronal image (B) shows strain (arrow) with tear of the medial collateral ligament

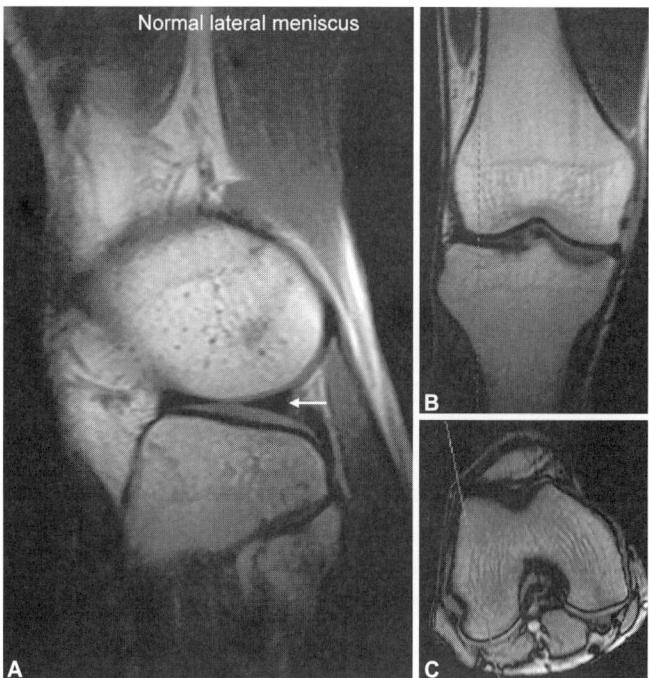

Figs 6.29A to C Sagittal section shows normal appearance of lateral meniscus. Localizers in coronal and axial planes (B and C) give the exact planes in which the sagittal section (A) shown has been taken

Double posterior cruciate ligament (PCL) sign: The double posterior cruciate ligament (PCL) sign is a low-signal-intensity band that is parallel and anteroinferior to the PCL on sagittal MR images. It is a highly specific indicator of a bucket-handle meniscal tear.

Kissing Contusions

Bone contusions are often identified at MRI in the acutely injured knee. Contusions of both surfaces of the joint are known as kissing contusions. Kissing

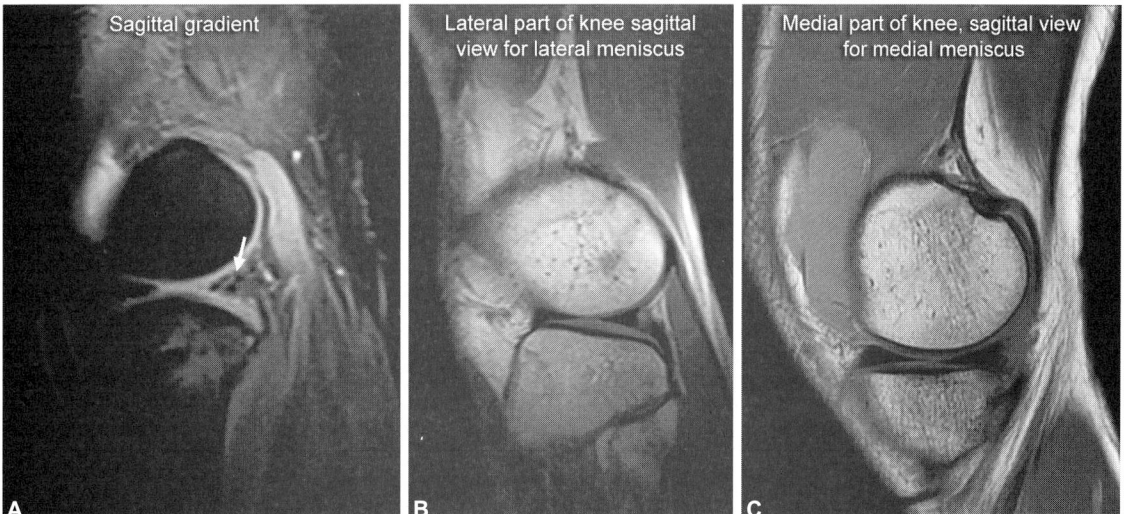

Figs 6.30A to C Sagittal gradient sequence (A) shows hyperintense signal in lateral meniscus of left knee extending into articular surface suggestive of Grade III lateral meniscal tear (arrow). Hint to recognize the medial or lateral meniscus on single sagittal section, when the fibular head is not included in the section. The tibial condyles always appear triangular in shape. The anterior margin of the lateral condyle (B) is vertical and the medial condyle (C) is almost an equilateral triangle in shape

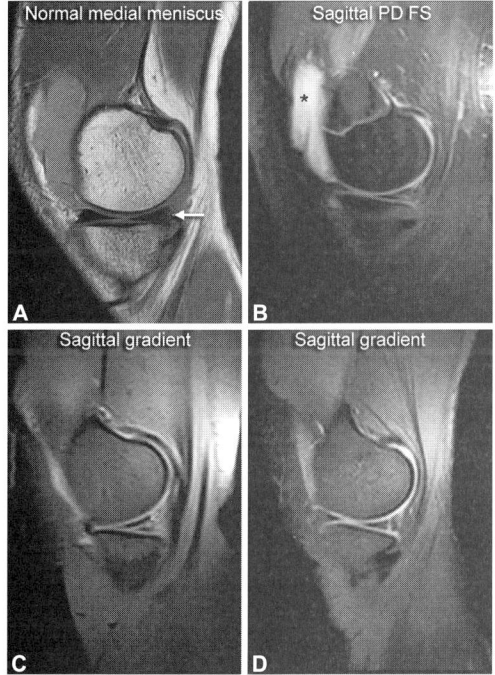

Figs 6.31A to D Sagittal section shows normal appearance of medial meniscus (A). Sagittal PD FS image (B) reveals linear hyperintense signal in the posterior horn of medial meniscus not reaching up to articular surface suggesting grade II tear with joint effusion (*). Sagittal GRE sequence (C) shows hyperintense signal in medial meniscus of left knee extending into articular surface (arrow) suggestive of grade III lateral meniscal tear. Sagittal gradient image (D) shows a meniscal tear as a vertical hyperintense signal in the posterior horn. It extends from the superior to the inferior articular surface and represents grade III medial meniscus tear

contusion is a significant injury often associated with ligamentous or meniscal injuries.

Classification of Kissing Contusions

In type I lesions there is a loss of signal intensity on T1W or proton density sequences and an increased signal on T2W, more evident in fat suppressed T2 or T2 FSE IR images; the area showing such variations in signal intensity is located primarily within the medullary cavity of the bone, without cortical interruption. Type I lesions are most common on the lateral femoral condyle.

Type II and type III lesions show the same signal intensity characteristics as type I, but type II is associated with interruption of the black cortical line, and type III is strictly located in the region of bone immediately adjacent to the cortex without any definite cortical interruption. Type III is seen on the lateral tibial condyle.

Bone contusions are considered to represent microtrabecular fractures, hemorrhage, and edema of the subcortical bone marrow are increasingly recognized through MR imaging of the acutely injured knee **(Figs 6.33A and B)**.

Parameniscal Cyst

A parameniscal cyst is a focal joint fluid collection located adjacent to a meniscus associated with a meniscal tear. Direct communication with the meniscal tear may or may not be demonstrated on MR

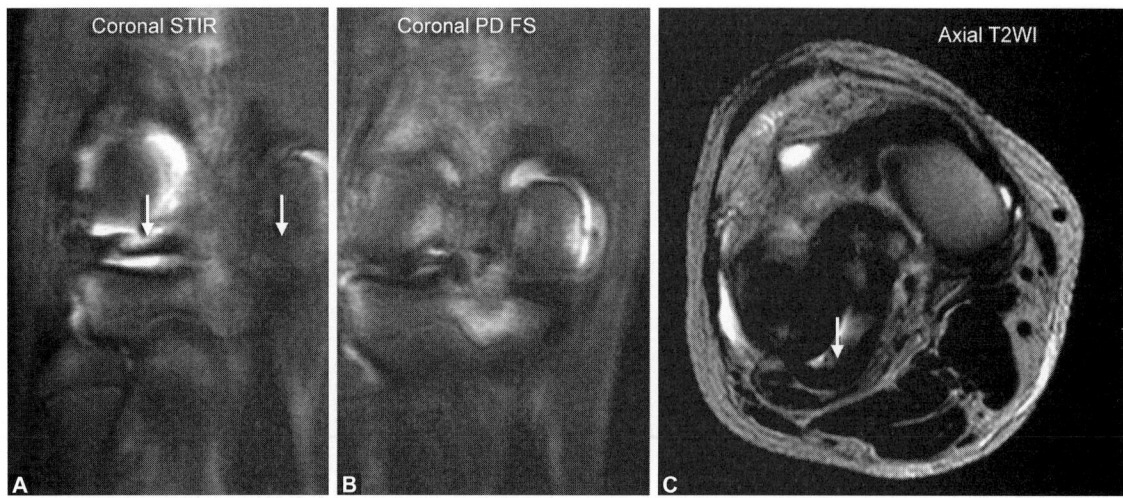

Figs 6.32A to C Coronal STIR (A), Coronal PD FS (B), and Axial T2 W (C) images show bucket handle tear involving the medial meniscus with meniscal flap (arrow) in the intercondylar region

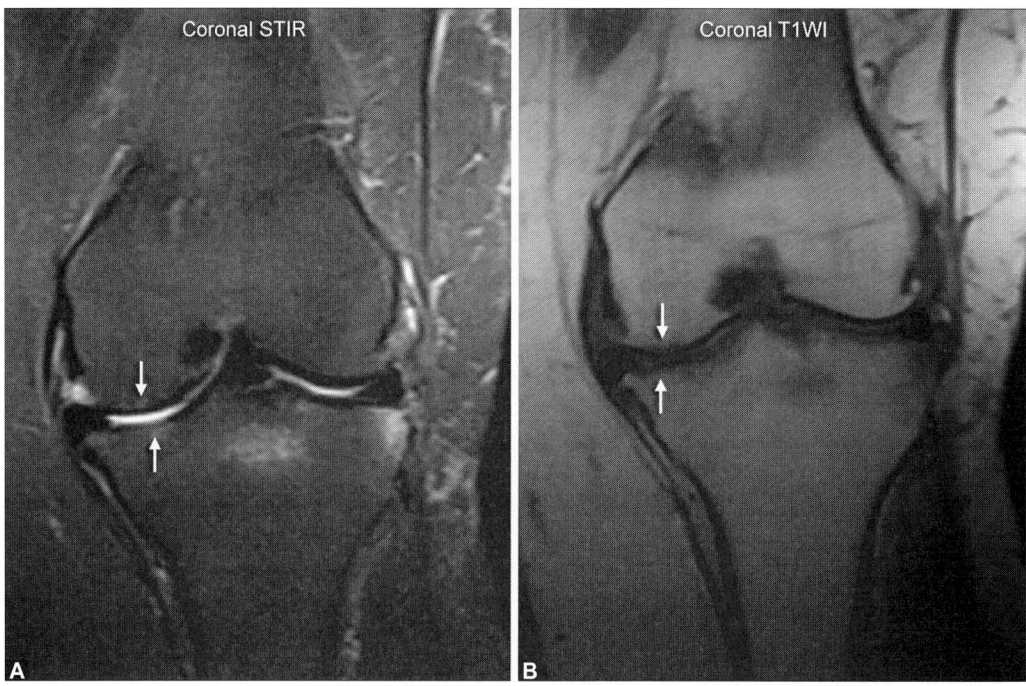

Figs 6.33A and B STIR coronal and T1 coronal images reveal bone contusion and marrow edema with kissing contusion involving the medial femoral and tibial condyles (arrows)

images. Meniscal cysts are typically demonstrated in all pulse sequences as well-defined cystic masses with fluid signal intensity **(Figs 6.34A to C)**. Occasionally they may demonstrate isointensity to skeletal muscles on T1-weighted images, due to hemorrhage or high protein content. In addition, low signal intensity on T2-weighted images may be secondary to water resorption by parameniscal tissues with residual desiccated cyst contents or due to hemosiderin deposition. Most parameniscal cysts are lobulated and internally septated and may rarely cause adjacent bone erosion. The most common medial parameniscal cyst is that adjacent to the posterior horn of the meniscus, since tears there are far more common. The most common location for a lateral parameniscal cyst is adjacent to the anterior horn or the body of the lateral meniscus. Since the lateral meniscus is not tightly bound to the joint capsule, parameniscal cysts originating from the anterior horn and body of lateral meniscus may penetrate the lateral supporting structures and extend even deep to the iliotibial tract.

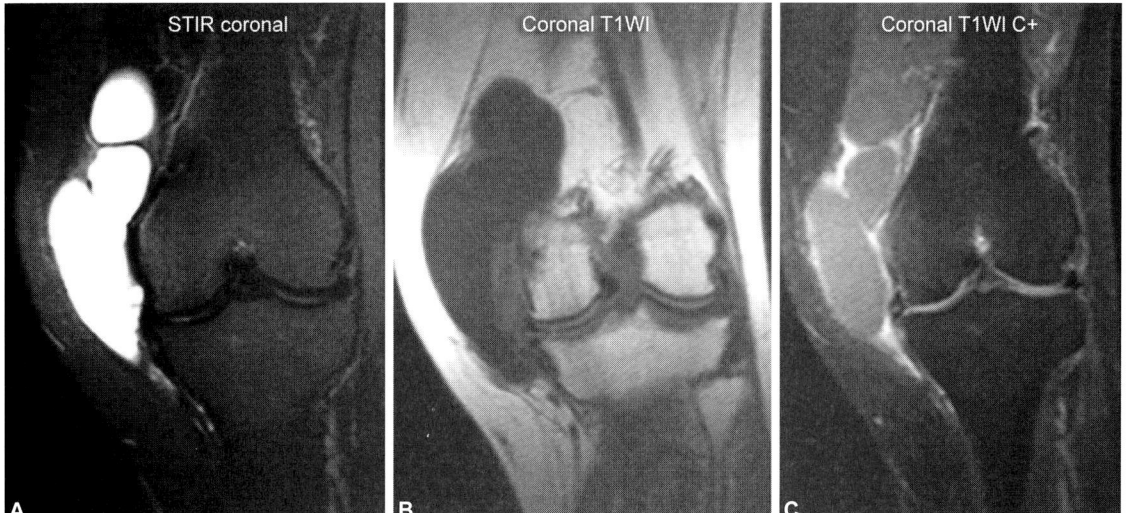

Figs 6.34A to C STIR coronal (A), T1 coronal (B), and postcontrast T1 coronal (C), images show Grade III tear involving the medial meniscus with parameniscal cyst

Pigmented Villonodular Synovitis

Pigmented villonodular synovitis (PVNS) is a proliferative disorder of the synovial membrane that most commonly involves the knee, hip, elbow and ankle. A brown fluid can frequently be aspirated from the joint, which reflects hemosiderin deposits from chronic hemorrhage or fresh blood from acute hemorrhage. Radiographs often show the findings of joint effusion, preservation of joint space, the absence of osteoporosis and the presence or absence of bone erosions and cysts. Bone erosions and subchondral cysts can be prominent, particularly in the hip, ankle, elbow and wrist. Many of the radiographic features of diffuse intra-articular PVNS are identical to those of idiopathic synovial chondromatosis. In PVNS calcification is not seen.

A giant cell tumor of a tendon sheath represents a nodular lesion of tendon sheaths, usually in the hand or foot, which may sometimes be confused with some forms of PVNS because of similar histologic findings. In PVNS, a diffuse or localized soft tissue mass is observed, with adjacent erosion of bone **(Figs 6.35A to G)**.

OSTEOMYELITIS

Osteomyelitis is an infection of bone and bone marrow, which may develop acute, subacute and chronic clinical stages. All cases do not show progression through all these phases, however; in some cases chronic osteomyelitis is present at the time of initial evaluation.

Four principal routes of contamination of bones and joints in osteomyelitis are from (a) hematogenous spread (b) spread from a contiguous source of infection (c) direct implantation of infectious material and (d) postoperative spread.

Owing to differences in vascular anatomy of tubular bones, hematogenous osteomyelitis may have different clinical and imaging patterns at different ages (infant, child, adult) which include sequestrum, a segment of necrotic bone separated from living bone by granulation tissue; involucrum, a layer of viable bone that has formed around necrotic bone; sinus tract, a tract leading to the skin surface from an infected site in bone; and Brodie's abscess a sharply delineated focus of infection in bone.

Chronic osteomyelitis shows areas of osteolysis, thin linear periostitis and sequestration. Scintigraphy and MR imaging are preferred methods in the early diagnosis of osteomyelitis, but MR imaging lacks specificity and bone abscesses cannot be distinguished from sterile fluid collections without intravenous contrast administration **(Figs 6.36A to D)**. Scintigraphy is useful in differentiation of osteomyelitis from cellulitis and in the recognition of renewed activity in chronic osteomyelitis. CT has been used to identify single or multiple sequestra, bone or soft tissue abscesses, and sinus tracts.

RHEUMATOID ARTHRITIS

Rheumatoid arthritis (RA) is a chronic systemic inflammatory disease and affects many organs, but predominantly involves the synovial tissues and joints. Etiology is unknown but may be due to genetic predisposition or reaction to antigen from Epstein-Barr virus. Highest incidence is between 40 and 50 years. The disease onset may be insidious or abrupt, the early features include tiredness, malaise and generalized aches. Arthritic symptoms generally

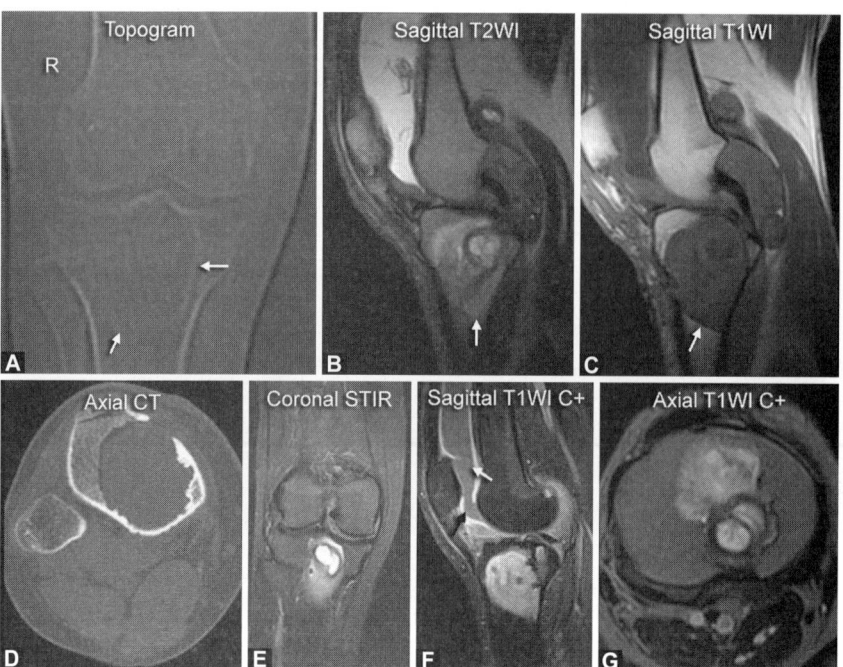

Figs 6.35A to G Topogram (A) reveal lytic lesion in the right tibia proximal metaepiphysis (arrows). Axial CT (D) reveal lytic lesion with soft tissue in the right proximal tibial metaepiphysis. Sagittal T2WI (B) shows heterogeneous hyperintense soft tissue intensity mass lesion in the proximal tibial metaepiphysis (arrow) which is heterogeneous hypointense on T1WI (C) with moderate joint effusion. Coronal STIR image (E) reveal abnormal hyperintense mass lesion in the proximal tibial metaepiphysis with surrounding marrow edema. Sagittal T1 and axial T1W postcontrast images (F and G) show abnormal postcontrast enhancement in the soft tissue lesion with abnormal peripheral synovial enhancement with moderate joint effusion (arrows)

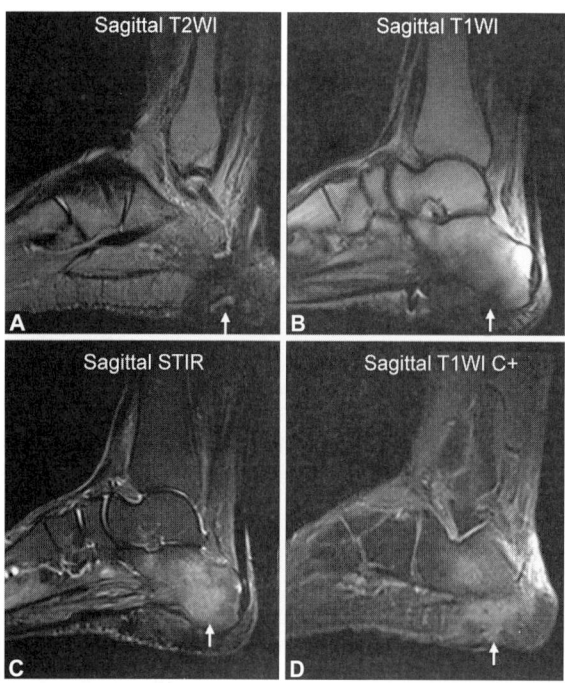

Figs 6.36A to D Sagittal T2WI image (A) reveal abnormal hyperintense signal in the heel soft tissue region (arrow), appearing hypointense on T1WI (B) with hypointense marrow edema in the calcaneum (arrow), sagittal STIR image (C) shows abnormal hyperintense marrow edema in the calcaneum (arrow), (D) postcontrast enhancement is seen (arrow)

first develop in the hands and wrists in a symmetric, proximal distribution. Feet and large joints may also be involved. It can be a disabling and painful condition, and can lead to substantial loss of functioning and mobility.

Radiological signs on X-rays:
A. Early signs include: (i) Periarticular soft tissue swelling (ii) widening of joint space (iii) regional osteoporosis (iv) bone erosion (v) giant synovial cyst (vi) subluxation.
B. Late signs include: (i) Subchondral cyst formation (ii) boutonniere deformities (iii) swan neck deformities (iv) Hitchhiker's thumb deformity.

Ultrasound can assess the soft tissue manifestation of RA, including effusion.

MRI is very sensitive for subtle and early feature of RA. Sequence used include are T1-weighted contrast-enhanced spin-echo with fat saturation and T2-weighted spin-echo or gradient-echo sequences. Features noted on MRI are synovial hyperplasia and hyperemia, pannus formation, decreased cartilage thickness, subchondral cyst and joint effusion.

Extra articular manifestation includes:
- Felty's syndrome—RA, splenomegaly and neutropenia
- Sjogren's syndrome—keratoconjunctivitis, xerostomia, RA

- Pulmonary manifestations—pleural effusion, rheumatoid nodule
- Subcutaneous nodule
- Rheumatoid vasculitis
- Lymphadenopathy

Diagnosis is based on a combination of clinical, radiological and serological criteria. The American College of Rheumatology revised criteria require that 4 out of 7 of the following are present:
1. Morning stiffness lasting at least 1 hour before maximal improvement
2. Soft tissue swelling of 3 or more joints observed by a physician
3. Swelling of the proximal interphalangeal, metacarpophalangeal, or wrist joints
4. Symmetric swelling
5. Rheumatoid nodules
6. The presence of rheumatoid factor; and
7. Radiographic erosions and/or periarticular osteopenia in hand and/or wrist joints.

NEUROPATHIC ARTHROPATHY

Neuropathic joint or Charcot joint is progressive degeneration and destruction of a weight bearing joint secondary to abnormal pain sensation. Any pathology that leads to loss of sensation in a joint can lead to a neuropathic arthropathy. Common conditions leading to neuropathic joints are diabetes, leprosy, syphilis, steroids, spinal cord injury, syringomyelia. Patient present with swollen, warm and usually painless joint. In 33% cases pain is present at presentation.

Etiology for Neuropathic

1. Neurotraumatic basis is absence of normal protective sensory feedback leads to repetitive trauma which goes unnoticed.
2. Neurovascular theory is loss of sympathetic tone in neuropathic patient leading to dysregulated autonomic nervous system reflexes, and sensation loss in joints which increased blood flow. The resulting hyperemia leads to increased osteoclastic resorption leading to bony destruction.

Neuropathic joint is described as hypertrophic joint with destruction and fragmentation, osseous sclerosis, and osteophyte formation. The atrophic form of neuropathic osteoarthropathy has an appearance of osseous resorption.

Early stage radiographic findings include persistent or progressive joint effusion, leading to narrowed joint space, soft-tissue calcification, minimal subluxation, preservation of bone density, and fragmentation subchondral bone.

In the late stage, there is evidence of destruction of articular surfaces, subchondral sclerosis, osteophytosis, intra-articular loose bodies, subluxation, dislocation of metatarsal bones, and rapid bone resorption demonstrating pencil-in-a-cup deformity or licked candy appearance. Complications in neuropathic arthropathy are osteomyelitis and bone ankylosis.

According to Yochum and Rowe, the "6 D's" to diagnose neuropathic arthropathy include: (a) Distended joint (b) Density increase (c) Debris production (d) Dislocation (e) Disorganization (f) Destruction.

7
Bone Tumors

WHO Classification of Bone Tumors

World Health Organization (WHO) accepted classification of bone tumors is given in **Tables 7.1A and B**. Advances in combined surgical and chemotherapy have lead to a significant increase in survival rates even for highly malignant tumors, including osteosarcoma and Ewing's sarcoma.

Bone tumors present radiological image which may be simple to diagnose such as bone cyst, fibrous dysplasia or osteogenic sarcoma or may be rather difficult to diagnose. Primary malignant tumors of bone are responsible for only 1% of all deaths from neoplasm. More common malignancy in bones is metastatic. Radiology not only to provides a diagnosis but also delineates soft tissue and extend of bony involvement **(Tables 7.2 and 7.3)**.

Bone sarcomas account for only 0.2% of all neoplasms, osseous neoplasms occur at a rate approximately one tenth that of their soft tissue counterparts. Osteosarcoma occurs predominantly in patients less than 20 years of age, of which 80% occur in long bones. Chondrosarcomas incidence rates show a gradual increase up to the age 75.

Benign cartilaginous dysplasias are the established precancerous conditions. Both osteosarcoma and malignant fibrous histiocytoma have been linked

Table 7.1A WHO classification of cartilage and osteogenic bone tumors

Cartilage tumors	Osteogenic tumors
• Osteochondroma	• Osteoid osteoma
• Chondroma	• Osteoblastoma
• Enchondroma	• Osteosarcoma
– Periosteal chondroma	– Conventional
– Multiple chondromatosis	- Chondroblastic
– Chondroblastoma	- Fibroblastic
• Chondromyxoid fibroma	- Osteoblastic
• Chondrosarcoma	– Telangiectatic
– Central, primary, and secondary	– Small cell
	– Low grade central
– Peripheral	– Secondary
– Dedifferentiated	– Parosteal
– Mesenchymal	– Periosteal
– Clear cell	– High grade surface

Table 7.1B Classification table of tumors of bone other than cartilage and osteogenic tumors

Fibrogenic tumors	*Smooth muscle tumors*
• Desmoplastic fibroma	• Leiomyoma
• Fibrosarcoma	• Leiomyosarcoma
Fibrohistiocytic tumors	*Lipogenic tumors*
• Benign fibrous histiocytoma	• Lipoma
• Malignant fibrous histiocytoma	• Liposarcoma
Ewing sarcoma/primitive neuroectodermal tumors	*Neural tumors*
• Ewing's sarcoma	• Neurilemmoma
Hematopoietic tumors	*Miscellaneous tumors*
• Plasma cell myeloma	• Adamantinoma
• Malignant lymphoma,	• Metastatic malignancy
Giant cell tumors	*Miscellaneous lesions*
• Giant cell tumor	• Aneurysmal bone cyst
• Malignancy in giant cell tumor	• Simple cyst
	• Fibrous dysplasia
	• Osteofibrous dysplasia
	• Langerhans cell histiocytosis
	• Erdheim–Chester disease
	• Chest wall hamartoma
Notochordal tumors	*Joint lesions*
• Chordoma	• Synovial chondromatosis
Vascular tumors	
• Hemangioma	
• Angiosarcoma	

Table 7.2 Differentiation between benign and malignant bone tumor

Benign tumors	Malignant tumors
Slow growth	Rapid growth
Asymptomatic to few symptoms	Pain, swelling, limitation of joint movement
Well-circumscribed margins, narrow transition zone	Ill-defined margins, wide transition zone
Noninvading	Invasion is seen into surrounding soft tissues
No metastasis	Metastasis takes place

Table 7.3 TMN classification of bone tumors

Primary tumor (T)	TX: Primary tumor cannot be assessed
	T0: No evidence of primary tumor
	T1: Tumor ≤ 8 cm in greatest dimension
	T2: Tumor > 8 cm in greatest dimension
	T3: Discontinuous tumors in the primary bone site
Regional lymph nodes (N)	NX: Regional lymph nodes cannot be assessed
	N0: No regional lymph node metastasis
	N1: Regional lymph node metastasis
Distant metastasis (M)	MX: Distant metastasis cannot be assessed
	M0: No distant metastasis
	M1: Distant metastasis
	M1a: Lung
	M1b: Other distant sites

Note: Regional node involvement is rare and cases in which nodal status is not assessed either clinically or pathologically could be considered N0 instead of NX or pNX.

to pre-existing condition of bone such as Paget's disease, radiation damage, bone infarction, fibrous dysplasia, chronic osteomyelitis, and some genetically determined syndromes.

The clinical features of bone tumors are non-specific; therefore a long period of time may elapse until the tumor is diagnosed. Pain, swelling and general discomfort are the cardinal symptoms that lead to the diagnosis of bone tumors. Limited mobility and spontaneous fracture are also important features.

Based on clinical and radiological signs, one should first diagnose benign lesions for which a subsequent biopsy may not be necessary such as metaphyseal fibrous defect, fibrous dysplasia, osteochondroma, enchondroma, simple bone cyst and vertebral hemangioma.

Aneurysmal Bone Cyst

Aneurysmal bone cysts are lytic bone lesions that occur in the distal parts of long bones or in spinal elements. Patients are usually less than 20 years of age. They contain a fibrous and vascular tissue in varying amount from only thin membranes to substantial areas of solid tissue. Their size can vary from tiny cysts to large cavities filing most of the lesion. CT gave much better anatomic delineation **(Figs 7.1A to E)** than the plain radiograph and the CT value of the cyst measured between 20–30HU. These cysts are most commonly filled with blood, but serosanguineous or even clear straw-colored fluid may be found. Some aneurysmal bone cysts may show fluid levels on CT-since the lesions contain collections of blood or fluid. Others are inhomogeneous, their CT images strongly resembling those of some giant cell tumors.

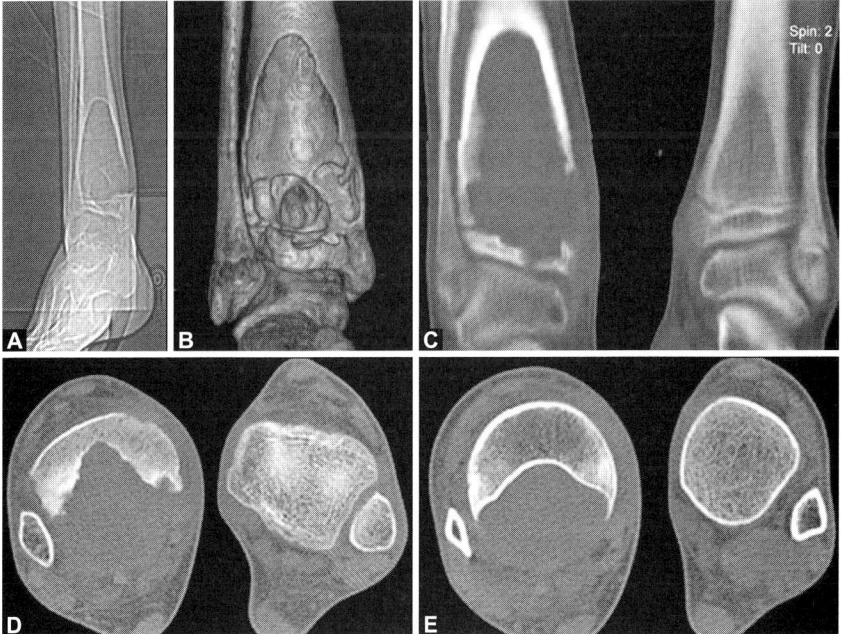

Figs 7.1A to E A 16-year-old male had history of painful swelling just above right ankle was subjected to CT, shows an eccentric expansile lytic lesion is seen in the distal diaphysis and metaphysis region of right tibia. Multiple septae are seen. The inner portion is sclerotic. No periosteal reaction is seen. The lesion does not cross the epiphyseal plate. Scanogram (A), volume-rendered image (B), coronal-reformatted image (C), axial images (D and E) *(For color version, see plate 2)*

Unicameral or Simple Bone Cyst

Bone cyst is a cavitary lesion of bone. Various types of bone cysts may be identified: simple or unicameral, epidermoid, aneurysmal, subchondral and ganglion. Bone cysts may occur after trauma and in osteoarthritis, rheumatoid arthritis, neurofibromatosis and calcium pyrophosphate dihydrate crystal deposition disease.

Unicameral bone cyst or simple bone cyst is an seen in the first two decades of life with M:F ratio of 2:1. It is situated in the metaphysis of the long bones commonly upper end of humerus or upper end of femur.

There are two types of cyst:
1. Active cyst is situated close to the epiphyseal plate
2. Inactive or latent cyst when the cyst has moved away from the growth plate.

The bone cyst is generally asymptomatic. Pain may occur, if a pathological fracture takes place. Joint deformities like shortening, lengthening, coxa vara, coxa valga may occur due to proximity of cyst to the growth plate.

Simple bone cysts are lesions of unknown cause that may result from venous obstruction with failure of drainage of the interstitial fluid in rapidly growing or remodeling bones. These cysts occur more commonly in long tubular bones, especially the metaphysis, and in the bony pelvis.

On X-ray, these lesions appear radiolucent and are located centrally, with cortical thinning and mild expansion of the bone. Bone cyst in patella is uncommon (**Figs 7.2A to G**). Pathological fractures are common. CT and MR imaging confirm the diagnosis of the bone cyst and shows no wall enhancement on post-contrast images. Complications of simple bone cysts include fractures, cementomas, and rarely malignant transformation.

On plain X-ray, it appears as a well-defined low density lesion with sclerotic borders located at the metaphysis which moves to the diaphysis as age advances. Overlying cortex is thinned out with or without cortical breach. Fallen fragment sign is due to fractured cyst when a piece of the bone migrates into the cavity and settles at the base. CT and MRI depict this signs better but patient should be subjective to CT and MRI only in equivocal cases.

Surgical excision is the treatment of choice. However, curettage and bone grafting, subtotal resection and bone grafting and total resection, and bone grafting is also carried out.

Osteoid Osteoma

Osteoid osteoma is a benign lesion frequently found in the appendicular skeleton. The tumors produce excess bone and secrete pain-causing prostaglandins, resulting in intense pain especially at night. A 22-year-old male presented with pain and tenderness in left thigh region since 4 months. Radiograph shows sclerosis and cortical thickening due to subperiosteal bone formation. The radiolucent nidus questionably

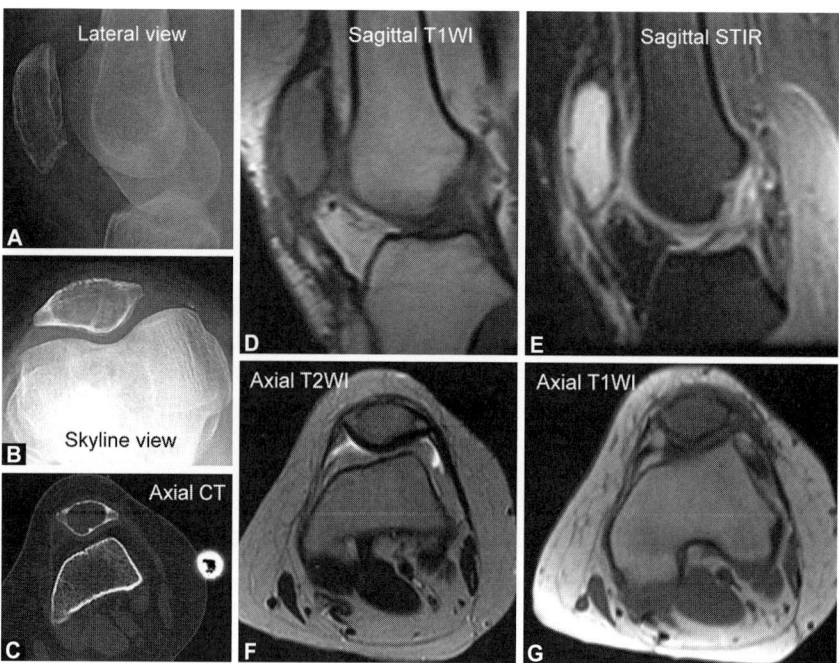

Figs 7.2A to G X-ray lateral (A) and skyline (B) views for patella show a large lucency with thinning of cortical bone in left patella; cyst is better appreciated on skyline view. Axial CT shows a large cystic lesion within the patella with a thin bony rim (C). Sagittal T1WI (D) shows reduced intensity in patella, appearing hyperintense on sagittal STIR image (E), confirms the finding of cyst. Axial T2WI (F) shows iso- to hyperintense signal in patella appearing hypointense on T1WI (G)

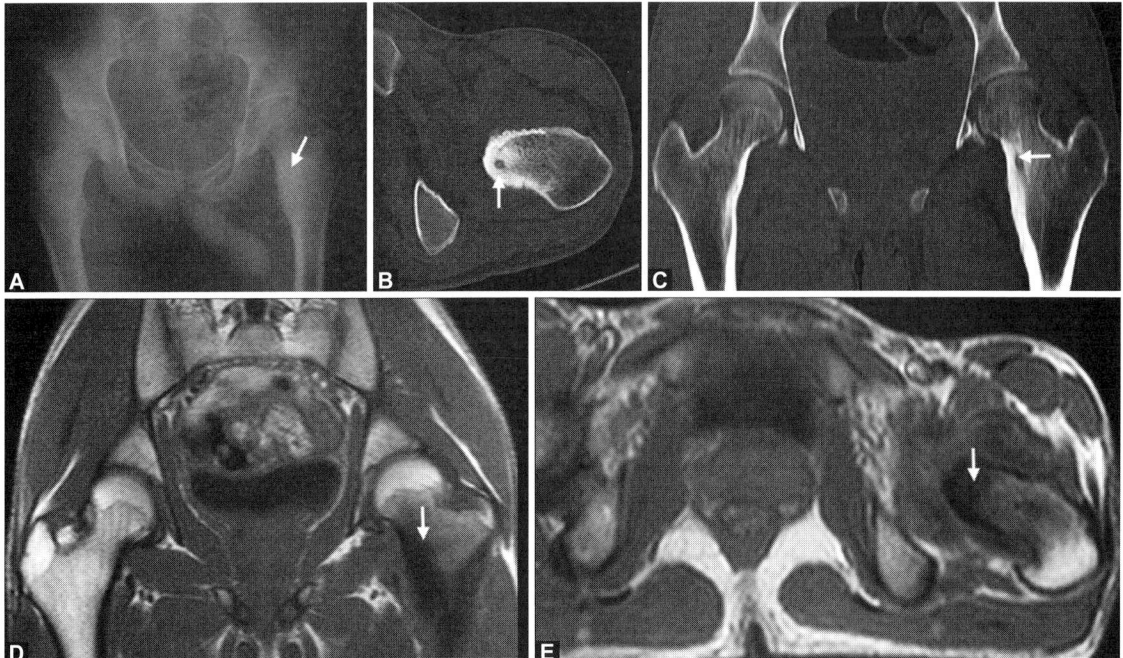

Figs 7.3A to E Plain radiograph (A) reveals an ill-defined region of increased cortical thickness (arrow) and CT axial (B) and coronal reformatted (C) reveals the presence small well defined calcified nidus and dense cortical thickening near lesser trochanter. MRI coronal (D) and axial (E) reveals hypointense cortical thickening along lesser trochanter with well-defined small hypointense lesion adjacent to it (arrow)

visualized. The location of the nidus, intranidal calcification, sclerosis, mature periosteal bone formation and location of original cortex precisely demonstrated by CT (**Figs 7.3A to C**). MRI also clearly showed the partially calcified nidus and associated cortical thickening. In addition, MR images (**Figs 7.3D to E**) revealed mild marrow and soft tissue edema in the vicinity of the nidus, which is not demonstrated by CT.

Osteochondroma

Osteochondroma is the most common benign tumor of bone seen in children and young adults. It has its origin from metaphysis with cartilage cap covering and bony attachment to underlying host bone. It is located at the sites of tendinous attachment around the metaphysis of long bones in the region of knee, ankle, hip, shoulder and elbow. An osteochondroma is a cartilage-covered bony excrescence (exostosis).

Patient is usually asymptomatic but may complain of pain, swelling, pathological fracture commonly secondary to complications. Clinical examination reveals a firm nontender swelling fixed to the bone around joints, decreased joint movements. Multiple osteochondromas occur as a manifestation of diaphyseal aclasia.

The radiographic appearance of this tumor is often diagnostic, and reflects its pathologic characteristics, that is, a lesion composed of cortical and medullary bone with an overlying hyaline cartilage cap. However, it is the continuity of this lesion with the underlying native bone cortex and medullary canal that is pathognomonic of osteochondroma (**Figs 7.4 and 7.5**). Fracture of osteochondroma is sometimes seen (**Figs 7.4A and B**).

Osteochondromas may be solitary or multiple, and they may arise spontaneously or as a result of previous osseous trauma. An osteochondroma can affect any bone performed in cartilage. Most solitary osteochondromas are discovered incidentally in children and

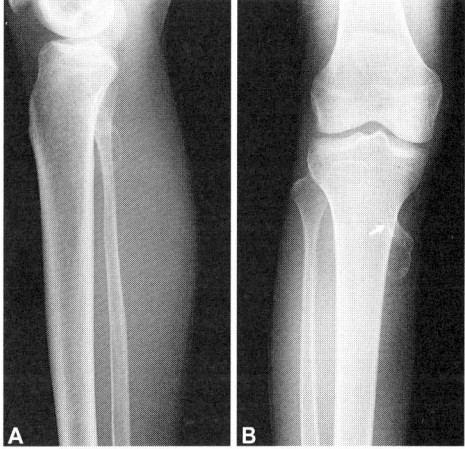

Figs 7.4A and B X-ray leg shows pedunculated osteochondroma seen arising from medial surface of proximal tibia

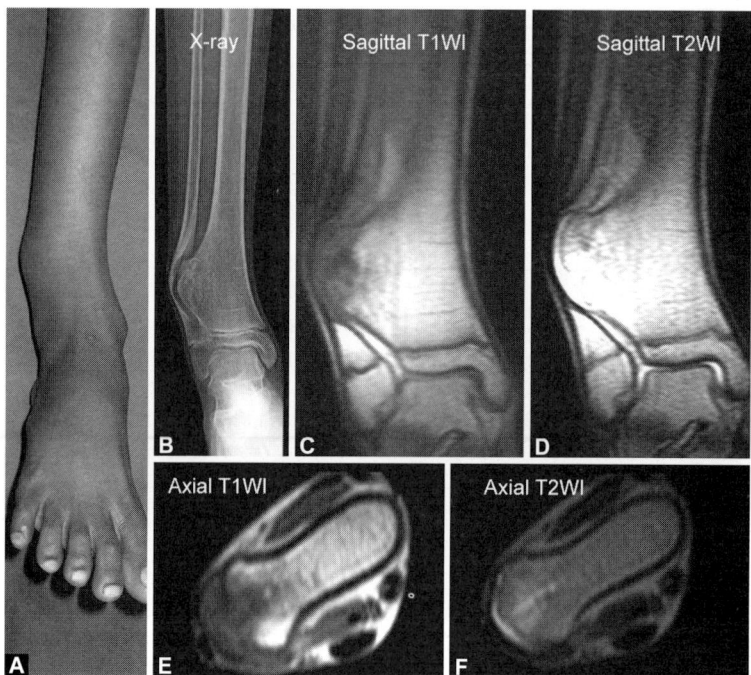

Figs 7.5A to F A 10-year-old female presented with pain and swelling in right lower leg. (A) and X-ray of both ankles anteroposterior view (B) reveals sessile bony outgrowth from right lower tibia, lateral aspect with continuity of cortex and medullary cavity with the parent bone, causing significant pressure erosion and thinning of the adjoining fibula. Mineralized areas in the cartilage cap remain low signal intensity with all MR pulse sequences. The high water content in no mineralized portions of the cartilage cap had intermediate-to-low signal intensity sagittal and axial on T1-weighted images (C and E) and very high signal intensity on sagittal and axial T2-weighted MR images (D to F) *(For color version, see plate 2)*

adolescents. Hereditary multiple exostoses (HME), also known as osteochondromatosis, is an inherited, autosomal dominant disorder in which multiple osteochondromas are seen throughout the skeleton. Complications of osteochondromas include fractures, bony deformities, neurologic and vascular injuries, bursa formation, and malignant transformation.

Most osteochondromas, solitary or multiple, arise from tubular bones and are metaphyseal in location. The lesion is composed of cortical and medullary bone protruding from and continuous with the underlying bone. The areas of osseous continuity between parent bone and osteochondroma may be broad—sessile osteochondroma, or narrow, with a bulbous tip—pedunculated osteochondroma. Identifying the characteristic cortical and medullary continuity between lesion and parent bone on radiographs is dependent on lesion type (sessile or pedunculated), location, and image projection. Pedunculated lesions usually point away from the nearest joint owing to the forces of the overlying tendons and ligaments.

Magnetic resonance imaging also demonstrates cortical and medullary continuity between the osteochondroma and parent bone, cortical bone remains low signal intensity with all pulse sequences, whereas the medullary component has an appearance of yellow marrow. MR imaging is the best radiologic modality for visualizing the effect of the lesion on surrounding structures and evaluating the hyaline cartilage cap **(Figs 7.5A to F)**.

Diaphyseal Aclasis (Chondromatosis)

Diaphyseal aclasis is also known as external chondromatosis syndrome, multiple exostoses, or multiple osteochondromatosis. Usually, presents during the first decade of life. It is characterized by multiple exostosis or bony protrusions and is inherited autosomal dominant disorder. Long bones are usually affected more severely and more frequently than the short bones but they also often involve the medial borders of the scapulae, ribs and iliac crests. The malignant change is more frequent compared to the solitary exostosis. Most of the osteochondromas are painless and the main concern is often cosmetic, they may rarely develop fracture following trauma **(Figs 7.6A and B)**.

Plain X-ray may be the only imaging study required **(Fig. 7.7)**. CT scan is useful in the assessment of osteochondromas in the pelvis, shoulder **(Fig. 7.8)** or spine. MRI scan is useful in the assessment of malignant transformation and for evaluating compression of the spinal cord, nerve roots and peripheral nerves.

Bone Tumors

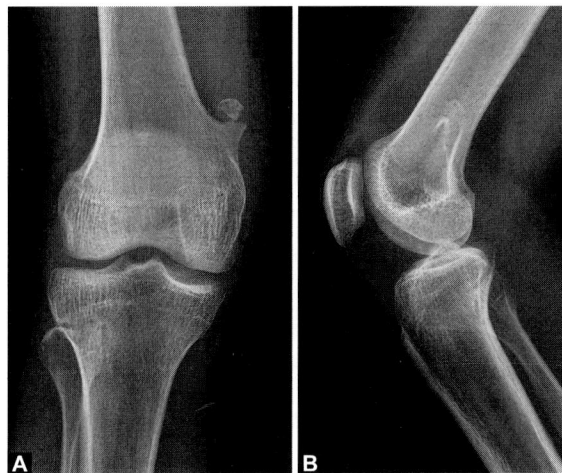

Figs 7.6A and B A 24-year-old male patient with history of trauma right knee shows pedunculated osteochondroma over medial supracondylar cortex of femur with fracture at its neck with displacement of bulbous tip.

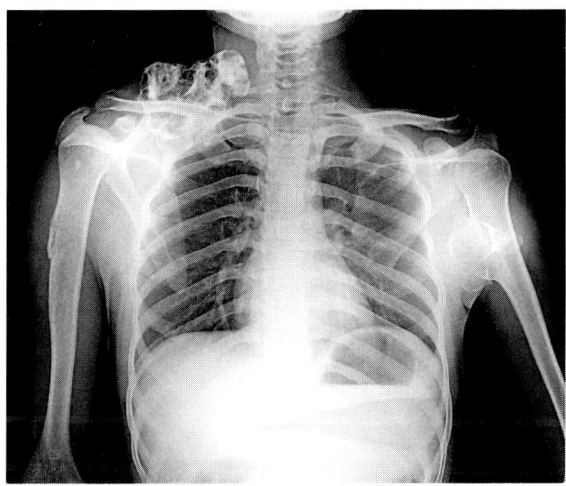

Fig. 7.7 X-ray chest shows a large bony outgrowth-exostosis arising from superior medial aspect of right scapula; it is not possible to say, if this large exostosis is pedunculated or sessile. Another exostosis is seen to arise from medial margin of upper shaft of left humerus and another small bony outgrowth from the lateral margin of upper 3rd shaft of right humerus. On CT-chest, the origin of lesion can be best evaluated

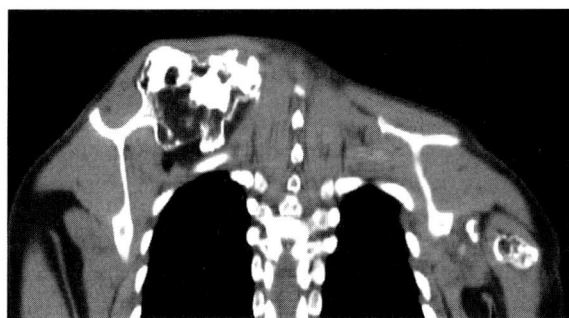

Fig. 7.8 On CT-chest coronal reconstruction, a large exostosis is seen to arise from the anterosuperior margin of right scapula. The exostosis has a pedicle which was not was not appreciated on posteroanterior chest, is clearly seen on CT

Tallus Chondroblastoma

These are rare cartilaginous tumor occurring in bone and seen in age range of 5–25 years. The tumor almost always arises in an epiphysis or apophysis but may extend into the joint or into the metaphysis, especially after skeletal maturity. Typical sites include the femur, humerus or tibia with approximately 50% occurring around the knee. Clinical presentation is usually with pain. There may be a joint effusion and reduced range of movement of the involved joint.

Radiographically, the lesion appears as a well-defined eccentrically located intramedullary rounded lucency. The tumor shows a sclerotic margin, may expand and erode the cortex and often contains punctate calcification within the matrix. If the lesion extends into the metaphysis, there may be associated periosteal new bone formation seen in the metaphyseal region. CT may better demonstrate the calcification within the lesion.

On MRI, it shows low signal intensity on T1WI and variable signal intensity on T2WI. Surrounding marrow edema may be evident **(Figs 7.9A to G)**.

Usually, chondroblastomas are benign, but occasionally, they exhibit a more aggressive course, invading soft tissues, adjacent bones and joint spaces. Metastases to the lung have been reported.

Giant Cell Tumor

Giant cell tumor (GCT) is usually a benign typically found in the metaepiphysis of long bones. It is locally aggressive tumor originates from undifferentiated cells of supporting tissues of bone marrow and is commonly occurs in young adults at 20–30 years of age. Tumor arises eccentrically in the metaphysis with tendency to approach subarticular cortex as they enlarge. About 70–80% occurs in the lower end of femur, upper end of tibia, fibula and distal end of radius.

Clinically presents as swelling near the joint on one side. Tenderness is moderate or absent. Egg-shell-crackling sensation may be present. There may be pathological fracture and limitation of joint movements in late stage.

Types are:
a. Benign GCT (more common)
b. Malignant GCT

X-ray shows well-defined multiloculated osteolytic lesion which expands the overlying cortex (soap bubble appearance) with no surrounding sclerosis (85% cases) **(Fig. 7.10)**. It may be associated with soft tissue component. Periosteal reaction is uncommon. MRI is best modality to diagnose recurrence following treatment. Pathological fracture may be present.

On surgery, en-bloc excision is the procedure of choice or curettage and bone grafting, curettage and acrylic cementation or cryosurgery.

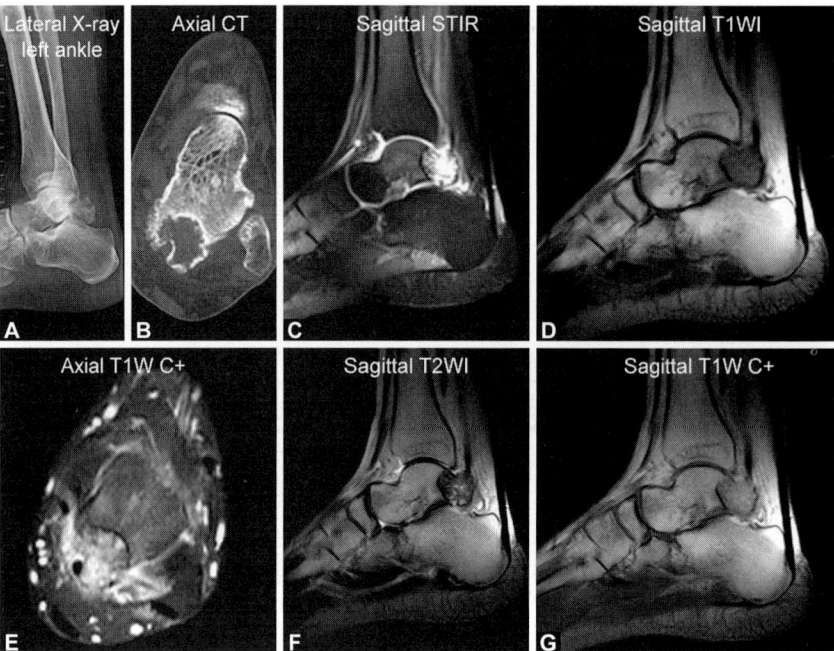

Figs 7.9A to G X-ray left ankle (A) in a 27-year-male with hard swelling and pain in left ankle reveals a lytic lesion in posterior aspect of left talus. Axial CT image (B) shows well-defined lytic lesion with sclerotic margin and cortical thinning. Sagittal STIR image (C) reveals well-defined lesion in posterior aspect of talus appearing hyperintense with associated mild marrow edema, it appears hypointense on T1WI (D). Sagittal (F) T2W image reveals well-defined lesion in posterior aspect of talus appearing hyperintense with hypointense margin. Postcontrast T1W axial (E) and sagittal (G) T1FS images shows significant enhancement of the lesion

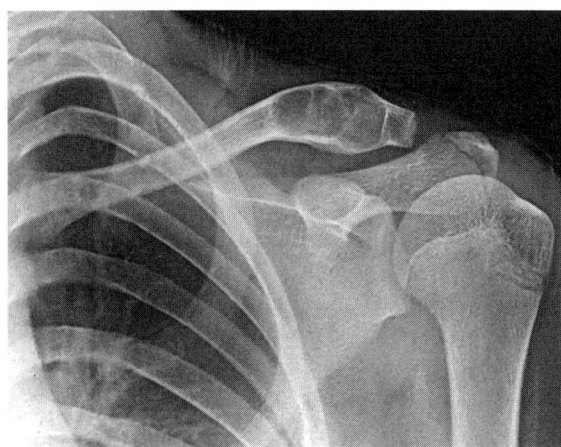

Fig. 7.10 X-ray shoulder PA view shows well-defined expansile lytic lesion involving lateral third of the clavicle suggestive of GCT, other differential is aneurysmal bone cyst

Hemangioma

Bone hemangiomas are benign, malformed vascular lesions, overall constituting less than 1% of all primary bone neoplasms. They occur most frequently in the vertebral column (30–50%) and skull (20%), whereas involvement of other sites (including the long bones, short tubular bones, and ribs) is rare. Hemangiomas are largely asymptomatic, usually found incidentally. On plain radiographs, hemangiomas are seen as dense lesions with prominent trabecular pattern. On MRI, hemangiomas are iso- to hyperintense on T1W images and appear hyperintense on STIR images. Postcontrast images show heterogeneous enhancement **(Figs 7.11A to F)**.

Lipoma

Lipoma is the most common benign tumor. It commonly occurs in head, neck, palm, sole and gastrointestinal tract. It can be localized or diffuse, single or multiple.

Sites of lipoma are subcutaneous, subfascial, intramuscular, intermuscular, parosteal, subserosal, submucosal, extradural and intra-articular.

Lipomas attain large size in thigh, shoulder, retroperitoneum and back. They presents as localized, lobular, nontender semifluctuant swelling. Submucosal lipoma can cause intestinal obstruction due to intussusceptions

On plain film, it appears as a lucency in contrast with surrounding soft tissues. CT provides a definitive diagnosis of lipoma as the characteristic attenuation of fat is (−) 50 to (−) 200 HU **(Figs 7.12A and B)**. It also helps to localize the origin and to identify malignant degeneration of a benign lesion.

Complications are sarcomatous degeneration into liposarcoma, myxomatous degeneration, saponification and calcification.

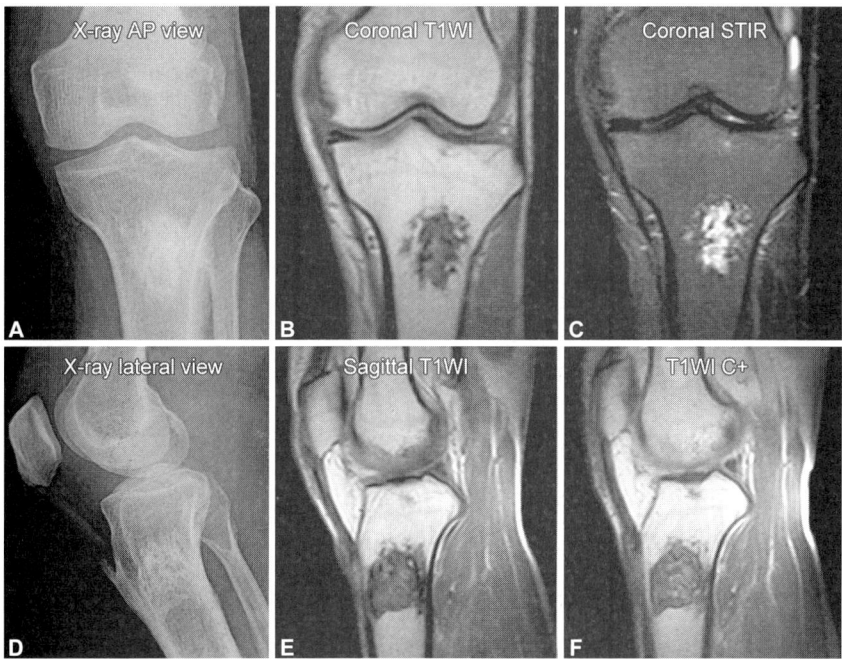

Figs 7.11A to F A 35-year-old male patient with history of mild pain left knee for 2 months on X-ray knee joint anteroposterior and lateral (A and B) views show heterogeneously dense intramedullary lesion in proximal tibial diaphysis. T1W coronal image (C) shows a well-defined iso- to hypointense lesion with irregular margins in proximal tibial diaphysis. This lesion appears hyperintense on coronal STIR image (D). There is no perilesional edema or medullary widening. On postcontrast T1WI, the lesion shows moderate heterogeneous enhancement (E and F). Findings are consistent with tibial hemangioma

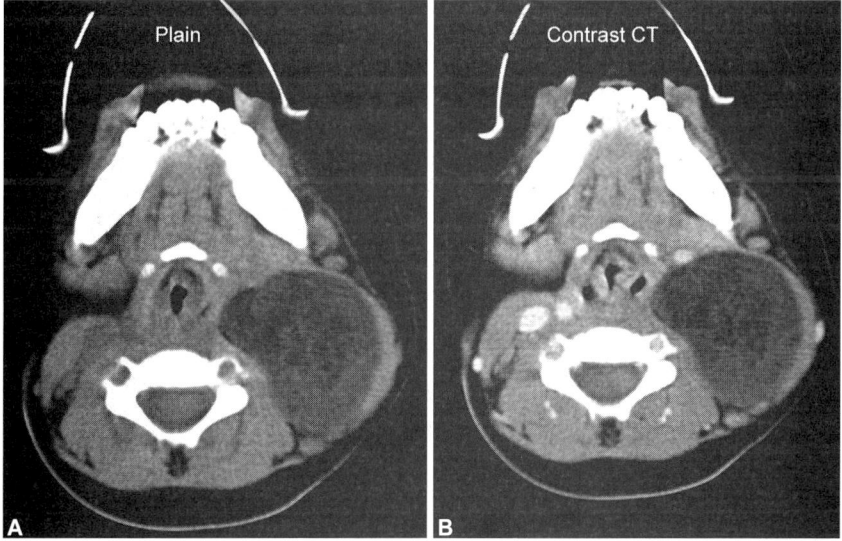

Figs 7.12A and B Large well-defined, fat attenuation (−70 to −9 HU) lesion noted in the left side and neck, just below the sternocleidomastoid muscle. The lesion is extending medially up to the left parapharyngeal space. Laterally, it is displacing sternocleidomastoid muscle. Multiple enlarged subcentimeter bilateral submandibular and submental nodes noted

Adamantinoma

Adamantinoma is a rare tumor typically involving the midshaft of tibia. Its pathogenesis is unknown but is histologically similar to ameloblastoma of the jaw. Most cases occur between 10 and 50 years of age. Male to female ratio is 5:4. Adamantinoma is locally aggressive or malignant lesion of bone composed of rows of epithelium-like cells in a dense fibrous stroma. Other bones that may be involved are the humerus, ulna, femur, fibula and radius. Local pain, tenderness and swelling of several months to years are the most common presenting complaint. The tumor continues to grow at a slow rate,

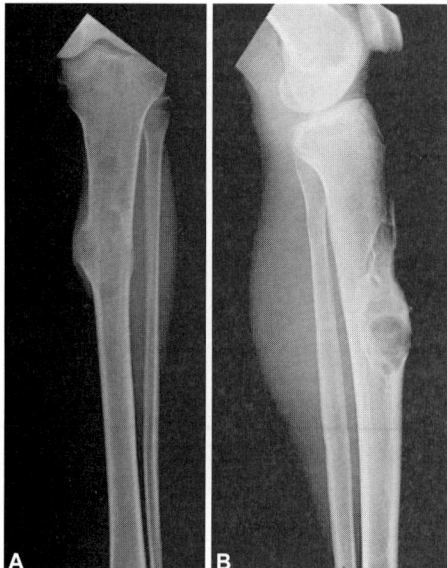

Figs 7.13A and B Anteroposterior and lateral X-ray left leg. A shows eccentric multiloculated osteolytic lesion in the tibial shaft with well-defined margin, causing expansion of the bone

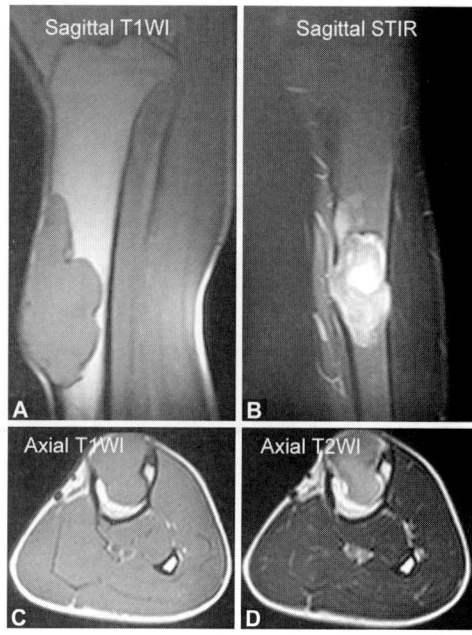

Figs 7.14A to D In 21-year-old male with pain and swelling left leg, on MR shows a lobulated, expansile, well-defined soft tissue lesion seen in diaphyseal region of tibia. It appears hypointense on T1WI (A and C) and hyperintense on STIR and T2WI (B and D)

but is characterized by local recurrence and eventual metastasis to lung. Extensive local resection is the usual form of treatment.

The lesion appears as a multilocular, slightly expansile, eccentric area of destruction with reactive bone sclerosis. Plain radiograph show central or eccentric osteolytic lesion in the shaft of the bone with well-defined margin, causing mild expansion of the bone **(Figs 7.13A and B)**. Multiloculated appearance and satellite lesions are useful diagnostic features. Periosteal reaction is uncommon. It grows at slow rate but is characterized by local recurrences and metastasis to lungs. Extensive local resection is the usual form of treatment. On MRI, these appear hypointense on T1 and hyperintense on STIR and T2WI **(Figs 7.14A to D)**.

Fibrolipomatous Hamartoma Median Nerve

Fat infiltration of the nerve is a rare benign lesion. The World Health Organization Tumor Classification describes fibrolipomatous hamartoma as lipomatosis of the nerve. It is also called as fibrolipomatous of nerve, lipofibromatous hamartoma, lipofibroma, fibro-fatty overgrowth, fatty infiltration of nerve, fibrofatty nerve enlargement, and neurolipoma. The etiology of this lesion by some authors is considered be a congenital tumor while others believe to be nerve irritation, inflammation, or prior trauma. There is usually a long history of a painless mass since childhood.

More than 80% of fibrolipomatous hamartomas arise exclusively in the median nerve. Other nerves, including the ulnar, radial, axillary, musculocutaneous, brachial plexus, and cranial nerves, and nerves in the lower extremity can be affected.

The reason for the predilection for the median nerve is not certain. However, the median nerve may easily become symptomatic due to encroachment of the flexor retinaculum. Men and women are equally affected and there is no familial predisposition.

Patients with fibrolipomatous hamartoma typically present in the third to fourth decades of life, with signs and symptoms associated with nerve compression in the distribution of the affected nerve.

Plain X-rays usually of normal appearance or show only a soft-tissue mass as in this case **(Figs 7.15A to C)**. The MRI features, especially the coaxial cable-like appearance on axial images are considered pathognomonic and should enable accurate diagnosis and differentiation from other possible diagnoses **(Figs 7.16A to C)**.

The treatment of fibrolipomatous hamartoma is controversial and depends on the extent of the nerve involvement. Treatment involves carpal-tunnel decompression by excising the transverse carpal ligament, followed by biopsy of the enlarged nerve [6] as was done in this case. This procedure results in clinical improvement.

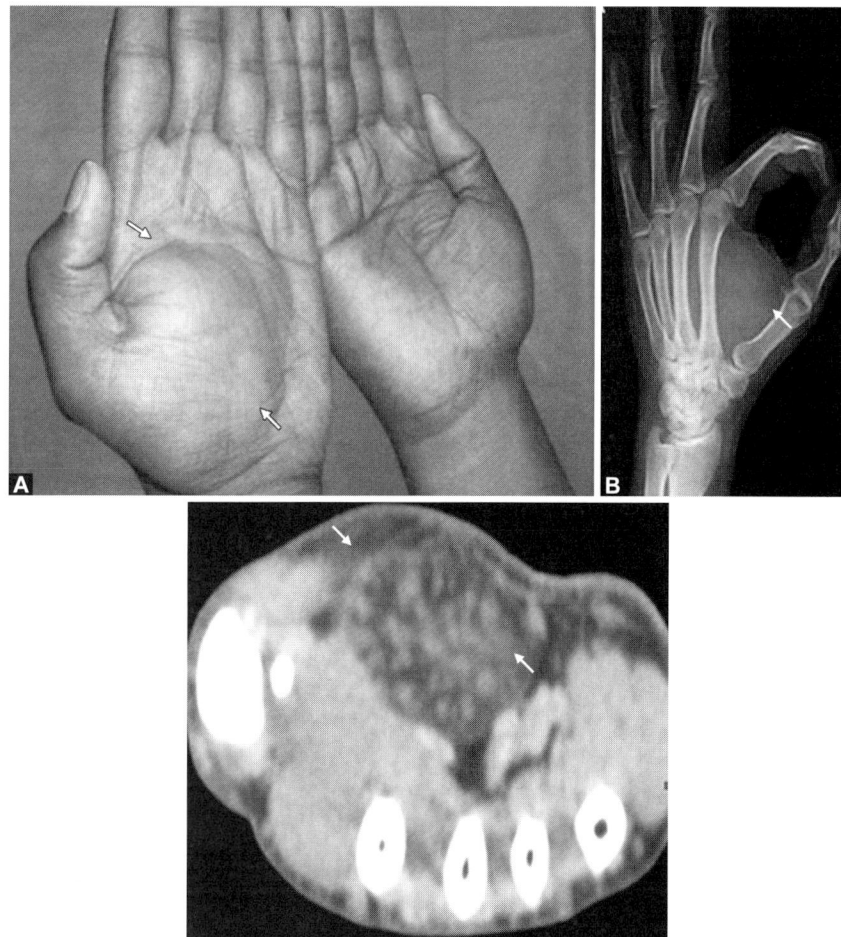

Figs 7.15A to C (A) Swelling over the thenar eminence of the left palm (arrows). (B) Oblique radiograph the left hand of patient showing soft tissue mass lesion in the thenar aspect of the left hand (arrows). (C) CT scan axial image of hand shows a well-defined heterogeneous lesion in ventral aspect anterior to the flexor tendons having fat density within it with cable-like appearance *(For color version, see plate 3)*

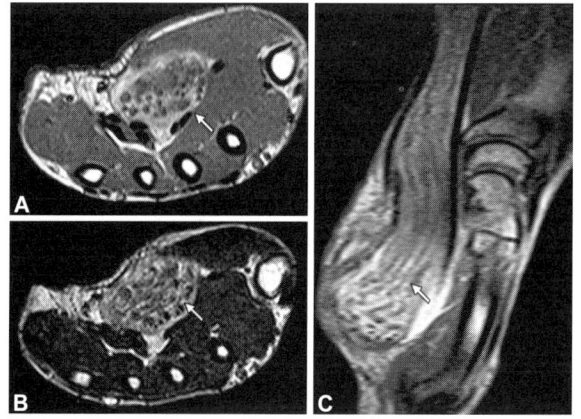

Figs 7.16A to C MRI T1W and T2W axial images of the left hand and T2W sagittal image of the left distal forearm and hand shows a well-defined fat containing lesion with linear hypointense structure representing the nerve fascicles

IMAGING FINDINGS IN PLASMA CELL TUMORS

Plasma Cell Tumor

A tumor that begins in plasma cells (white blood cells that produce antibodies). Multiple myeloma, monoclonal gammopathy of undetermined significance (MGUS), and plasmacytoma are types of plasma cell tumors.

Multiple Myeloma

In multiple myeloma, abnormal plasma cells (myeloma cells) build up in the bone marrow, forming tumors in many bones of the body. These tumors may prevent the bone marrow from making enough

healthy blood cells. Normally, the bone marrow produces stem cells (immature cells) that develop into three types of mature blood cells:
- Red blood cells that carry oxygen and other materials to all tissues of the body.
- White blood cells that fight infection and disease.
- Platelets that help prevent bleeding by causing blood clots to form.

As the number of myeloma cells increases, fewer red blood cells, white blood cells, and platelets are made. The myeloma cells also damage and weaken the hard parts of the bones. Sometimes multiple myeloma does not cause any symptoms.

Plasmacytoma

In this type of plasma cell neoplasm, the abnormal plasma cells (myeloma cells) collect in one location and form a single tumor, called a plasmacytoma. A plasmacytoma may form in bone marrow or may be extramedullary (in soft tissues outside of the bone marrow). Plasmacytoma of the bone often becomes multiple myeloma. Extramedullary plasmacytomas commonly form in tissues of the throat and sinuses; these usually can be cured.

Macroglobulinemia

In macroglobulinemia, abnormal plasma cells build-up in the bone marrow, lymph nodes, and spleen. They make too much M protein, which causes the blood to become thick. The lymph nodes, liver, and spleen may become swollen. The thickened blood may cause problems with blood flow in small blood vessels.

Radiographic Features

The classic radiographic appearance of multiple myeloma is that of multiple, small, well-circumscribed, lytic, punched-out, round lesions within the skull, spine, and pelvis. The lesions tend to vary slightly in size. In addition, the bones of myeloma patients are, with few exceptions, diffusely demineralized. Because myeloma is a disease of the medullary compartment of the bone, more subtle lesions can be detected by the appearance of endosteal scalloping that is seen as slight undulation to the inner cortical margin of bone. This finding is suggestive of myelomatous involvement. Plasmacytoma are typically seen as well-defined, "punched-out" lytic lesions with associated extra-pleural soft-tissue masses, similar in appearance to most metastatic lesions. In advanced plasmacytoma, there is often marked erosion, expansion, and destruction of bone cortex, sometimes with thick ridging around the periphery, creating a soap-bubble appearance.

Computed Tomography

Computed tomography (CT) may demonstrate subtle lytic lesions or small soft-tissue masses, particularly of the sternum, that are not visible at radiography. CT scanning can also guide percutaneous biopsies, especially of osseous or extraosseous lesions that are suspected of being plasmacytomas.

Magnetic Resonance Imaging

Magnetic resonance imaging (MRI) is useful for imaging multiple myeloma because of its superior soft-tissue contrast resolution. The typical appearance of a myeloma deposit is a round, low signal intensity (relative to muscle) focus on T1-weighted images, which becomes high in signal intensity on T2-weighted sequences. Myeloma lesions tend to enhance with gadolinium administration. In addition, diffuse areas of marrow replacement may be seen, resulting in large regions of low T1-weighted signal. Use of short-inversion-time inversion recovery and contrast-enhanced fat suppression techniques may improve the sensitivity of MR imaging.

Nuclear Imaging

Myeloma is a disease that results in overactivity of osteoclasts, with resultant liberation of bone and suppression of osteoblasts. Nuclear medicine bone scans rely on osteoblastic activity (bone formation) for diagnosis. As such, standard technetium-99m (^{99m}Tc) bone scans have underestimated the extent and severity of disease and should not be used routinely.

Tibial Plasmacytoma

Plasmacytoma is the term used when a solitary lesion is detected in the bone caused by isolated focus of atypical plasma cells. A high level of clinical and radiological suspicion helps in identifying this condition.

Plasmacytomas are rare forms of plasma cell dyscrasias. About 50% of plasmacytomas may transform into multiple myeloma in 2–8 years time. Factors that indicate the high possibility of transformation to multiple myeloma include size more than 5 cm in diameter, osteopenia, angiogenesis on bone marrow sample and lastly an elderly patient. Plasmacytomas are radiosensitive tumors and can be treated by a course of radiation therapy. Steroid therapy is helpful when combined with radiotherapy. Pathological fractures need appropriate orthopedic interventions. The mean survival period of cases detected with bone plasmacytoma is about 10 years.

CT scan helps in showing the extent of bone destruction and to estimate the risk of fracture. Spinal cord compression from pathological fracture can occur

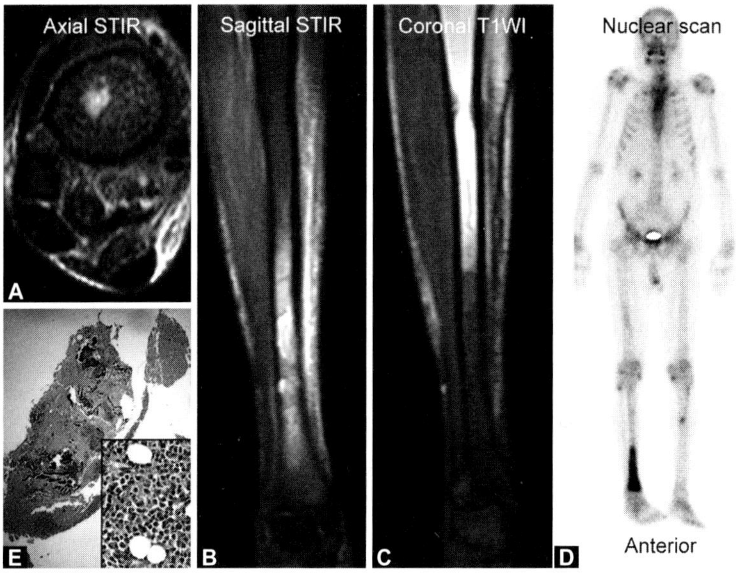

Figs 7.17A to E A 65-year-old male presented with vague pain right leg of 6 months duration on STIR axial (A) and sagittal (B) images of right leg lower third of tibia shows hyperintense signal. Coronal T1W (C) image shows the lesion to be hypointense. Whole body nuclear scan (D) shows avid uptake of tracer in right leg lower third of tibia. High power view of the sheets of plasma cells (E) shows eccentric nucleus with typical cart wheel nuclear chromatin and dense eosinophilic cytoplasm confirming the diagnosis of plasmacytoma *(For color version, see plate 3)*

if the plasmacytoma is located in the vertebra. Error of mistaking a pathological fracture from plasmacytoma as an osteoporotic fracture should be avoided. MRI is a very sensitive imaging tool to diagnose plasmacytoma, and bone marrow involvement is suggested by diffuse hypointense signal on T1W images and hyperintense signal on STIR images **(Figs 7.17A to C)**. Post-contrast enhancement is also seen. Bence-Jones proteinuria and M-band on serum electrophoresis are absent in cases of plasmacytoma. Nuclear scan show increase uptake **(Fig. 7.17D)**. Sheets of atypical plasma cells with eccentric nucleus seen on hematoxylin and eosin stains helps in confirming the diagnosis of plasmacytoma **(Fig. 7.17E)**.

Multiple Myeloma

A tumor derived from cells normally found in bone marrow. Various forms are recognized, the most common of which is plasma cell myeloma. Plasma cell myeloma is a malignant plasma cell dyscrasia characterized by widespread or localized osteolysis resulting from infiltration of the bone marrow by plasma cells. Solitary lesions are termed plasmacytoma. Among the rheumatologic manifestations of plasma cell myeloma are neurologic findings (sciatica, brachial neuralgia, peripheral neuropathy), polyneuropathy, organomegaly, endocrinopathy, M proteins and skin changes (POEMS) syndrome, amyloidosis, gout and infection (lung, urinary tract, osteomyelitis, septic arthritis).

Solitary myeloma (plasmacytoma) can occur as a solitary lesion of bone. This disorder differs in several ways from plasma cell myeloma. In some patients with solitary plasmacytoma, serologic tests are negative or abnormal patterns of serum electrophoresis disappear after excision of the tumor. Solitary plasmacytoma is also rarer than multiple myeloma, affects younger patients, is commonly accompanied by neurologic manifestations, and can simulate giant cell tumor on radiological examination. On radiographs, a multicystic expansile lesion or a purely osteolytic focus without expansion may be observed. Solitary plasmacytoma can also appear as a radiodense vertebral body (ivory vertebral body). In some cases, amyloid may be deposited, and the resulting calcification may resemble a chondrosarcoma on radiographs.

Sclerosing myeloma may be associated with osteosclerosis and POEMS (polyneuropathy, organomegaly, endocrinopathy, monoclonal gammopathy, and skin changes) syndrome.

The classic radiographic appearance of multiple myeloma is that of multiple, small, well-circumscribed, lytic, punched-out, round lesions within the skull, spine, and pelvis. The lesions tend to vary slightly in size. In addition, the bones of myeloma patients are, with few exceptions, diffusely demineralized. Because myeloma is a disease of the medullary compartment of the bone, more subtle lesions can be detected by the appearance of endosteal scalloping that is seen as slight undulation to the inner cortical margin of bone. This finding is suggestive of myelomatous involvement **(Fig. 7.18)**.

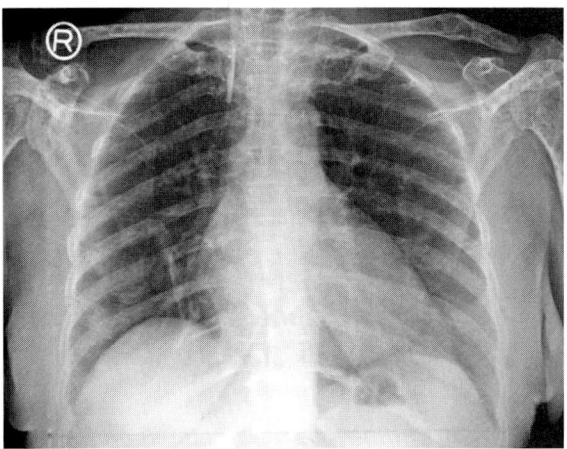

Fig. 7.18 On chest X-ray the ribs show generalized reduction in bone density with wide spread destructive foci. The lesions are more prominent and larger in size in the left clavicle and proximal part of humerus X-ray skull

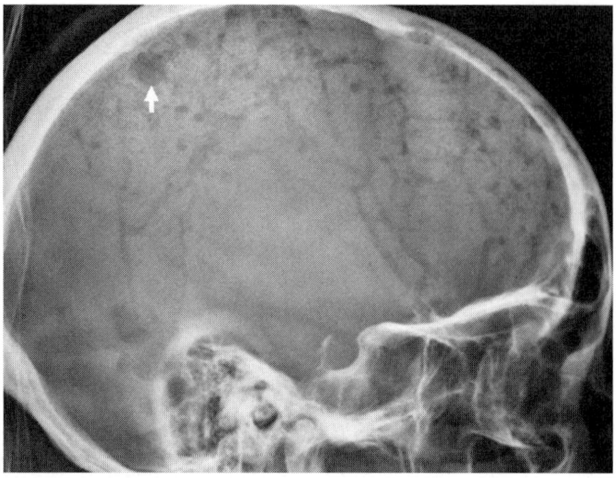

Fig. 7.19 X-ray skull shows multiple widespread osteolytic rounded circular defects of varying diameter from 2–15 mm with no surrounding bone reaction or sclerosis

Computed Tomography

Computed tomography (CT) is a sensitive imaging modality in detecting the osteolytic effects of multiple myeloma and has a higher sensitivity than plain radiography at detecting small lytic lesions. CT findings in multiple myeloma consist of punched-out lytic lesions, expansile lesions with soft tissue masses, diffuse osteopenia, fractures, and, rarely osteosclerosis (**Fig. 7.19**).

Magnetic Resonance Imaging

Whole-body MR (WBMR) has emerged as the most sensitive imaging modality to date at detecting diffuse and focal multiple myeloma in the spine, as well as the extra-axial skeleton. Due to its ability to visualize large volumes of bone marrow without inducing radiation exposure and in an acceptable amount of time. MR imaging has become a favored imaging method for evaluating disease within the bone marrow. MR also has prognostic significance; the number and pattern of lesions detected on MRI correlates very well with treatment outcome and overall survival. It is important to note that MRI predominantely reflects marrow infiltration, which may or may not be associated with bone destruction.

Whole-body MR, CT, and PET/CT can provide valuable complimentary information when used in the correct setting. As the availability of these techniques increase, so too will their use. This is becoming increasingly important as clinicians strive to best assess the appropriateness and effectiveness of new and changing treatment regimes. Newer and more sensitive imaging techniques including CT and MR whole-body imaging and functional imaging modalities including PET/CT and [99] Technetium-2-methoxy-isobutyl-isonitrile open up new avenues in assessing not only morphological disease activity, but also functional disease activity which may be of use in assessing response to treatment as well as tailoring treatment modalities to individual patients.

Pigmented Villonodular Synovitis

Pigmented villonodular synovitis (PVNS) is uncommon disease characterized by hyperplasic synovium, bloody effusion and bone erosions. It usually affects individuals in the age group of 20–45 years. There is no gender predilection. Knee is most common joint affected followed by hip. Etiology of this condition is not fully known, however inflammatory and benign neoplastic etiology is suggested for it.

Radiograph of affected joint is normal in early stage and reveals relatively dense periarticular soft tissue swelling. Joint space is normal until late in course of disease. Bone erosions with sclerotic margin are seen in affected bones in later stages. CT shows small erosions in affected bones in periarticular region.

MRI reveals diffuse nodular synovial thickening which shows high signal intensity on T2W and STIR images. In comparison to muscle, synovium is low to intermediate signal intensity on T1WI (**Figs 7.20A to F**). Hemosiderin appears low signal intensity on T1W and T2W images and is best seen on gradient images (**Figs 7.21A to F**). On postcontrast images lesion enhances peripherally. Hyperplasic synovium tissue may extend in adjacent bursa. Subchondral lesion/erosion is of variable signal intensity depending on fluid/synovium/hemosiderin.

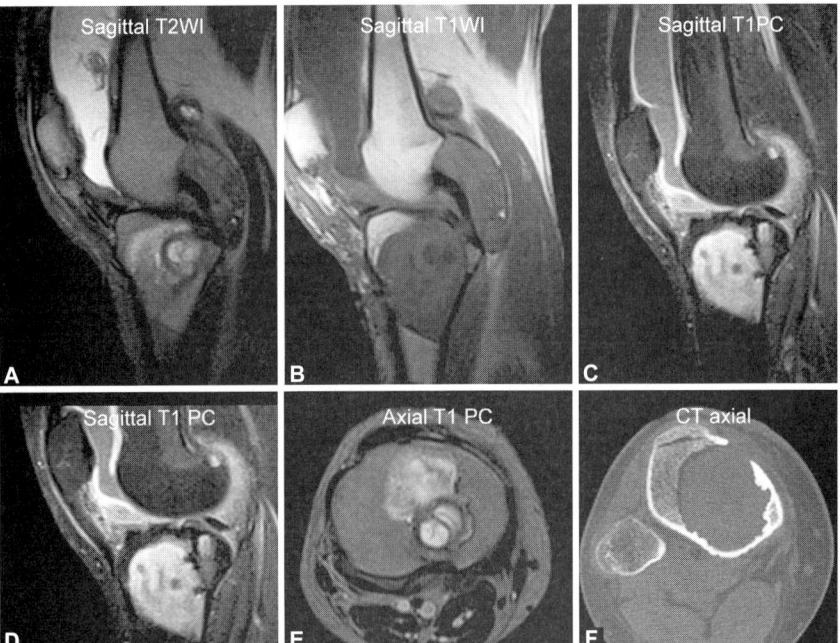

Figs 7.20A to F Sagittal T2WI (A) shows heterogeneous hyperintense soft tissue mass in proximal tibial metaphysis and along posterior aspect of knee joint which is hypointense on T1WI (B) and shows heterogenous post contrast enhancement (C to E) Moderate joint effusion and enhancing synovial thickening also noted (A to C), lytic lesion with cortical erosion is seen in proximal tibia on axial CT image (F)

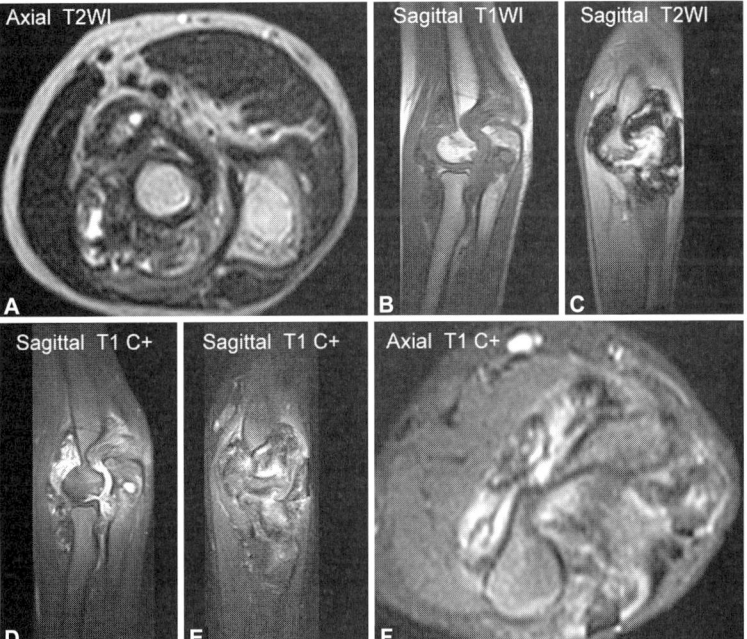

Figs 7.21A to F Significant synovial thickening and soft tissue in right elbow joint showing heterogeneous mixed signal with hypointense areas on T2WI (A and C) and appearing iso to hypointense on T1WI (B) Multiple hypointense areas were also seen on GRE images (not shown in figure) Erosions are seen in distal end of humerus and proximal ends of radius and ulna

IMAGING AND ASSOCIATIONS OF FIBROUS DYSPLASIA

Fibrous Dysplasia (Figs 7.22A to E)

It is a developmental abnormality of unknown cause in which osteoblasts fail to differentiate and mature normally. It may affect a single, a few or many bones. When the polyostotic variety is associated with endocrine dysfunction, typically manifested by precocious female sexual development and cutaneous pigmentation, the disease is known as the Albright's syndrome.

The cutaneous findings consist of café-au-lait spots, caused by increased amounts of melanin in the basal cells of the epidermis. The spots resemble those in neurofibromatosis but usually are fewer, contoured more irregularly and darker in color.

Most patients have monostotic lesions, predominating in one of the ribs or the femur, tibia, gnathic bone, calvaria or humerus; polyostotic fibrous dysplasia more frequently involves the skull and facial bones, pelvis, spine and shoulder girdle. The ilium is involved only infrequently with solitary lesions. When multiple bones are affected, then lesions may be unilateral or bilateral and may affect several bones of a single limb or both limbs, with or without axial skeletal involvement. The polyostotic variety shows significantly more severe and extensive bone involvement, and patients with this form more typically have pain, a limp, a pathologic fracture and deformity.

In skull and facial bones, hypertelorism, displacement of the globe, exophthalmos, diplopia and visual impairment may be seen, and distortion of the sphenoid wing and temporal bone may lead to compromise of the internal auditory nerve. Radiographs show radiolucent or sclerotic lesions, with osseous expansion almost always occurring in an outward direction. The outer table of the cranial vault is convex, and a localized zone of relative radiolucency surrounded by a sclerotic rim may be seen (doughnut lesion).

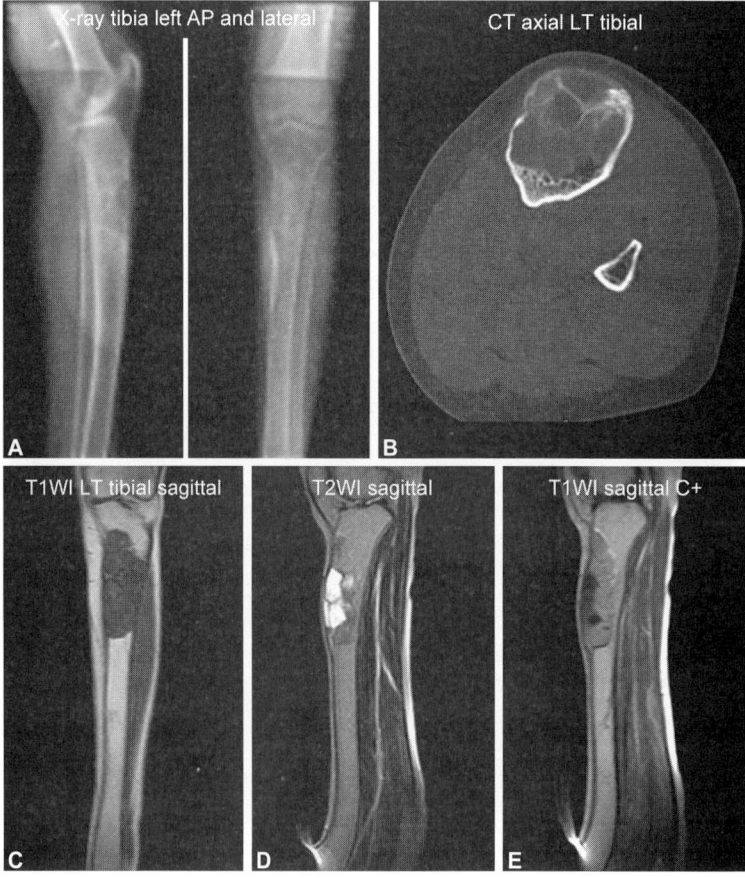

Figs 7.22A to E (A) Plain X-ray left tibia shows expansile lesion in proximal one-third of left tibial diaphysis, partly extending in metaphysis without cortical reaction and thining and break of cortex in anteromedial aspect; (B) CT scan axial plane shows expansile lesion with ground-glass appearance and internal septae; (C to E) In T1 sagittal, T2 sagittal, T1 contrast planes show well-demarcated mildly expansile solid-cystic lesion in proximal one-third of left tibial diaphysis, partly extending in metaphysis on anteromedial aspect. Thinning of adjoining anterior, medial and lateral cortex is noted with cortical breaks at multiple places with minimal adjacent anterior extraosseous soft tissue extension. Posterior cortex is intact. The solid component show T1 hypointense and T2 mildly hyperintense signal intensity with moderate postcontrast enhancement. The hypointense septae also show postcontrast enhancement with no enhancement of cystic spaces. No periosteal reaction noted. No adjoining marrow infiltration or edema seen

In the spine, radiographic features include expansile radiolucent lesions with multiple internal septations in the vertebral body and sometimes the pedicles and vertebral arch. Rarely, paraspinal soft tissue extension and vertebral collapse may lead to angular deformity and spinal cord compression.

Lesions in the long tubular bones are usually intramedullary and diaphyseal, radiolucent and hazy (ground-glass appearance). A zone of reactive sclerosis may also be present. Other occasional findings are endosteal erosion with focal cortical thinning and bone expansion, internally trabeculated configuration, and matrix that may be focally calcified or ossified.

A severe coxa vara deformity may be caused by pronounced curvature of the femoral neck and proximal portion of the femoral shaft (Shepherd's Crook deformity). Fractures are encountered frequently after minor injuries, as are stress fractures.

Other sites of involvement include the ribs, innominate bones, clavicle, scapula, sacrum, and carpal and tarsal bones. When the ribs are involved, unilateral, fusiform expansion of one or more bones is characteristic.

CT scanning and MR imaging are extremely valuable for an accurate assessment of the extent of bone involvement. The signal intensity characteristics of fibrous dysplasia vary. On T1-weighted spin-echo MR images, the lesions are of low signal intensity, whereas on T2-weighted images the lesions may be of low-, intermediate- or high-signal intensity.

Rarely, the skeletal lesions of fibrous dysplasia may undergo malignant transformation, most often to osteosarcoma or fibrosarcoma. Generally, such lesions have been irradiated.

Hypophosphatemic rickets and osteomalacia have also been noted in patients with either monostotic or polyostotic fibrous dysplasia, both with and without the Albright's syndrome.

Polyostotic Fibrous Dysplasia (Figs 7.23A to E)

A developmental abnormality of unknown cause in which osteoblasts fail to differentiate and mature normally. It may affect a single, a few or many bones. When the polyostotic variety (and rarely the monostotic type) is associated with endocrine dysfunction, typically manifested by precocious female sexual development and cutaneous pigmentation, the disease is known as the Albright's syndrome.

The cutaneous findings consist of café-au-lait spots, caused by increased amounts of melanin in the basal cells of the epidermis. The spots resemble those in neurofibromatosis but usually are fewer, contoured more irregularly and darker in color.

Developmental abnormality of bones, of unknown cause, in which there is failure of normal ossification and deposition of fibrous tissues. Three varieties are described monostotic, polyostotic and McCune Albright syndrome, i.e. polyostotic fibrous dysplasia with sexual precocity and skin pigmentation.

Radiologically, the appearances of the areas of fibrous dysplasia vary. Typically, there is an area of rarefaction with ground glass density, and sometimes patchy sclerosis as it resolves. They tend to occur in the diaphyses of the bone. There may be expansion of the bone, thinning of the cortex and endosteal scalloping, with a short transition zone to normal bone. In the skull vault it typically affects the sphenoidal and petrous bones, which are thickened and sclerotic and expands to obliterate the normal cavities. In the skull vault the areas may be lucent. In the pelvis, typically fibrous dysplasia lesions are lytic, and particularly occur in the iliac bones. Coxa vara commonly occurs with femoral neck involvement. Areas of fibrous dysplasia show avid activity on radionuclide scans.

Polyostotic fibrous dysplasia, in which the patient often has café-au-lait spots, typically affects multiple bones. It may be unilateral, bilateral, affect both sets of limbs or the axial skeleton. Complications of deafness and blindness occur if there is skull vault involvement secondary to pressure on the cranial nerves. Fractures through the areas of fibrous dysplasia occur and heal poorly. A further complication is insufficiency or stress fracture.

CT scanning and MR imaging are extremely valuable for an accurate assessment of the extent of bone involvement. The signal intensity characteristics of fibrous dysplasia vary. On T1-weighted spin-echo MR images, the lesions are of low signal intensity, whereas on T2-weighted images the lesions may be of low, intermediate or high signal intensity.

On scintigraphy, lesions of fibrous dysplasia show increased uptake. MRI appearances are variable but tend to have low density on T1- and T2-weighted sequences but may be of higher signal intensity on T2.

Rarely, endocrine manifestations have been described which include rickets and osteomalacia. These may occur in patients with or without McCune-Albright syndrome (*See* fibrous dysplasia).

Most patients have monostotic lesions, predominating in one of the ribs or the femur, tibia, gnathic bone, calvaria or humerus; polyostotic fibrous dysplasia more frequently involves the skull and facial bones, pelvis, spine and shoulder girdle. The ilium is involved only infrequently with solitary lesions. When multiple bones are affected, the lesions may be unilateral or bilateral and may affect several bones of a single limb or both limbs, with or without axial skeletal involvement. The polyostotic variety shows significantly more severe and extensive bone involvement, and patients with this form more typically have pain, a limp, a pathologic fracture and deformity.

In skull and facial bones, hypertelorism, displacement of the globe, exophthalmos, diplopia and visual impairment may be seen, and distortion of

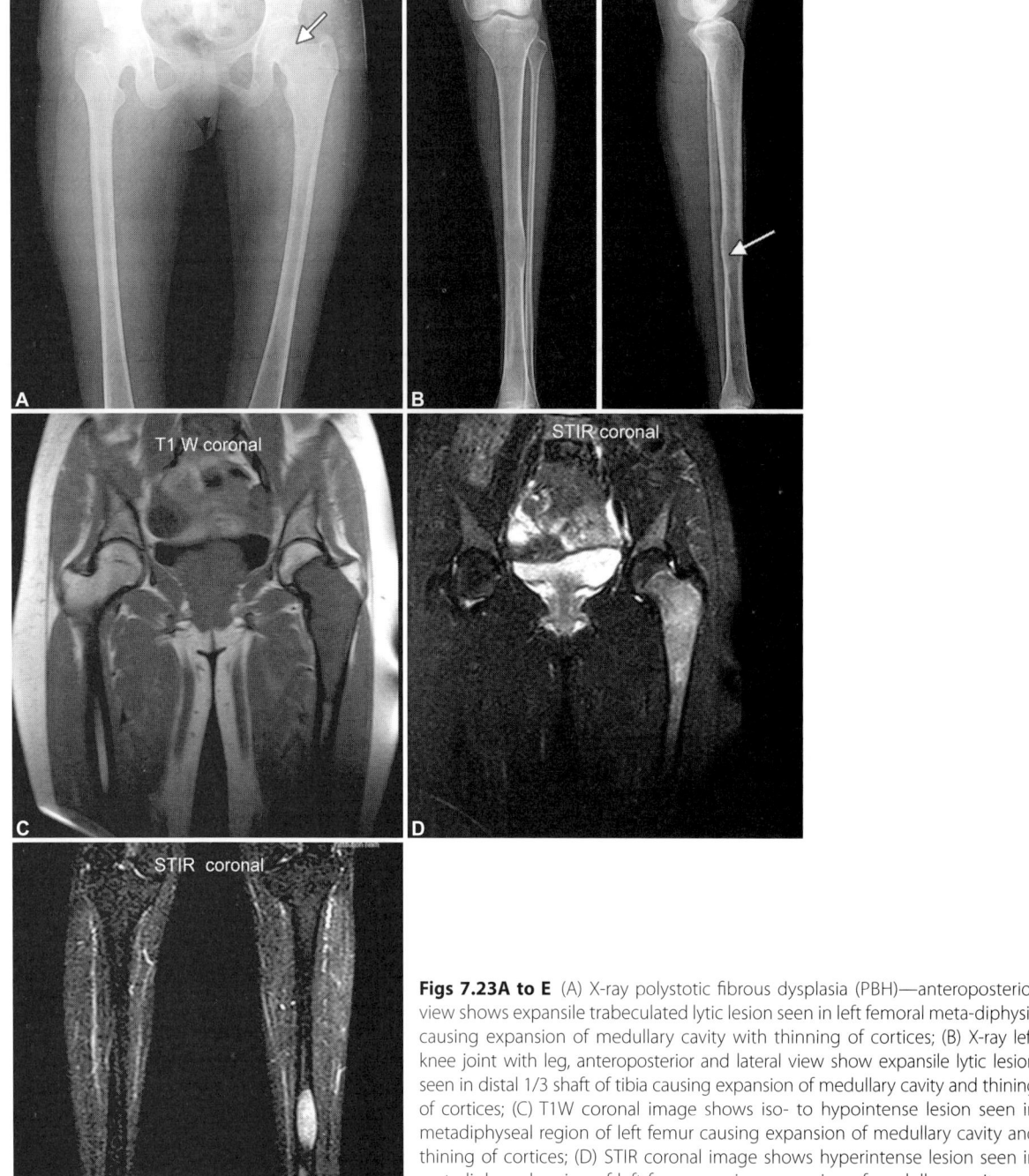

Figs 7.23A to E (A) X-ray polystotic fibrous dysplasia (PBH)—anteroposterior view shows expansile trabeculated lytic lesion seen in left femoral meta-diphysis causing expansion of medullary cavity with thinning of cortices; (B) X-ray left knee joint with leg, anteroposterior and lateral view show expansile lytic lesion seen in distal 1/3 shaft of tibia causing expansion of medullary cavity and thining of cortices; (C) T1W coronal image shows iso- to hypointense lesion seen in metadiphyseal region of left femur causing expansion of medullary cavity and thining of cortices; (D) STIR coronal image shows hyperintense lesion seen in metadiphyseal region of left femur causing expansion of medullary cavity and thining of cortices; (E) STIR coronal image shows hyperintense lesion seen in distal 1/3 of left tibia causing expansion of medullary cavity and thinning of cortices

the sphenoid wing and temporal bone may lead to compromise of the internal auditory nerve. Radiographs show radiolucent or sclerotic lesions, with osseous expansion almost always occurring in an outward direction. The outer table of the cranial vault is convex, and a localized zone of relative radiolucency surrounded by a sclerotic rim may be seen (doughnut lesion).

In the spine, radiographic features include expansile radiolucent lesions with multiple internal septations in the vertebral body and sometimes the pedicles and vertebral arch. Rarely paraspinal soft tissue extension and vertebral collapse may lead to angular deformity and spinal cord compression.

Lesions in the long tubular bones are usually intramedullary and diaphyseal, radiolucent and hazy (ground-glass appearance). A zone of reactive sclerosis may also be present. Other occasional findings are endosteal erosion with focal cortical thinning and bone expansion, internally trabeculated configuration, and matrix that may be focally calcified or ossified.

A severe coxa vara deformity may be caused by pronounced curvature of the femoral neck and proximal portion of the femoral shaft (Shepherd's-crook deformity). Fractures are encountered frequently after minor injuries, as are stress (insufficiency) fractures.

Other sites of involvement include the ribs, innominate bones, clavicle, scapula, sacrum, and carpal and tarsal bones. When the ribs are involved, unilateral, fusiform expansion of one or more bones is characteristic.

Rarely, the skeletal lesions of fibrous dysplasia may undergo malignant transformation, most often to osteosarcoma or fibrosarcoma. Generally, such lesions have been irradiated.

Hypophosphatemic rickets and osteomalacia have also been noted in patients with either monostotic or polyostotic fibrous dysplasia, both with and without the McCune-Albright syndrome.

Ameloblastoma

An ameloblastoma or adamantinoma of the jaw is a benign locally agressive tumor arising from the mandible, or from the maxilla. Ameloblastomas are the second most common odontogenic tumor after odontoma. They are slow growing and tend to present in the 3rd to 5th decades of life, with no gender predilection.

Ameloblastomas typically occur as hard painless lesions near the angle of the mandible in the region of the 3rd molar tooth although they can occur anywhere along the alveolus of the mandible and maxilla. When the maxilla is involved, the tumor is located in the premolar region, and can extend up in the maxillary sinus.

Although benign, it is a locally aggressive neoplasm with a high rate of recurrence. Approximately, 20% of cases are associated with dentigerous cysts and unerupted teeth.

Ameloblastomas arise from ameloblasts (part of the odontogenic epithelium, responsible for enamel production and eventually crown formation. Three variants are described:
1. Simple
2. Luminal
3. Mural

It is classically seen as a multilocualted, expansile "soap-bubble" lesion on X-rays, with well-demarcated borders and no matrix calcification. Occasionally erosion of the adjacent tooth roots can be seen which is highly specific. When larger it may also erode through cortex into adjacent soft tissues. On MRI ameloblastomas demonstrate a mixed solid and cystic pattern, with a thick irregular wall, often with papillary solid structures projecting into the lesion. These components tend to vividly enhance.

Ameoloblastomas tend to be treated by surgical en-bloc resection. Local curettage is associated with a high rate of local recurrence. Differential diagnosis include:
a. Dentigerous cyst
b. Odontogenic keratocyst

Solitary Bone Cyst of the Mandible

A solitary bone cyst of the mandible (aka traumatic bone cyst of jaw, hemorrhagic cyst of the mandible, extravasation cyst, progressive bone cavity and unicameral bone cyst) is an uncommon nonepithelial lined lucent mandibular lesion. Trauma has been suggested as the etiology along with other non-substantiated theories such as cystic degeneration of a preexisting tumor or of the fatty marrow in the area.

The lesion is mainly diagnosed in young patients most frequently during the second decade of life. Some reports suggest that it is more common in males while others report equal distribution between males and females. Majority of them are located in the mandibular body between the canine and the third molar. The second most common site is the mandibular symphysis. Fewer cases are reported in the ramus, condyle and the anterior maxilla. Traumatic bone cavity is not unique to the jawbones; it is also described in the long bones and is known as a simple solitary bone cyst occurring mostly in the humerus or femur, close to the epiphyseal plate. The long bone counterpart is more common in males by a ratio of 2.5:1.

The lesion is asymptomatic in the majority of cases and is often accidentally discovered on routine radiological examination usually as an unilocular radiolucent area with a "scalloping effect".

They are usually unilocular and radiolucent, typically above the alveolar canal and in many cases with a scalloped superior border spreading between the roots of vital teeth. Large, expansile and multilocular traumatic bone cavities have been described, but are rare. Expansion is not characteristic of TBC but it is described in about 26% of the cases. They are otherwise asymptomatic. The margins of these lesions range from very well-defined to corticated to punched out radiolucency. Pathologic fractures associated with traumatic bone cavity have been described in the jaws, but are rare. They are however more common with those of the long bones. The definite diagnosis of traumatic cyst is invariably achieved at surgery. Since material for histological examination may be scant or non-existent, it is very often difficult for a definite histological diagnosis to be achieved.

Loose Bodies in Shoulder Joint

CT scan of left shoulder shows two loose bodies in the joint. These on becoming symptomatic can cause painful joint movement and delimit range of movement **(Fig. 7.24)**.

Osteochondritis Dissecans

Osteochondritis Dissecans of Tibial Plafond

- Coronal CT scan shows osteochondral lesion with loose body at lateral aspect of tibial plafond (distal articular surface of tibia) **(Fig. 7.25A)**.
- Sagittal reconstructed image shows osteolysis at lateral aspect of tibial plafond in a case of osteochondritis dissecans **(Figs 7.25B and C)**.

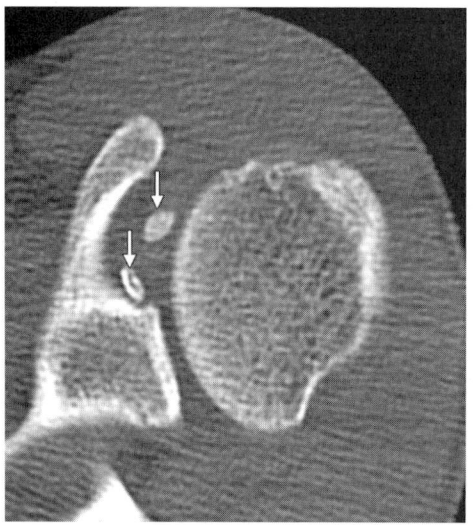

Fig. 7.24 Loose bodies in shoulder joint

- Axial image shows osteolysis at lateral aspect of tibial plafond **(Fig. 7.25C)**.

On conventional radiographs, osteochondritis dissecans of the tibial plafond appears lucent and may contain a loose bony fragment. CT and MR imaging are able to show the exact location and extent of the lesion.

Odontogenic Fibromyxoma of the Maxilla

Odontogenic fibromyxoma are slow growing benign tumors of the maxilla, occurring between 20 to 40 years of age, rarely in children and over 50 years of age. They are myxoma with abundant collagen fibers. Their size varies and may reach 4 cm **(Figs 7.26A to D)**. They do not metastasize via the lymphatics. Present with swelling of the affected region and the displacement of dentition, and pain is seen less often. Its origin is likely from the dental follicle. Total enucleation prevents recurrence.

MALIGNANT TUMORS

Osteosarcoma

Osteosarcoma is a malignant neoplasm of bone composed of proliferating tumor cells that in most instances produce osteoid or immature bone. Osteosarcomas can be classified according to location of the tumor within the bone (intramedullary, intracortical, surface, periosteal, or parosteal); degree of cellular differentiation (high or low grade); histologic composition, number of foci of involvement (single or multicentric); and status of the underlying bone.

Osteosarcomas generally involve the long tubular bones about the knee. A metaphyseal location predominates. The bone involvement shows a mixed

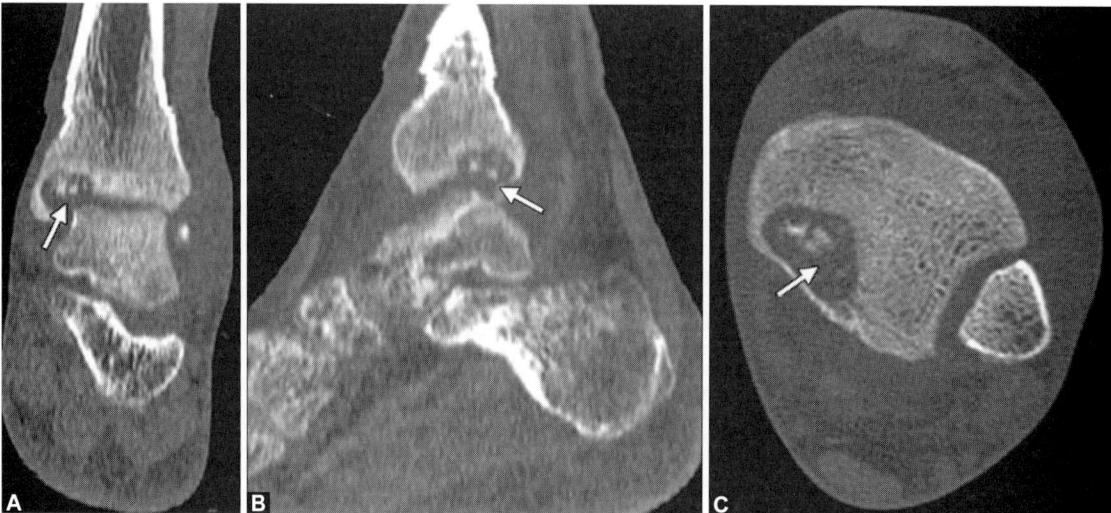

Figs 7.25A to C (A) Coronal CT scan shows osteochondral lesion with loose body at medial aspect of tibial plafond (distal articular surface of tibia). (B) Sagittal reconstructed image shows osteolysis at medial aspect of tibial plafond in a case of osteochondritis dissecans. (C) Axial image shows osteolysis at medial aspect of tibial plafond

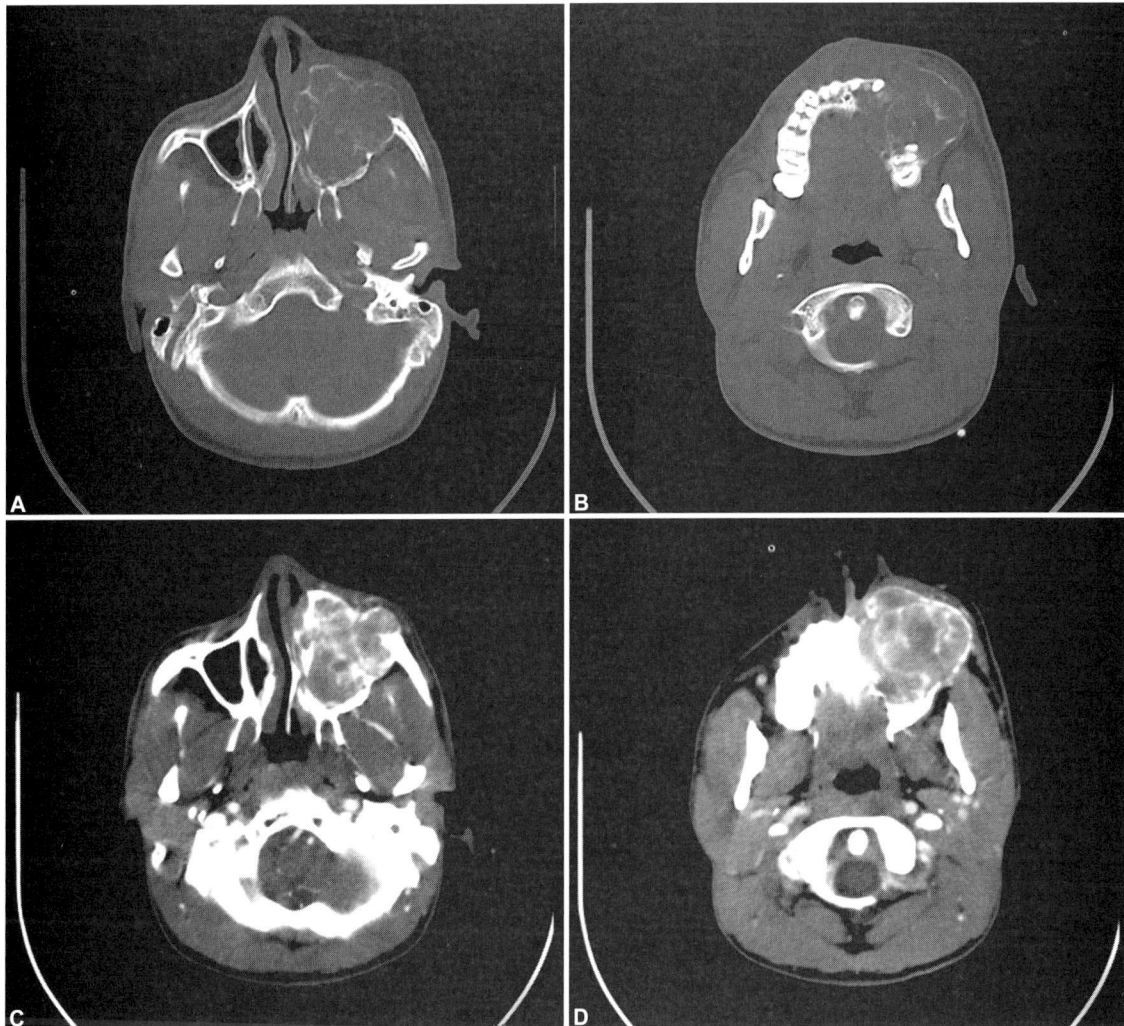

Figs 7.26A to D (A) A well-defined, expansile soft tissue density lesion noted arising from the maxillary sinus and maxillary bone. There are multiple thin radiodense septae within the lesion. There is erosion and thinning of the cortex; (B) A well-defined, expansile soft tissue density lesion noted arising from the maxillary sinus and maxillary bone. There are multiple thin radiodense septae within the lesion. It is partially eroding and destructing the left alveolar process of maxilla; (C) A well-defined, expansile, moderately enhancing soft tissue density lesion noted arising from the maxillary sinus and maxillary bone. There are multiple thin radiodense septae within the lesion. There is erosion and thinning of the cortex; (D) A well-defined, expansile, moderately enhancing soft tissue density lesion noted arising from the maxillary sinus and maxillary bone. There are multiple thin radiodense septae within the lesion. It is partially eroding and destructing the left alveolar process of maxilla

pattern consisting of both osteolysis and osteosclerosis. Osteosarcomas in the tubular bones are usually evident as poorly defined intramedullary metaphyseal lesions that extend through the cortex and produce a sizeable soft tissue component. A periosteal reaction (Codman's triangle or sunburst pattern) and sometimes a pathologic fracture are additional features. In other skeletal sites, the radiographic features of osteosarcoma are similar.

MR imaging is superior to CT scanning in defining the intraosseous and extraosseous extent of the tumor. On T1-weighted spin-echo images the tumor is typically of low signal intensity, whereas on T2-weighted images, it is usually of high-signal intensity **(Figs 7.27A to C)**.

Radiological Features of Osteosarcoma

Osteosarcoma is the most common primary malignant tumor of bone. It is an aggressive malignant neoplasm arising from primitive transformed cells of mesenchymal origin that exhibit osteoblastic differentiation and produce malignant osteoid. It is the most common histological form of primary bone cancer. It is the 2nd most common primary malignant bone tumor. Peak incidence in males occurs in 10–20 years of age with 3 cases/million population/year. Metaphysis of long bone is affected and 60% of cases are about the knee.

Predisposing conditions: It is associated with old age, Paget's disease, radiation exposure, bone infarcts, or

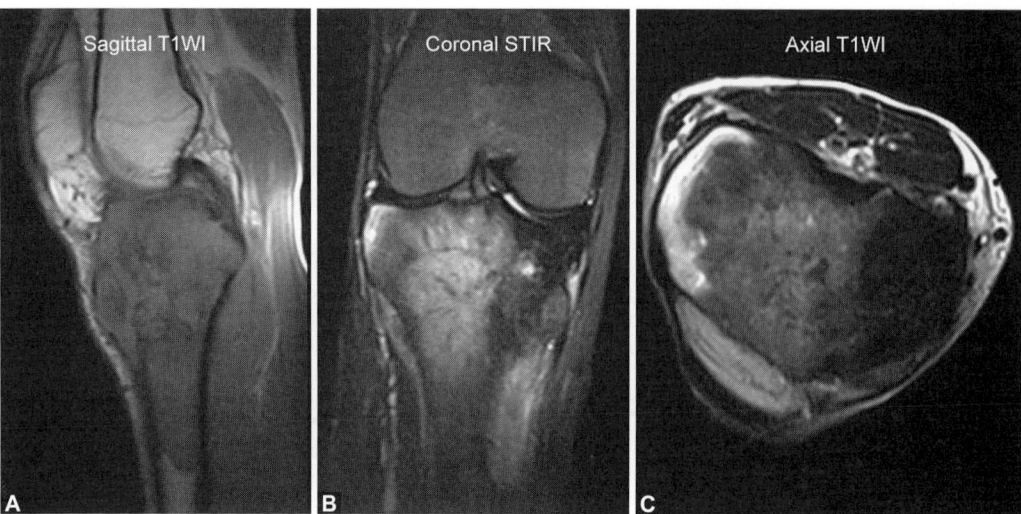

Figs 7.27A to C Sagittal T1W (A) shows heterogenous signal intensity lesion appearing predominantly hypointense in proximal tibial epimetaphysis and hyperintense on STIR coronal images (B). Axial T1W image (C) shows heterogeneous signal intensity lesion appearing predominantly hypointense

chondrosarcomas. Potential etiologies include viral, mutations (RB), p53, ionizing radiation.

Varieties of Osteosarcoma

- *Classic osteosarcoma (conventional) (75%)* affects long tubular bones, particularly, the metaphysis, with mixed osteolysis and osteosclerosis and marked periosteal reaction.
- *Telangiectatic osteosarcoma (2.5–12.5%):* Lytic tumors consisting of large cystic cavities filled with blood.
- *Small cell osteosarcoma (1–4%):* Similar to classic osteosarcoma, primarily osteolytic with a poor prognosis
- Multifocal osteosarcoma
- *Extraskeletal (Extraosseous osteosarcoma):* When osteosarcoma occurs at multiple sites. It occurs as a large soft-tissue tumor that is not necessarily close to bone.

  X-rays and CT show a large soft tissue mass dominated by an osteoid matrix which appears dense centrally. The non-mineralized portions of these tumors have a similar appearance to muscle, and are hypointense on T1WI and hyperintense on T2WI.
- *Gnathic:* On X-rays, these tumors are sclerotic with areas of lytic bone destruction and periosteal reaction with long thin spicules of bone extending into a soft tissue mass. MRI shows both intramedullary involvement and soft tissue mass. Lesions have low-to-intermediate signal intensity on T1WI and high signal intensity with T2WI.
- *Surface:* These lesions include parosteal, periosteal, high-grade surface, intracortical, and a recently described osteochondroma-like parosteal osteosarcoma: (1) *Parosteal osteosarcoma* slowly enlarges and invades surrounding soft tissues, resulting in irregular, indistinct borders, and can be seen both on plain films as well as on cross-sectional imaging; (2) *Periosteal osteosarcoma* arises from the inner layer of the periosteum. X-rays show an elongated incompletely mineralized lesion with cortical thickening, erosion and peripheral periosteal reaction. CT shows the aggressive tumor with chondroid areas, spiculated periosteal bone, and possible soft tissue mass; (3) *High-grade surface osteosarcoma* has a similar clinical and radiographic appearance to periosteal osteosarcoma; (4) *Intracortical osteosarcoma* arises in the cortex, usually in the femur or tibia, and has a predilection for the diaphysis; (5) *Osteochondroma-like parosteal osteosarcoma* shows a dense exophytic juxtacortical lesion adjacent to the surface of a long bone on X-rays. No aggressive periosteal reaction or unossified soft tissue masses are present. MRI will show the central portion of the lesion to follow a fat signal, suggestive of mature bone as well as a thin cartilaginous cap, which should be less than 5 mm in thickness.
- *Secondary osteosarcoma* is associated commonly with Paget's disease and radiotherapy. A hyaline cartilaginous cap that involutes after growth can undergo malignant degeneration, resulting in lesions such as osteosarcoma. The cartilage cap thickness is related to malignant degeneration. X-rays show bone destruction, osteoid matrix and MRI is used for measurement of hyaline cartilage cap thickness
  - *Conventional osteosarcoma (OS) (central osteosarcoma):* The tumor is seen in second and third decades. In patients over the age of

40 years, osteosarcoma is usually secondary to a pre-existing disorder of bone, such as Paget's disease. Similarly, osteosarcoma of the jaws occurs in an older age group than that of the appendicular skeleton and carries a better prognosis. Male : female ratio is 2:1. The typical lesion affects the metaphyseal region of the growing end of a long bone and about 75% are found in the distal femur or the proximal tibia. Other sites commonly affected include the proximal humerus and femur. Involvement of the pelvis and scapula is less common, while it is indeed rare for the spine, hands or feet to be affected.

Malignant tumor manufacturing tumor bone is an osteosarcoma. Unfortunately, even if tumor bone is present, it cannot always be differentiated radiologically from reactive woven bone. In many cases, the radiological appearance is typical and reflects the underlying pathological process. Osteosarcoma usually arises in the metaphysis of a long bone. The early medullary changes are minimal, although a non-specific laminar periosteal reaction may be evident. The medullary lesion shows a permeating pattern with a wide zone of transition between normal and affected bone. Mineralization of the tumor osteoid leads to a characteristic medullary density. As the tumor reaches the cortex, it traverses it and finally destroys it. Extraosseous extension occurs early. The soft-tissue mass enlarges and, like the intraosseous element, is first uncalcified but later shows ill-defined cloud-like bone within it. The density in the extracortical tissue is increased by periosteal reaction. This is usually irregular, perpendicular to the cortex or producing a characteristic but not specific sunburst spiculations following the line of extended Sharpey's fibers.

In Ewing's sarcoma, if such spicules form, they are fewer and more delicate. Reactive (Codman's) triangles may form at the margin of the lesion, due to subperiosteal extension of tumor. They signify rapid soft-tissue extension outside the cortex, whether due to tumor, blood, and pus.

Imaging findings: On X-rays, most lesions show a mixture of lytic and sclerotic areas. Lesions show moth-eaten, with ill-defined edges, or permeative lesion. Soft tissue extension of osteosarcoma is seen as a soft tissue mass. Cloud like areas of sclerosis, resulting from malignant osteoid production and calcification are seen within the mass. Periosteal reaction is commonly seen with spectrum of changes like Codman's triangles, multilaminated, spiculated, and sunburst spiculation. CT helps to diagnose when the radiographic appearances are confusing. Superior identification of matrix mineralization is achieved by CT which, in addition, may clearly define both the extent of soft-tissue mass and its relationship to adjoining structures. In MRI, the intraosseous and extraosseous extent of the tumor is assessed. MR shows the intraosseous disease and the longitudinal distance of bone involvement, the involvement of adjacent epiphyses, and the presence or absence of skip metastases. Epiphyseal involvement is seen as abnormal signal intensity similar to that of the metaphyseal tumor within the epiphysis in association with focal destruction of the growth plate. Skip metastases are tumor foci that are anatomically separate from the primary lesion and occur within the same bone. The relationship of extraosseous tumor to neurovascular structures is well shown on STIR and fat-suppressed T2WI. The neurovascular bundle can be seen as free from tumor, abutting tumor or unequivocally involved. Joint involvement can also be seen. MRI may contribute little to the histological diagnosis; but important for staging by defining the extent of the tumor. Both medullary and soft-tissue extension is demonstrated accurately. Skip metastases, although rare, can be identified, and it is essential to image the whole bone. Osteosarcoma shows increased uptake of radioisotope on bone scans obtained by use of technetium-99m and methylene diphosphonate

- *Telangiectatic osteosarcoma:* It accounts for less than 5.0% of all osteosarcoma cases and most commonly occurs in the 1st and 2nd decades of life. The tumor occurs most often in metaphyses of long bones, with the femur being the most common site. In these tumors, hemorrhagic, cystic, or necrotic spaces occupy more than 90% of the tumor, with only a small fraction of solid tissue. Therefore, at low power, telangiectatic osteosarcoma mimics aneurysmal bone cyst. With minimal bone matrix, it gives a characteristic radiolucent appearance of the tumor. At high magnification, the presence of cells with significant nuclear pleomorphism and a high mitotic rate as well as the presence of osteoid matrix, enable one to make a specific histologic diagnosis. X-ray appearance of telangiectatic osteosarcoma include aggressive growth pattern with cortical destruction and minimal peripheral sclerosis with asymmetric expansion, geographic lysis of bone. Pathologic fracture is common. CT features of telangiectatic osteosarcoma include a soft-tissue mass with attenuation lower than that of muscle, osteoid matrix mineralization, fluid levels, and thick peripheral and nodular septal enhancement. The enhancing thick rim and septa correspond to viable high-grade sarcomatous tissue in hemorrhagic or necrotic spaces; osteoid matrix mineralization occurs only in the viable neoplastic tissue in these areas. Osteoid matrix mineralization is often subtle on radiographs and of limited extent because viable tumor cells make up only a small component of the lesion compared with the volume of cystic spaces. This osteoid is easily detected at CT than at radiography. On MR, hemorrhage shows high signal intensity on T1-weighted images and variable signal intensity on T2-weighted images. Fluid levels are frequently identified. Differential diagnoses include ABC, and giant cell tumor, metastases. Distinguishing ABC from telangiectatic OS can be challenging because of histologic and radiologic similarities. Similar to telangiectatic OS, ABC can be hypervascular and demonstrates progressive osteolytic bone expansion and hemorrhage with fluid levels at CT or MR imaging. However, ABC typically shows only an enhancing thin peripheral rim and septa without nodularity or osteoid matrix mineralization. Furthermore, the pattern of growth in ABC is frequently less aggressive, and is well-defined

- *Small cell osteosarcoma:* Small cell osteosarcoma constitutes approximately 1% of all OS cases and affects patients in the 2nd and 3rd decades of life. These lesions are commonly located in the metaphyseal region of long bones and most frequently involve the femur, rarely the lesion purely diaphyseal. Production of osteoid matrix by tumor cells confirms points towards the diagnosis of osteosarcoma. Exclusion of the *EWS-ETS* chromosome 22 rearrangements associated with the Ewing sarcoma family of tumors is crucial, because small cell osteosarcoma and Ewing sarcoma can appear very similar to each other at histologic analysis. The radiographic features of small cell osteosarcoma include permeative lytic bone destruction in all cases, a soft-tissue mass, and periosteal reaction. In small cell osteosarcoma, calcification in the intramedullary cavity or an associated extraosseous soft-tissue mass at radiography or CT is frequent helpful diagnostic clue that the lesion is an osteoid matrix producing small cell OS. Diagnostic considerations include Ewing's sarcoma, lymphoma, and conventional osteosarcoma. In particular, Ewing's sarcoma is difficult to differentiate from small cell osteosarcoma because of its histologic and radiologic resemblance to the latter. Calcifications rarely occur in Ewing's sarcoma and are therefore useful for distinguishing between small cell osteosarcoma and Ewing's sarcoma. Other features that allow differentiation of Ewing's sarcoma from small cell osteosarcoma include cortical thickening and cortical saucerization. Cortical saucerization is caused by local periosteal destruction by tumor and surrounding periosteal reaction, whereas pressure erosion is bone remodeling by a mass outside the bone. Lymphoma of bone is a permeative lytic lesion commonly associated with extraosseous masses; like Ewing's sarcoma, lymphoma is able to spread outside of bone without osseous destruction. However, calcifications are uncommon in lymphoma, although sequestrum is occasionally found at pretherapy cross-sectional imaging. In general, histopathologic appearances and immunohistochemical findings readily allow distinction between small cell osteosarcoma and its differential diagnostic entities.

- *Surface osteosarcoma/juxtacortical osteosarcoma:* It is primarily associated with the periosteum, with variable medullary canal involvement. The term juxtacortical osteosarcoma was initially used to describe parosteal osteosarcoma. Juxtacortical osteosarcoma is now classified into three main subtypes; parosteal, periosteal, and high-grade surface.

    - *Parosteal osteosarcoma:* It is the most common type of juxtacortical osteosarcoma, accounting for approximately 5% of all cases and typically manifesting in the 2nd to 4th decades of life. The tumor usually occurs in the metaphyses of long bones and the posterior aspect of the distal femur is the most frequent site. The prognosis for parosteal osteosarcoma is better than that for conventional osteosarcoma. Anatomically, parosteal osteosarcoma originates from the outer fibrous layer of the periosteum. At radiography, the classic appearance is a lobulated and exophytic mass with central dense ossification adjacent to the bone. A cleavage plane separating the tumor and adjacent normal cortex (also known as the string sign) cortical thickening with a relative lack of aggressive periosteal reaction is often apparent, due to focal expansion of the inner portion of the tumor and fusion with the cortex. At magnetic resonance (MR) imaging, the ossified tumor is predominantly low in signal intensity on both T1- and T2-weighted images, similar to the appearance of the cortex. Differential diagnostic considerations for parosteal osteosarcoma include benign entities such as osteochondroma, myositis ossificans, and periosteal chondroma and malignant entities such as fibrous malignancy, periosteal chondrosarcoma, and other subtypes of juxtacortical osteosarcoma.

- *Periosteal osteosarcoma:* Periosteal osteosarcoma is the second most common type of juxtacortical osteosarcoma. It typically affects patients in the 2nd or 3rd decade of life, with a characteristic location along the diaphyses of long bones, most commonly the tibia. The prognosis for periosteal osteosarcoma is better than that for conventional osteosarcoma but worse than that for parosteal osteosarcoma. Periosteal osteosarcoma arises from the inner, germinative layer of periosteum. Common radiographic findings include a soft-tissue mass with periosteal reaction, cortical erosion, and cortical thickening with rare intramedullary extension. Periosteal reaction often extends perpendicularly from the inner cortex to the outer margin of the tumor. The predominantly chondroid matrix of this tumor results in a lesion that is low in attenuation on CT images and hyperintense on T2-weighted MR images, with smaller foci of low signal intensity on MR images representing calcified matrix or hair-on-end periosteal reaction. Considerations in the radiologic diagnosis of periosteal osteosarcoma include other types of juxtacortical osteosarcoma and periosteal chondroid tumors. Parosteal osteosarcoma is a densely ossified juxtacortical mass that lies outside the cortex and occurs in metaphyses, whereas periosteal osteosarcoma is usually more lytic in appearance, causing cortical erosion and periosteal reaction, and occurs in diaphyses. Differentiation of high-grade surface osteosarcoma from periosteal osteosarcoma may be difficult at imaging, as both can occur in diaphyses and cause periosteal reaction and bone destruction. However, high-grade surface osteosarcoma often involves the entire circumference of the cortex and is more likely to show medullary invasion. Furthermore, the presence of a high histologic grade, identical to that of conventional osteosarcoma, throughout the entire tumor is diagnostic of high-grade surface osteosarcoma. Periosteal chondroid tumors are juxtacortical soft-tissue masses with well-defined borders, typically metaphyseal in location, and contain curvilinear calcifications along the periphery of the cartilage lobules; in contrast, periosteal osteosarcoma is a broad-based soft-tissue mass, commonly diaphyseal in location, and produces a cortical erosion and periosteal reaction perpendicular to the cortex
- *High-grade surface osteosarcoma:* High-grade surface osteosarcoma is rare, accounting for 0.4% of all osteosarcoma cases, and is the least common type of juxtacortical osteosarcoma. The tumor affects patients in the 2nd and 3rd decades of life. Common locations include the diaphyses and metaphyses of long bones, with the femur being the most common site. The prognosis for high-grade surface osteosarcoma was initially considered worse than that for other types of juxtacortical osteosarcoma and similar to that for conventional osteosarcoma; however, more recent studies have shown an improved prognosis that is better than that for conventional osteosarcoma, probably due to aggressive chemotherapy and surgical resection. At pathologic analysis, high-grade surface osteosarcoma arises from the surface of bone; however, unlike the other forms of juxtacortical osteosarcoma, it is entirely high grade, with a high-mitotic activity identical to that of conventional osteosarcoma. At radiography, dense ossification and periosteal reaction are seen in the majority of cases; cortical erosion and thickening are also seen frequently. The rate of intramedullary invasion is variable among small studies, occurring in anywhere from 8–48% of cases, but its presence has not been found to decrease the survival rate. Imaging mimics of high-grade surface osteosarcoma include parosteal osteosarcoma, periosteal osteosarcoma, and conventional osteosarcoma. High-grade surface osteosarcoma may resemble either parosteal osteosarcoma with ill-defined and fluffy bone formation or periosteal osteosarcoma when it is diaphyseal and associated with cortical destruction and periosteal reaction, depending on degrees of osteoblastic and chondroblastic differentiation. Circumferential bone involvement can be more extensive in high-grade surface osteosarcoma than in other forms of juxtacortical osteosarcoma. When medullary invasion is a prominent feature, it may be difficult to distinguish this tumor from conventional osteosarcoma with a large extraosseous component. However, to make the diagnosis of high-grade surface osteosarcoma, the bulk of the lesion must be external to the bone at radiography.
- *Secondary osteosarcoma:* Malignant tumors are said to arise in bone affected by Paget's disease in about 1% of cases. It is difficult to

gauge the exact incidence, because many cases of Paget's disease are asymptomatic or diagnosed by chance. Clinically, the possibility of a sarcoma arising in Paget's disease should be considered when alteration occurs in the character of bone pain, either an increase in severity or more precise localization, and if a pathological fracture develops. The presence of a soft-tissue mass and further rise in the serum alkaline phosphatase may be observed. The skull, pelvis and long bones are typical sites. Men are more commonly affected, even allowing for the increased male incidence of Paget's disease. Histologically, tumors may be classified as osteosarcoma, fibrosarcoma and chondrosarcoma. However, the tumor is very aggressive and the outcome is poor. On imaging in order of frequency, the lesion is lytic, mixed or sclerotic. The tumor grows rapidly with an extensive soft-tissue component. The margins of the lesion within bone are ill defined, with extensive cortical destruction. Periosteal new bone formation is uncommon.

Radiation, induced sarcomas are a group of osteogenic sarcomas that occur secondary to radiation exposure. They arise in the body when the radiation dose exceeds 30 Gy and after 7-10 latent years. The diagnosis is not difficult radiologically because highly aggressive and lytic nature. They arise in sites subjected to radiations as in pelvis after treatment of cervical cancer.

- *Primary multifocal osteosarcoma:* The demonstration of more than one osteosarcoma of bone in a patient at presentation is rare. Histologically, each lesion is a typical osteosarcoma and generally similar in size. Recently, the concept has been favored that synchronous multifocal osteosarcoma is one extreme of a spectrum of metastatic osteosarcoma, particularly, if there is a single dominant tumor with many smaller lesions. Children between the ages of 5 and 10 years are predominantly affected, although involvement of adolescents and adults has been reported. The radiological appearance is characteristic, with densely osteoblastic lesions, all of much the same size and maturity, involving the metaphyses of long bones. Early in their evolution, the lesions appear dense and relatively benign, resembling giant bone islands, with clear demarcation of their margins. Soon, however, they show the typical spread into the soft tissues. The similar size of all the lesions and the absence of metastatic lesions in the lungs differentiate the disease from metastatic osteosarcoma. Lung metastases, however, soon appear and the disease is inevitably fatal.
- *Extraosseous osteosarcoma:* This rare neoplasm presents the same histological pattern as other osteosarcomas. Usually, presentation is with a large soft-tissue tumor that is not necessarily close to bone. The radiological appearances are non-specific and although mineralization of the matrix may suggest the diagnosis, other soft-tissue sarcomas, such as chondrosarcoma, fibrosarcoma or synovial sarcoma, also calcify. Visceral osteosarcoma is an even rarer occurrence, but has been reported in the kidney.

Ewing's Sarcoma

Ewing's sarcoma is a small, round-cell, malignant bone tumor which accounts for between 10% and 15% of primary malignant bone tumors. Its peak incidence is between 10 and 15 years; it is rare under 5 years or over 30 years of age. It is more common in males. It is the second most common malignant bone tumor in children, osteogenic sarcoma being the most common. It occurs in long bones (50%) and flat bones (40%). The femur is most frequently involved with other common sites being the pelvis, ribs, tibiae, humeri and scapulae. Long bones are more commonly involved in young children. Presentation is usually with pain and a palpable soft tissue mass, sometimes with fever. Anemia and leukocytosis also occur and may lead to an incorrect diagnosis of osteomyelitis.

On plain films, there is destruction of the bone with cortical erosions and poor transition to normal bone. The periosteal reaction, when involving the central diaphysis that occurs in 50% of cases, is often laminated, producing an onion-skin appearance. Bone sclerosis is unusual. In many cases, there are perpendicular spiculations producing a 'hair on end' appearance in the center of the tumor. The laminated appearance occurs towards the edge of the tumor where there may be a Codman's triangle. There is usually a soft tissue mass rarely containing calcification **(Figs 7.28A to E)**.

MRI is the investigation of choice as it shows the extent of tumor in the bone marrow, the soft tissue component and any skip lesions. The signal is intermediate on T1 and increased on T2 with heterogenicity, if there is reaction from the bone. It is more homogeneous where there is little bone reaction. The soft tissue component is less prominent in the long bones compared with osteogenic sarcoma but may be large in the flat bones. Following treatment, changing volume is an indicator of necrosis and is a strongly favorable prognostic factor. Initial staging should also include skeletal scintigraphy to detect bony metastases and chest CT.

Osseous Lymphoma

Primary lymphoma of bone is a rare malignant condition. It has also been called reticulum cell sarcoma or malignant lymphoma of the bone and more

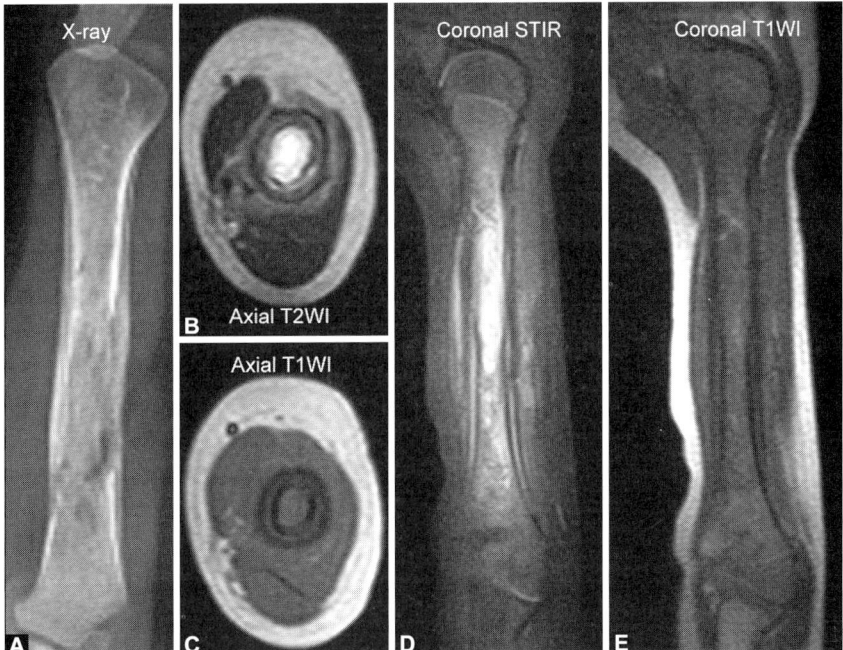

Figs 7.28A to E In a 2-year-old child with history of left arm swelling, X-ray of upper arm shows widening of humerus with cortical erosion and periosteal reaction involving most of the shaft. Irregular lucent areas seen within. Coronal STIR (B) and T1W (C) Axial T1W (D) and T2W (E) images show periosteal reaction with marrow edema in the diaphysis of the humerus

recently osteolymphoma. The vast majority of cases are of the non-Hodgkin type, with Hodgkin disease accounting for very few of cases. Distinguishing primary bone lymphoma from other bone tumors is important because the former has a better response to therapy and a better prognosis. Primary bone lymphomas most commonly are large cell or mixed small and large cell lymphomas of the B-cell lineage.

Radiography

Patterns of osseous lymphoma are:
- *Lytic-destructive pattern:* The lytic-destructive pattern is the most common radiographic appearance of primary bone lymphoma. The lytic pattern may be permeative—characterized by numerous small, elongated rarefactions that are parallel to the long axis of the bone and relatively uniform in size or moth-eaten—a pattern of many medium to large areas of radiolucency in a poorly marginated area of bone. Periosteal reaction may be either lamellated or layered, wherein layers of periosteal bone are seen parallel to the long axis of the bone (also called onion-peel appearance), or broken, when discontinuous or interrupted periosteal new bone is seen. The latter appearance of disrupted periosteal bone is believed to be a helpful radiographic sign that indicates a poorer prognosis.
- *Blastic-sclerotic pattern:* Primarily blastic-sclerotic lesions are rare in primary bone lymphoma compared with metastatic bone lymphoma. However, a mixed lytic lesion with sclerotic areas can be seen. Sclerotic changes in primary bone lymphoma may seem scarce, since of the two types of lymphoma, it is Hodgkin disease of bone (the less common subtype of primary bone lymphoma) that tends to be sclerotic and even in Hodgkin disease, lytic lesions predominates). Sclerotic areas can, however, develop in an originally lytic pattern after therapy (irradiation and chemotherapy).
- *Subtle or "Near-normal" findings:* A third pattern seen and described in primary bone lymphoma is the near absence of detectable abnormalities on plain radiographs. A remarkably normal-appearing radiographs may show striking abnormalities on radionuclide bone scans and MR images. As a result, in patients with symptoms but negative radiographic findings, further assessment with a second, more sensitive modality such as scintigraphy or MR imaging is essential.

MRI

Bone marrow replacement T1-weighted pulse sequences are the best for demonstrating marrow changes, as T1-weighted images reveal areas of low signal intensity within the marrow On T2-weighted images, these areas generally appear bright. Peritumoral edema and reactive marrow change can also produce high signal intensity on T2-weighted images. However, if fibrosis is present in a lesion, it may show low signal intensity. Short inversion-time inversion recovery (STIR) images, which are obtained with heavily T2-weighted pulse sequences, similarly, delineate the normal from abnormal marrow. When contrast material is administered, MR images can demonstrate areas of enhancement within the lesion.

Soft-tissue Involvement

Nearly, all cases that have a permeative pattern on plain radiographs are associated with soft tissue masses on MR images. Interestingly, the pattern of extensive marrow disease and surrounding soft-tissue masses but without extensive cortical destruction is seen nearly exclusively in round cell tumors such as primary bone lymphoma, multiple myeloma, and Ewing's sarcoma.

Cortical Erosion

Both MR imaging and CT demonstrate cortical erosion, although the former permits early detection.

Nuclear Imaging

Bone scintigraphy is more sensitive than conventional radiography. The pattern of extensive abnormality within a bone on a bone scan, accompanied by normal findings on conventional radiographs, suggests a round cell tumor, such as primary lymphoma of bone (PLB). A scintigraphic pattern that is suggestive is a combination of lesions in the skull, distal femur, and proximal tibia. Gallium-67 (^{67}Ga) citrate and thallium-201 (^{201}Tl) also are positive in patients with PLB. Whole-body ^{67}Ga scanning can help with initial staging by identifying or excluding soft-tissue foci of disease.

Liposarcomas

Liposarcomas is malignant tumor that arises in fat cells in deep soft tissue, such as that inside the thigh or in the retroperitoneum. Most frequent in middle-aged and older adults (age 40 and above), liposarcomas are the second most common of all soft-tissue sarcomas following malignant fibrous histiocytomas. Patients usually note a deep-seated mass in their soft tissue. Only when the tumor is very large do symptoms of pain or functional disturbances occur.

MRI is the imaging modality of choice (**Figs 7.29A to D**) after conventional X-rays.

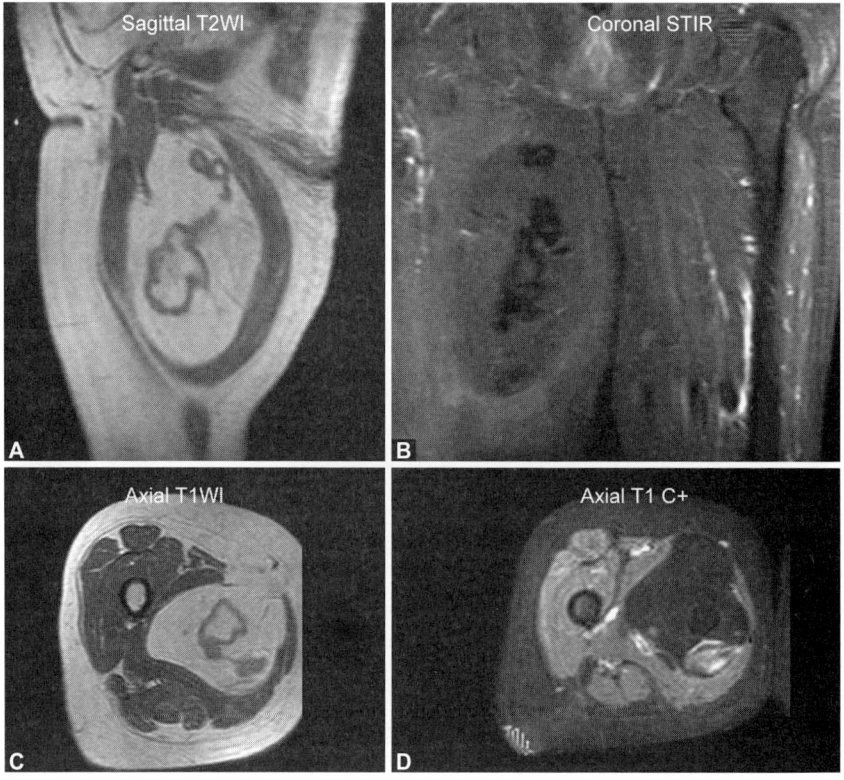

Figs 7.29A to D A 45-year-old female with history of swelling along the medial aspect of thigh. A large well-defined fat intensity hyperintense lesion is seen in the medial aspect of thigh between the adductor and gracilis muscles sagittal T2 W (A) and on axial T1 (C) images. It is mildly heterogeneous with few central septations. On fat saturation images, there is homogeneous suppression of fat (coronal STIR, C). Mild postcontrast enhancement (D) is seen. No evidence of invasion or infiltration. Neurovascular bundle appears normal

Sacrococcygeal Teratoma
(Figs 7.30A and B)

A teratoma is a germ cell tumor, 40% of which are found in the sacrococcygeal region. A mature teratoma is benign, but on imaging, it is impossible to exclude malignant components. In the neonate histological malignancy is present in up to 30%. The malignant component is usually due to embryonal carcinoma, yolk sac carcinoma or choriocarcinoma. Though histologically malignant, if the tumor is completely excised the prognosis is good. If elements are left behind, or the diagnosis is delayed, the incidence of malignancy increases. Elevated alpha-fetoprotein levels can indicate malignancy but unfortunately in the neonatal period, this is normally high and does not fall to normal levels until 9 months of age.

A sacrococcygeal tumor in the neonate usually presents as an external mass and where there is a presacral component, the infant may also have urinary frequency or retention, or constipation. These are the symptoms in children who present later. Any intra-abdominal extent of disease renders the lesion more likely to be malignant.

The plain film will usually show a rounded mass extending externally in the buttock region. Calcification may be present and there are sometimes formed structures such as bone or occasionally teeth in solid lesions. The spectrum varies from being completely solid through mixed solid and cystic lesions to an almost completely cystic mass.

Full evaluation is best performed by MRI. If there is invasion of the soft tissues or bone, it implies malignancy, but the majority of the teratomas do not show this feature, and the diagnosis has to be made by histology.

Skeletal Metastasis

Primary tumors which originate in other organs and involve the skeletal structures of the body either by hematogenous, lymphatic route or by direct invasion are called metastasis. Metastasis are generally multiple commonly found in the axial skeleton and sites of residual red marrow. The common sites are vertebrae, pelvic bones, proximal femora and humerii, skull and ribs **(Figs 7.31 and 7.32)**. It is unusual for metastasis to involve bones distal to the elbows or knees.

The common primary neoplasm which spread to bones is carcinoma breast, lungs, prostate, kidney and thyroid.

Occult primary is a primary malignancy in which there are no localizing signs suggestive of the site of primary tumor and has not been detected by any of the available investigative protocols. However, the metastatic lesions have been detected on clinical, radiological and biomedical parameters. Histopathology may suggest the likely site of primary.

Spinal metastases can be vertebral, intradural extramedullary or intradural. Spread of malignant cells to the region can occur via various routes including hematogenic (arterial or venous via Batson's plexus). Direct invasion is typically from paraspinal, retroperitoneal or pulmonary malignancies. Lymphatic spread is along the root sleeves. Subarachnoid spread is from intracanalicular seeding of primary and secondary CNS neoplasms. Having said that breast cancer, lung cancer and melanoma are also relatively common sources of intradural disease.

Breast, lung, prostrate, lymphoma, kidney and melonoma are among the common primaries to metastasize to spine.

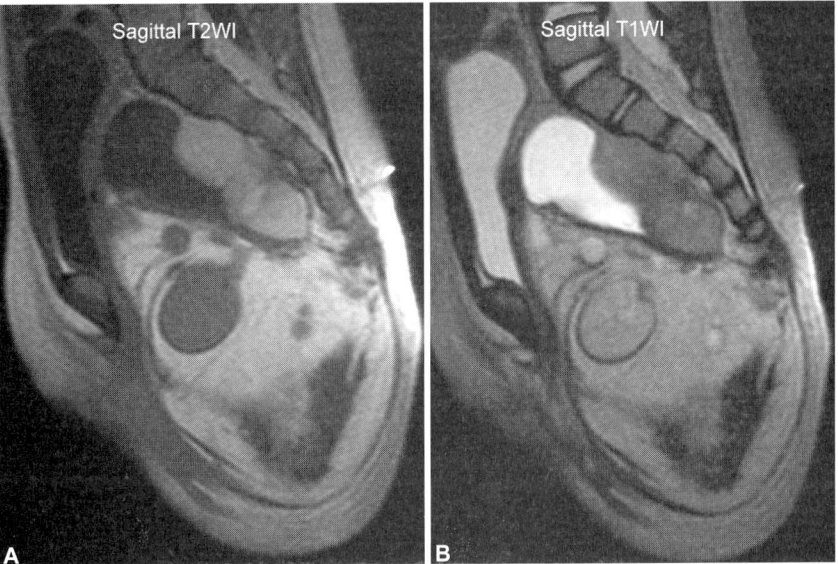

Figs 7.30A and B In one year female having buttock swelling since birth, and finds difficulty to walk on MR shows a large 12 x 6 cm. well-defined heterogeneous lesion in the pelvis posterior to the bladder. It is predominantly fatty with cystic and soft tissue component. Superiorly it extends up to the pelvic inlet, inferiorly into the right ischiorectal fossa and laterally extends up to the lateral pelvic wall. The coccygeal vertebrae reveal altered narrow signal. There is no intraspinal extension

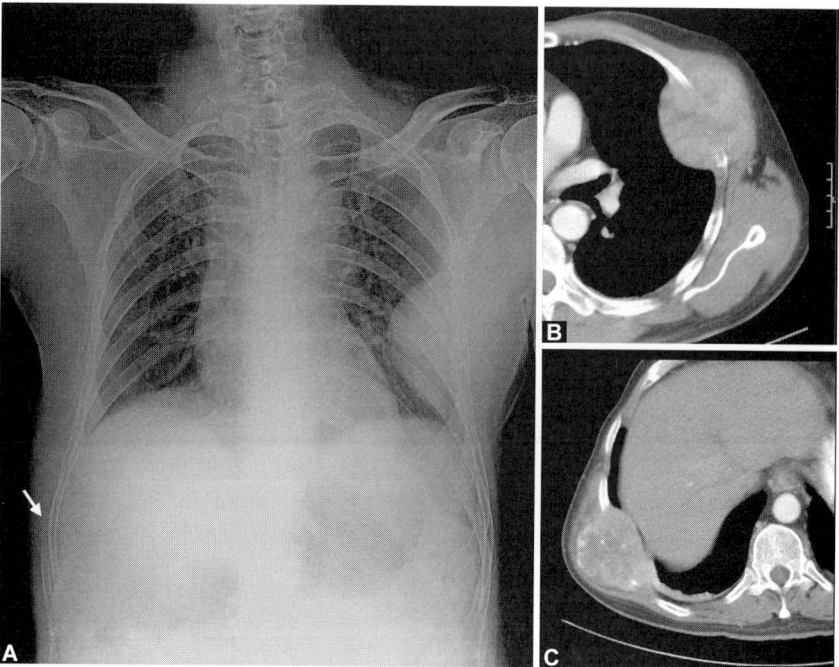

Figs 7.31A to C X-ray chest (A) shows a large (8 × 6 cm) well-defined mass lesion abutting the left lower chest wall with broad base towards the chest wall with partial destruction lateral aspect 4th rib on the left. Contrast CT chest shows moderately enhancing metastatic bone lesion which is rounded well-defined having a large soft tissue component from the left 4th rib (B) and right 10th rib (C) laterally, the ribs are partially destroyed, few small scattered calcific densities are seen in the lesions

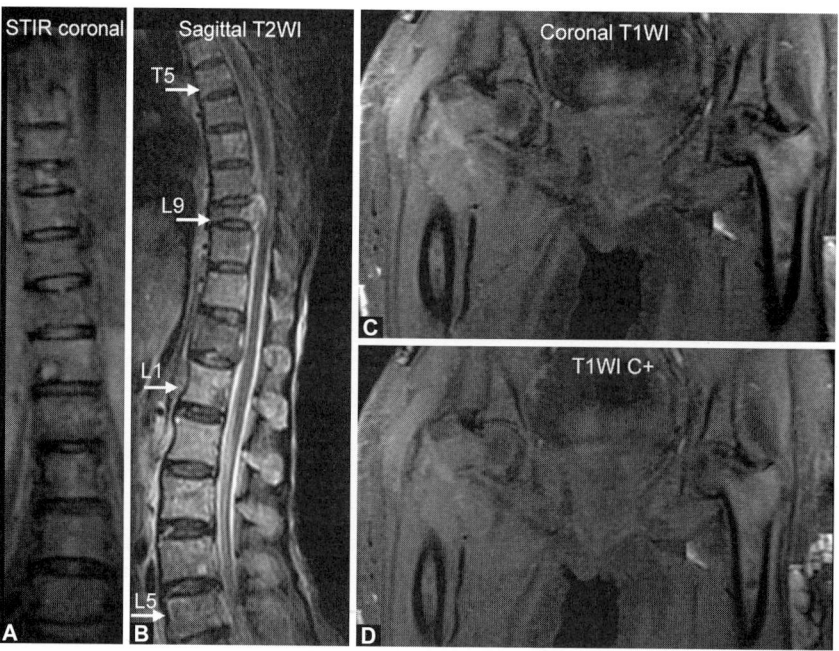

Figs 7.32A to D Sagittal STRI and T2WI MR images show collapse and retropulsion of D9 vertebrae and lesions at multiple levels (A and B). Coronal T1WI shows fracture right neck of femur with soft tissue component and hematoma (C). Postcontrast coronal T1WI shows the mass enhancing mass (D)

MRI is sensitive to metastatic disease and is able also assess for cord compression **(Figs 7.32A to D)**. The signal intensity of the metastatic deposits will vary according to the degree of mineralization.

Osteoblastic metastases will have T1: hypo-intense and T2: hypointense.

Mixed sclerotic and lytic extradural bone lesions will have T1: hypointense and T2: hypo- or/and hyperintense.

Lytic extradural bone lesions will have T1: intermediate to hypointense and T2: hyper- or isointense. T1 C+: enhancement is usually present.

8
Soft Tissues

Classification of Soft Tissue Tumors

The World Health Organization (WHO) classification system for cancer represents the common nomenclature for cancer worldwide. This common lexicon is critical for the performance of clinical trials, which are increasingly international in scale, and for translational research to be comparable. The WHO system helps to assure doctors and researchers that we are on the same diagnostic page in such undertakings.

The grading of soft tissue tumors has always been a controversial issue. While the WHO does not strictly state a preference in grading systems, one of the major modifications that have been made to the current WHO classification **(Table 8.1)** is the designation of two distinct types of intermediate malignancy in terms of biological potential: the "locally aggressive" and the "rarely metastasizing."

The large majority of soft tissue tumors are benign, with a very high cure rate after surgical excision. Malignant mesenchymal neoplasms amount to less than 1% of the overall human burden of malignant tumors but they are life-threatening and may pose a significant diagnostic and therapeutic challenge.

Benign mesenchymal tumors outnumber sarcomas by a factor of at least 100. At least one-third of the benign tumors are lipomas, one-third fibrohistiocytic and fibrous tumors, 10% vascular tumors and 5% nerve sheath tumors.

Lipomas are painless, rare in hand, lower leg and foot and very uncommon in children, multiple (angio) lipomas are sometimes painful and most common in young men.

Soft tissue sarcomas may occur anywhere but three fourths are located in the extremities (most common in thigh) and 10% each in the trunk wall and retroperitoneum. There is a slight male predominance. Like almost all other malignancies, soft tissue sarcomas become more common with increasing age; the median age is 65 years.

The etiology of most benign and malignant soft tissue tumors is unknown. In rare cases, genetic and environmental factors, irradiation, viral infections and immune deficiency have been found associated with the development of usually malignant soft tissue tumors.

Benign soft tissue tumors outnumber sarcomas by at least 100 to 1, although it is almost impossible to derive accurate numbers in this regard. Most benign lesions are located in superficial (dermal or subcutaneous) soft tissue. By far the most frequent benign lesion is lipoma, which often goes untreated.

Most soft tissue sarcomas of the extremities and trunk wall present as painless, accidentally observed tumors, which do not influence function or general health despite the often large tumor volume. The seemingly innocent presentation and the rarity of soft tissue sarcomas often lead to misinterpretation as benign conditions.

MRI is the modality of choice for detecting, characterizing, and staging soft tissue tumors due to its ability to distinguish tumor tissue from adjacent muscle and fat, as well.

Considering the prognostic and therapeutic importance of accurate diagnosis, a biopsy is necessary and most appropriate to establish malignancy, to assess histological grade, and to determine the specific histological type of sarcoma, if possible. A treatment plan can then be designed that is tailored to a lesion's predicted pattern of local growth, risk of metastasis, and likely sites of distant spread.

Most benign soft tissue tumors do not recur locally. Those that do recur do so in a nondestructive fashion and are almost always readily cured by complete local excision.

In malignant tumors in addition to the potential for locally destructive growth and recurrence, malignant soft tissue tumors' (known as soft tissue sarcomas) have significant risk of distant metastasis, ranging in most instances from 20% to almost 100%, depending upon histological type and grade. Some (but not all) histologically low grade sarcomas have a metastatic risk of only 2–10%, but such lesions may advance in grade in a local recurrence, and thereby acquire a higher risk of distant spread (e.g. myxofibrosarcoma and leiomyosarcoma).

Subcutaneous Lipoma

Lipoma, a benign tumor composed of mature fat cells, which may occur in any tissue that contains fat. Lipomas of soft tissue are seen more commonly in the subcutaneous tissues of the back, extremities and thorax. Lipomas are the most common soft-tissue tumor. Lipomas are slow growing, benign fatty tumors. They form soft, lobulated masses enclosed by

Table 8.1 WHO classification of soft tissue tumors

Adipocytic tumors		
Benign	Intermediate (locally aggressive)	Malignant
Lipoma Lipomatosis Lipomatosis of nerve Lipoblastoma Angiolipoma Myolipoma Chondroid lipoma Extrarenal angiomyolipoma Extra-adrenal myelolipoma Spindle cell/Pleomorphic lipoma Hibernoma	Atypical lipomatous tumor/well differentiated liposarcoma	Dedifferentiated liposarcoma Myxoid liposarcoma Round cell liposarcoma Pleomorphic liposarcoma Mixed-type liposarcoma Liposarcoma (not otherwise specified)

Fibroblastic/myofibroblastic tumors		
Benign	Intermediate (locally aggressive)	Malignant
Nodular fasciitis Proliferative fasciitis Proliferative myositis Myositis ossificans fibro-osseous pseudotumor of digits Ischemic fasciitis Elastofibroma 8820/0 Fibrous hamartoma of infancy Myofibroma/Myofibromatosis 8824/0 Fibromatosis colli Juvenile hyaline fibromatosis Inclusion body fibromatosis Fibroma of tendon sheath 8810/0 Desmoplastic fibroblastoma 8810/0 Mammary-type myofibroblastoma 8825/0 calcifying aponeurotic fibroma 8810/0 Angiomyofibroblastoma 8826/0 Cellular angiofibroma 9160/0 Nuchal-type fibroma 8810/0 Gardner fibroma 8810/0 Calcifying fibrous tumor Giant cell angiofibroma 9160/0	Superficial fibromatoses (palmar/plantar) Desmoid-type fibromatoses 8821/1 Lipofibromatosis *Intermediate (rarely metastasizing)* Solitary fibrous tumor 8815/1 and hemangiopericytoma 9150/1 (including lipomatous hemangiopericytoma) Inflammatory myofibroblastic tumor 8825/1 Low grade myofibroblastic sarcoma 8825/3 Myxoinflammatory fibroblastic sarcoma 8811/3 Infantile fibrosarcoma 8814	Adult fibrosarcoma Myxofibrosarcoma Low grade fibromyxoid sarcoma hyalinizing spindle cell tumor Sclerosing epithelioid fibrosarcoma

Fibrohistiocytic tumors		
Benign	Intermediate (rarely metastasizing)	Malignant
Giant cell tumor of tendon sheath 9252/0 Diffuse-type giant cell tumor 9251/0 Deep benign fibrous histiocytoma 8830/0	Plexiform fibrohistiocytic tumor 8835/1 Giant cell tumor of soft tissues 9251/1	Pleomorphic (MFH)/Undifferentiated pleomorphic sarcoma 8830/3 Giant cell MFH/Undifferentiated pleomorphic sarcoma with giant cells Inflammatory MFH/Undifferentiated pleomorphic sarcoma with prominent inflammation

Skeletal muscle tumors		
Benign		Malignant
Rhabdomyoma a. Adult type b. Fetal type c. Genital type		Embryonal rhabdomyosarcoma (including spindle cell, botryoid, anaplastic) Alveolar rhabdomyosarcoma (including solid, anaplastic) Pleomorphic rhabdomyosarcoma

Vascular tumors		
Benign	Intermediate (locally aggressive)	Malignant
Hemangiomas of	Kaposiform hemangioendothelioma	Epithelioid hemangioendothelioma
a. Subcut/deep soft tissue		Angiosarcoma of soft tissue
b. Capillary	Intermediate (rarely metastasizing)	
c. Cavernous	Retiform hemangioendothelioma	
d. Arteriovenous	Papillary intralymphatic angioendothelioma Composite hemangioendothelioma	
e. Venous		
f. Intramuscular		
g. Synovial 9120/0	Kaposi sarcoma	
Epithelioid hemangioma 9125/0		
Angiomatosis		
Lymphangioma 9170/0		
Tumors of uncertain differentiation	Intermediate (rarely metastasizing)	Malignant
Benign	Angiomatoid fibrous histiocytoma 8836/1	Synovial sarcoma 9040/3
Intramuscular myxoma (including cellular variant)		Epithelioid sarcoma 8804/3
Juxta-articular myxoma	Ossifying fibromyxoid tumor (including atypical/malignant)	Alveolar soft part sarcoma 9581/3
Deep ('aggressive') angiomyxoma pleomorphic hyalinizing angiectatic tumor	Mixed tumor	Clear cell sarcoma of soft tissue 9044/3
	a. Myoepithelioma	Extraskeletal myxoid chondrosarcoma ("chordoid" type)
Ectopic hamartomatous thymoma	b. Parachordoma	
		Primitive neuroectodermal tumor (PNET), extraskeletal Ewing tumor pPNET (p stands for peripheral)
		Desmoplastic small round cell tumor
		Extra-renal rhabdoid tumor
		Malignant mesenchymoma
		Neoplasms with perivascular epithelioid cell differentiation (PEComa) clear cell myomelanocytic tumor
		Intimal sarcoma 880
		synovial 9120/0
		Epithelioid hemangioma 9125/0
		Angiomatosis
		Lymphangioma 9170/0
Smooth muscle tumors		
Angioleiomyoma 8894/0		
Deep leiomyoma 8890/0		
Genital leiomyoma 8890/0		
Leiomyosarcoma (excluding skin) 8890/3		
Pericytic (perivascular) tumors	Chondro-osseous tumors	
Glomus tumor (and variants) 8711/0	Soft tissue chondroma 9220/0	
malignant glomus tumor 8711/3	Mesenchymal chondrosarcoma 9240/3	
Myopericytoma 8713/1	Extraskeletal osteosarcoma 9180/3	

a thin, fibrous capsule. Lipomas may rarely undergo sarcomatous change. On USG lipoma are well-defined masses of fat signature, although blood vessels, muscles, and fibrous tissue may be seen along with fat.

On MRI they are seen with signal intensity characteristics similar to subcutaneous fat; hyperintense on T1-weighted images and moderately intense on T2-weighted images. Fat suppression techniques are extremely useful in differentiating them from other soft tissue tumors **(Figs 8.1A to C)**.

Macrodystrophia Lipomatosa

Macrodystrophia lipomatosa is a congenital local gigantism of the hand and foot, characterized by proliferation of all mesenchymal components, particularly fibroadipose tissue **(Figs 8.2A to E)**. Macrodystrophia lipomatosa comes to clinical attention because of cosmetic reasons, mechanical problems secondary to degenerative joint disease or development of neurovascular compression.

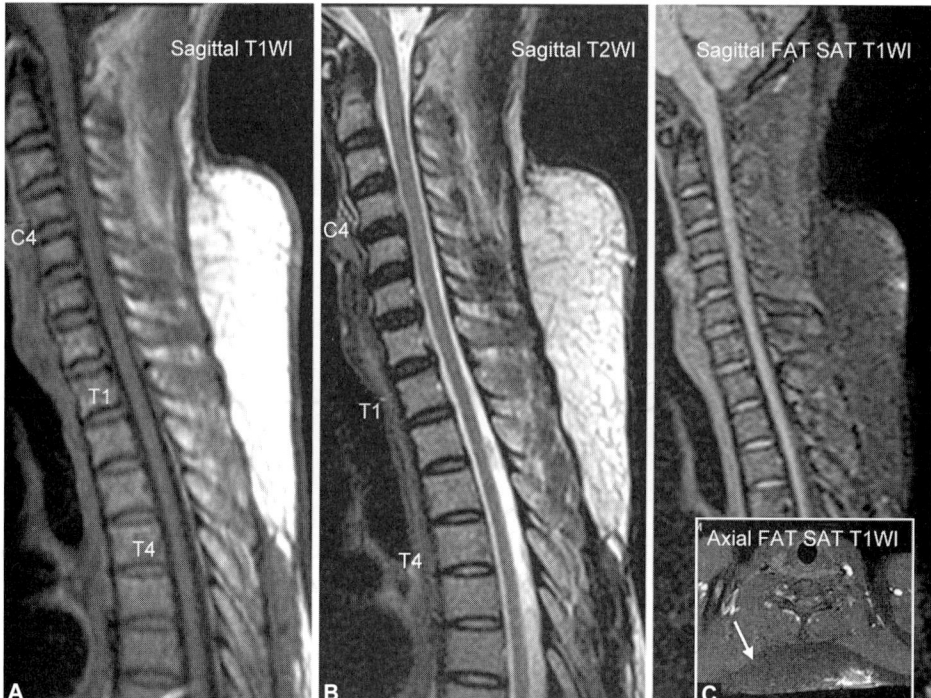

Figs 8.1A to C A large well-defined subcutaneous hyperintense lesion is seen on T1W and T2W images (A and B) in the posterior midline cervico-dorsal region (14 × 4 × 9 cm). It gets suppressed on (Fat-Saturated) Fat Sat T1W images (C) and in inset in C (arrow). Fat planes between the muscles and this lesion are well maintained. No evidence of deep extension

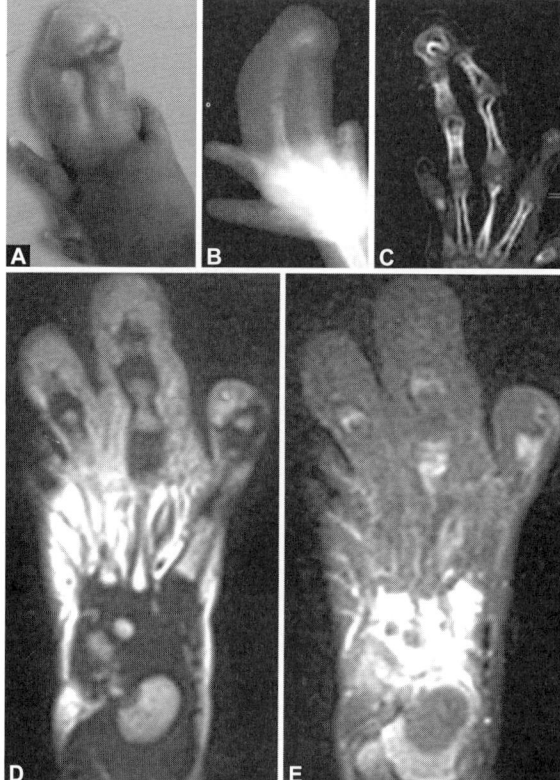

Figs 8.2A to E Clinical photograph (A) of right hand shows enlarged, fused ring and middle finger; plain radiograph (B); coronal reformatted CT (C) shows soft tissue swelling and proliferation of fat on palmar aspect of the ring and middle fingers, along with dorsal angulation and syndactyly. T1 coronal MRI (D) reveals proliferation of fatty tissue on plantar aspect of the second and third toes of right foot with signal intensity similar to that of subcutaneous fat as seen by fat suppressed STIR coronal image (E)

Liposarcoma

Liposarcoma is malignant tumor that arises in the fat cells in deep soft tissue, such as that inside the thigh or in the retroperitoneum. They are typically large bulky tumors which tend to have multiple smaller satellites extending beyond the main confines of the tumor. Most frequent in middle-aged and older adults (above 40 years), liposarcomas are the second most common of all soft-tissue sarcomas following malignant fibrous histiocytomas. Patients usually note a deep seated mass in their soft tissue. Only when the tumor is very large symptoms of pain or functional disturbances occur.

Liposarcoma is a tumor derived from primitive cells that undergo adipose differentiation. It is largely a disease of adults, with peak incidence between 40 years and 60 years of age, and it shows a slight predominance in men. When liposarcomas occur in the pediatric population, they tend to present in the second decade of life. In either event, the deep soft tissues of the extremities, particularly those of the thigh, are the most common location, accounting for more than 50% of liposarcomas. Its presentation in this location is most commonly that of a slow growing, painless mass. Often these tumors are first noticed following a minor trauma.

MRI is obtained, both with and without contrast enhancement. The MRI **(Figs 8.3 and 8.4)** findings in liposarcoma can be quite distinct, and suggest the diagnosis even before biopsy report. This largely depends on how closely the tumor resembles normal fat and how well-differentiated it is.

Fibrolipomatous Hamartomas of Median Nerve

Fibrolipomatous hamartomas are benign tumors usually affecting infants and less commonly children and young adults. This uncommon lesion is also known as neural fibrolipoma, lipofibromatous hamartoma, perineural lipoma and intraneural lipoma. The median nerve is overwhelmingly the most commonly affected nerve (80% of cases), followed by the ulnar and radial nerves, and brachial plexus. The most common presentation is that of a soft, slowly enlarging and often asymptomatic mass on the volar wrist or forearm often present since infancy. Occasionally nerve compression will lead to symptoms of pain, paresthesia or carpal tunnel syndrome. There is equal prevalence among males and females. Although the pathogenesis has not been definitively elucidated, it is postulated that a congenital abnormality of

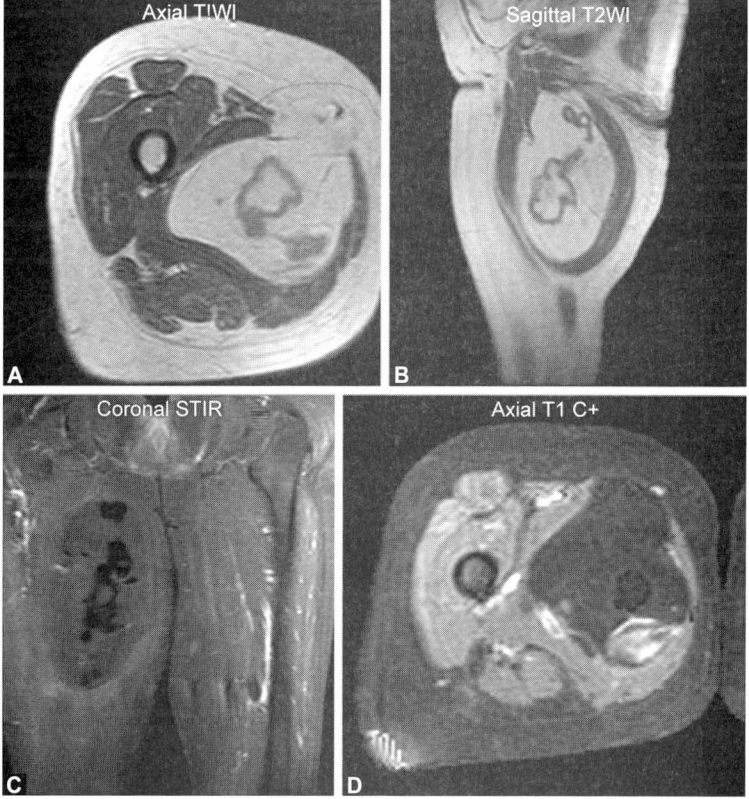

Figs 8.3A to D A 45 years old female with history of swelling along the medial aspect of right thigh. A large well-defined fat intensity hyperintense lesion is seen in the medial aspect of thigh between the adductor and gracilis muscles on axial T1 (A) and sagittal T2WI (B). It is mildly heterogeneous with few central septations. On coronal STIR fat saturation image (C) there is homogeneous suppression of fat. Mild enhancement is seen on postcontrast image (D). No evidence of invasion or infiltration. Neurovascular bundle appears normal

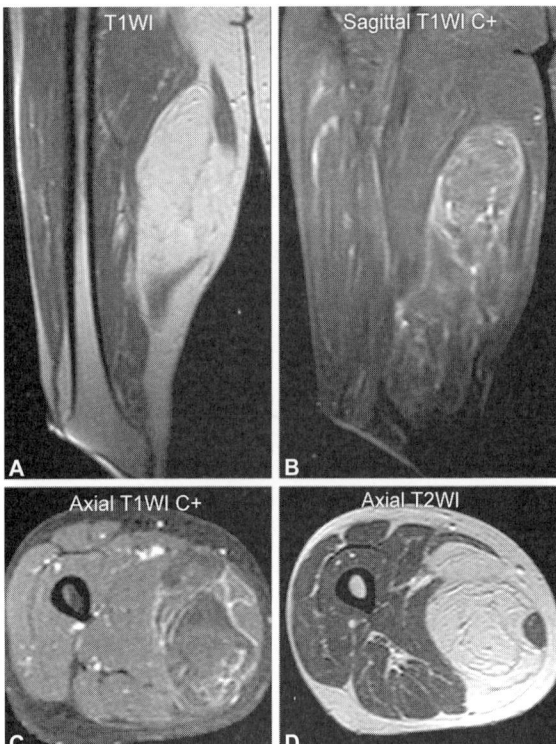

Figs 8.4A to D Large well-defined T1 hyperintense lesion is seen along the medial aspect of thigh between the adductor group muscles and the gracilis muscle on T1WI (A) and T2WI (D). Multiple septae are seen within it. No evidence of fluid component or calcification. Postcontrast images (B and C) show mild patchy enhancement

growth of fibrofatty tissues causes infiltration of the endoneurium, perineurium and epineurium resulting in fusiform nerve enlargement.

Computed tomography (CT) and MRI imaging findings of fibromatous hamartomas show fusiform nerve enlargement, which is caused by thickening of nerve bundles and fatty and fibrous proliferation. Enlarged nerve bundles look like serpentine or tubular structures. The MRI characteristics of fibromatous hamartomas are pathognomonic presenting high signal intensity from fat on T1 and T2-weighted sequences which will drop out on fat suppressed images surrounding the bands of enlarged nerve fascicles (**Figs 8.5A to F**).

Baker's Cyst

Baker's cyst is a synovial cyst in the posterior aspect of the knee related to a knee effusion leading to distension of the gastrocnemius or semimembranosus bursa. This entity is also termed as popliteal cyst.

The cysts may or may not communicate with the neighboring joint. Baker's cysts may dissect between the muscles of the leg or rupture, with extravasation of fluid, producing clinical manifestations similar to thrombophlebitis.

Ultrasonography, CT, and MR imaging are useful in the diagnosis of a Baker's cyst. On MR imaging it is low signal on T1 and high signal on T2 (**Figs 8.6A to C**). The joint connection can be seen on axial images. MR imaging may provide the most detailed information regarding the distribution and extent of the process and the degree of synovial inflammation.

Complete Tear Tendoachilles

Achilles tendon attaches the triceps surae muscle to the tuberosity of the calcaneum. It is covered by a fascia rather than a tendon sheath.

Chronic tendinitis involving the Achilles tendon leads to thickening or focal enlargement. Involved portions of the tendon are of low signal intensity on MR images. When intratendinous foci of increased signal intensity are observed in T2-weighted MR images, an accompanying partial tear of the Achilles tendon is likely. Complete or partial tears of the tendon, typically occurring in sedentary persons who attempt strenuous activity. It is characterized by discontinuity of some or all of the tendon fibers. Regions of increased signal intensity on T2-weighted MR images (**Figs 8.7A to D**), and blood and edema within a tendinous gap are seen. Ultrasonography is helpful in evaluating this injury. Predisposing factors include chronic tendinitis, rheumatoid arthritis, systemic lupus erythematosus and administration of corticosteroid preparations.

Superficial bursitis about the Achilles tendon accompanied by retrocalcaneal bursitis and a soft tissue mass at the site of insertion of the tendon is known as Haglund's syndrome.

Neurogenic Tumors

Neurogenic tumors are relatively common and account for approximately 12% of all benign and 7–8% of all malignant soft tissue neoplasms. Their characteristic imaging findings include a specific clinical presentation or location, relationship to a nerve, and certain lesion shape and signal intensity patterns. Schwannoma (neurilemmoma, neurinoma) is a slow-growing neurogenic tumor that is believed to arise from the Schwann cells of a peripheral nerve. Therefore, the lesion usually develops eccentrically to the nerve fibers and is encapsulated by the perineurium. Schwannoma most frequently affects patients 20–50 years of age and accounts for approximately 5% of all benign soft tissue neoplasms. Men and women are affected equally. Although the head and neck, the flexor surfaces of the extremities (particularly the ulnar and peroneal nerves), and the mediastinum and retroperitoneum represent the most common sites of involvement, schwannomas can occur almost anywhere. Pain and neurologic symptoms are uncommon unless the lesion is large. Long-standing tumors that are relatively large can

Soft Tissues ❖ 107

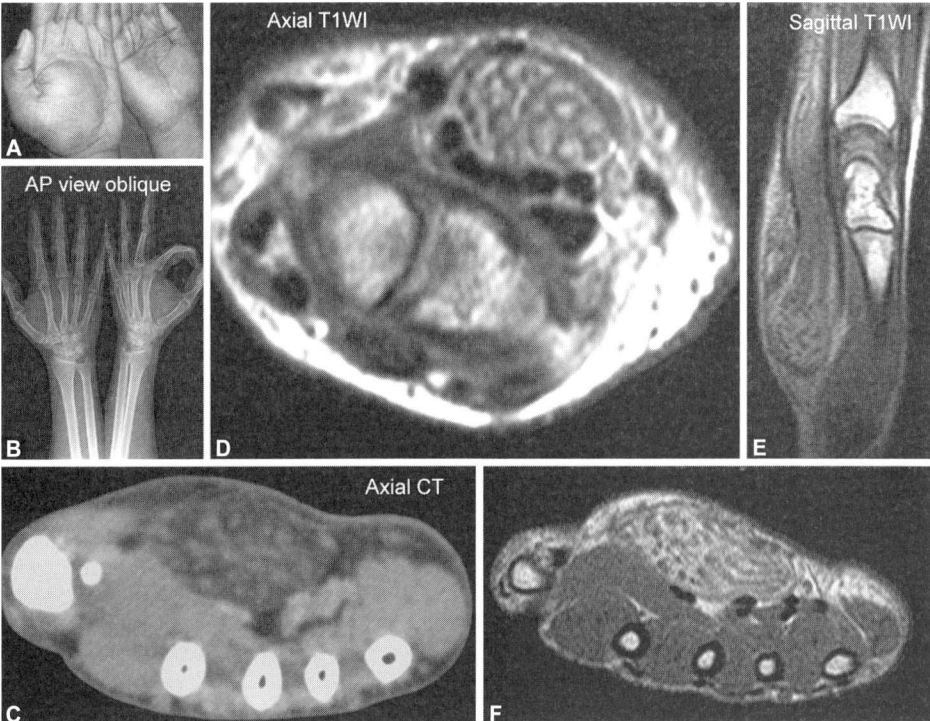

Figs 8.5A to F Photograph of hands show swelling of the left thenar eminence (A). X-ray AP and oblique views (B) of left hand show soft tissue swelling in the region of thenar eminence. Axial CT section shows a well-defined heterogeneous lesion seen in ventral aspect distal to wrist, anterior to the flexor tendons having fatty density within the lesion (C). Axial T1WI and sagittal T1WI (D and E) shows well-defined oval lesion on ventral aspect just distal to wrist appearing hyperintense with flow voids within it. In the fatty lesion, flow voids are seen abutting the flexor tendons with polka dot appearance (D to F) because of enlarged median nerve with fat infiltration in between fascicles of median nerve *(For color version, see plate 3)*

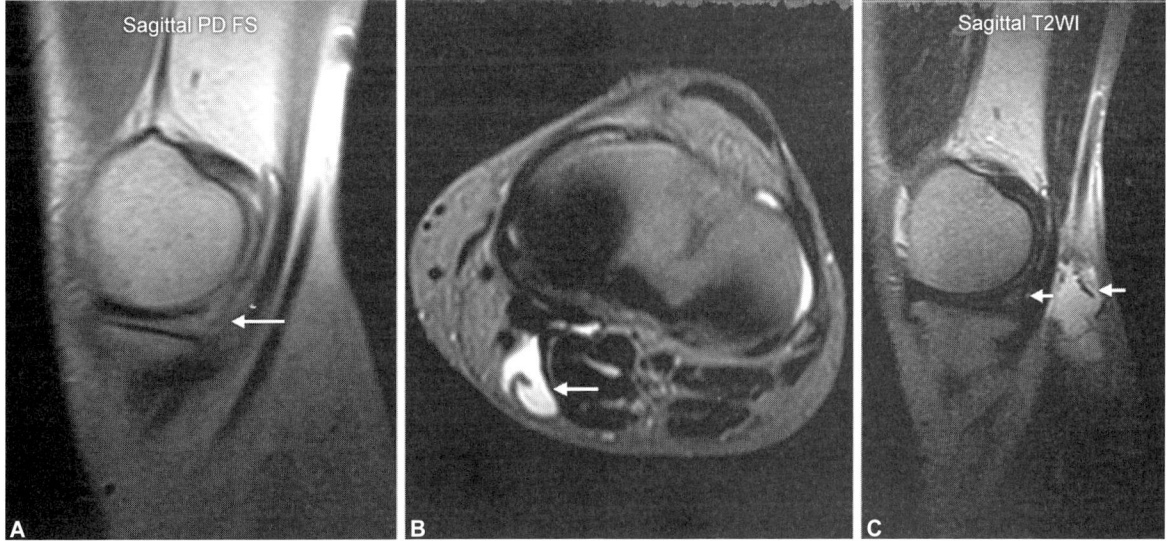

Figs 8.6A to C Sagittal PD FS image shows Grade II tear in the posterior horn of the medial meniscus (arrow) (A). Sagittal T2W (C) axial T2W (B) image shows loculated collection posteriorly with septae suggesting Baker's cyst (arrows)

undergo degenerative changes such as cyst formation, calcification, hemorrhage, and fibrosis.

STIR images **(Fig. 8.8A)** show fusiform hyperintense mass in continuity with the neurovascular bundle, a finding that is virtually diagnostic of peripheral nerve sheath tumor. A sagittal T1-weighted image **(Fig. 8.8B)** shows the fusiform mass is surrounded by a thin margin of fat (split fat sign) **(Fig. 8.8C)**. This appearance results as the mass within the neurovascular bundle enlarges and displaces the adjacent intramuscular fat.

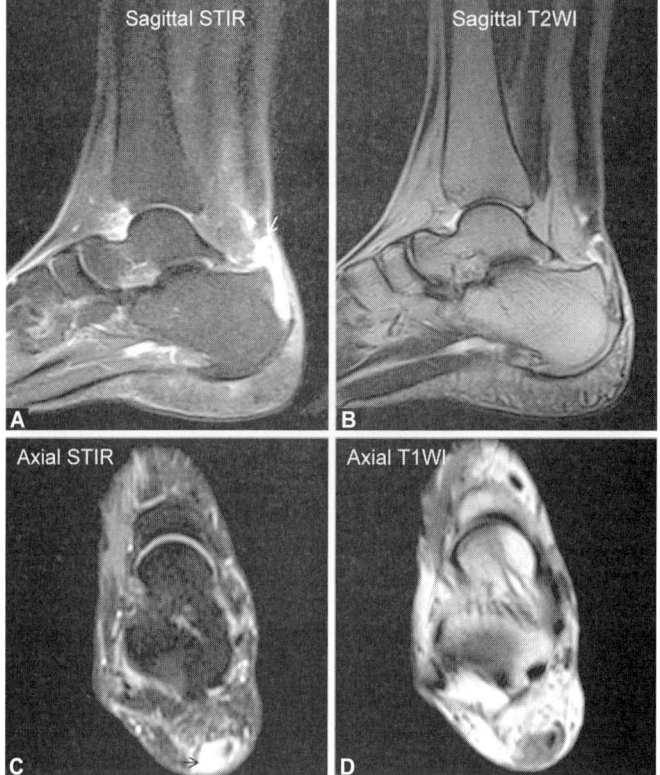

Figs 8.7A to D Sagittal STIR (A) and sagittal T2WI (B) shows full thickness tear (arrow) of the tendo achilles. Axial STIR (C) and axial T1WI (D) image shows the tear with fluid surrounding it

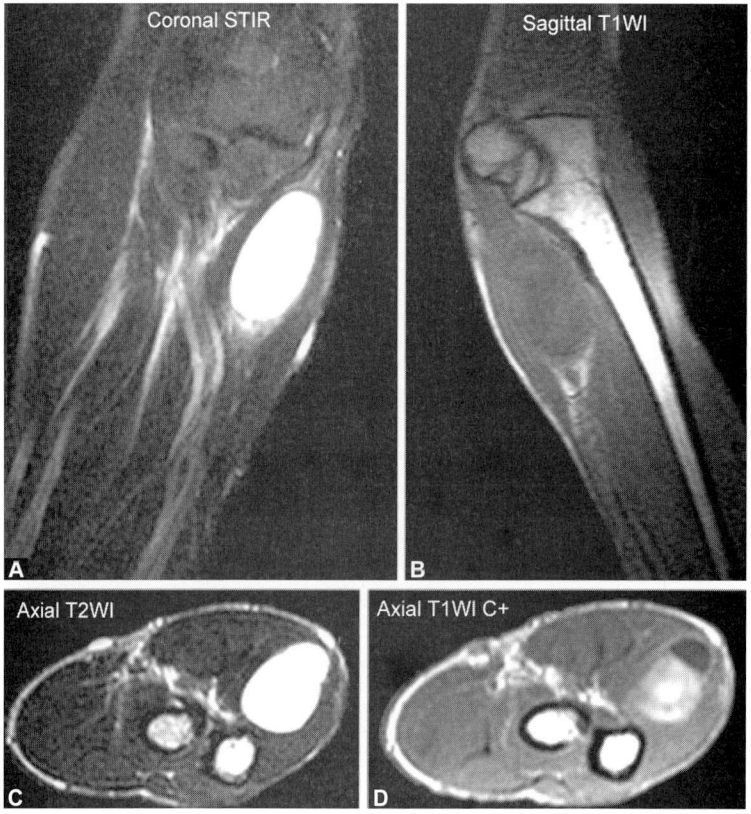

Figs 8.8A to D An oval well-defined hyperintense lesion on STIR and T2WI (A and C), appearing isointense on T1WI (B) is seen in the anterior aspect of right forearm in the intermuscular fat plane and shows moderate postcontrast enhancement (D)

On contrast-enhanced images **(Fig. 8.8D)**, small nerve sheath tumors often show intense and relatively homogeneous enhancement.

Large lesions may demonstrate predominantly peripheral, central or heterogeneous nodular enhancement.

Bilateral Nasolabial Cyst

Nasolabial cysts is a rare odontogenic cyst occurring in the nasal ala. On CT shows a well-defined homogeneous low density soft tissue lesion at the nasolabial region **(Figs 8.9 to 8.12)**.

Soft-tissue Calcifications

Costal Cartilage Calcification

Costal cartilage calcification can help distinguish the sex. Calcification of costal cartilage may be seen above

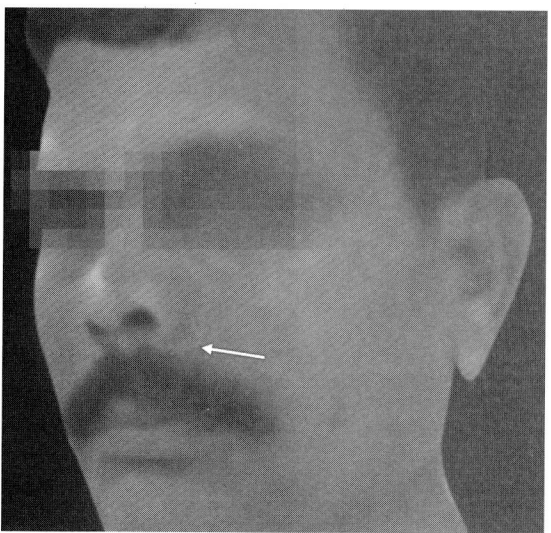

Fig. 8.9 Photograph of patient shows swelling (arrow) on left side in the nasolabial region *(For color version, see plate 4)*

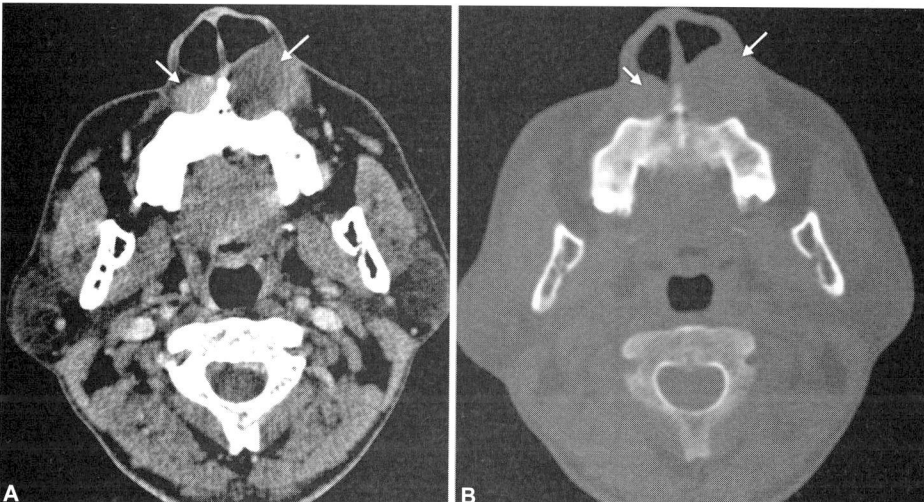

Figs 8.10A and B Axial CT image in soft tissue window (a) shows bilateral nasolabial cyst (arrow) and (b) in bone window shows scalloping of the alveolar margin

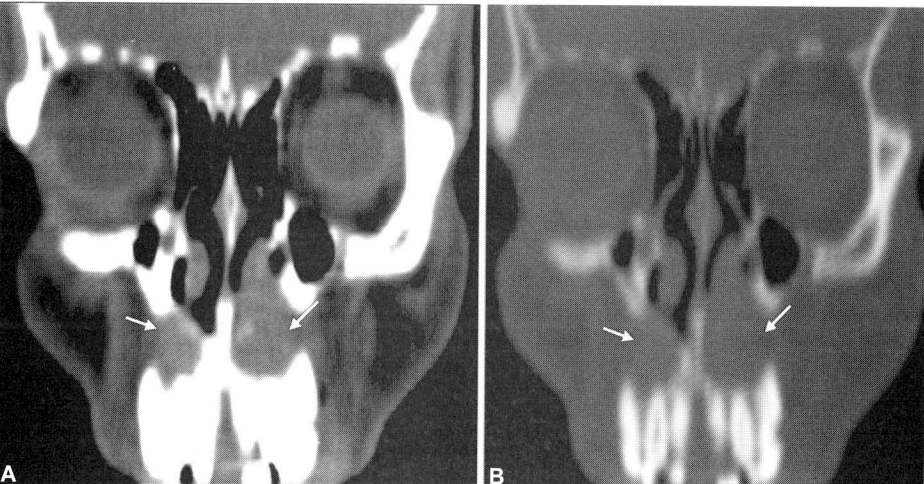

Figs 8.11A and B Coronal reformatted CT image soft tissue window (a) shows bilateral nasolabial cyst (arrow) and (b) in bone window shows scalloping of the alveolar margins.

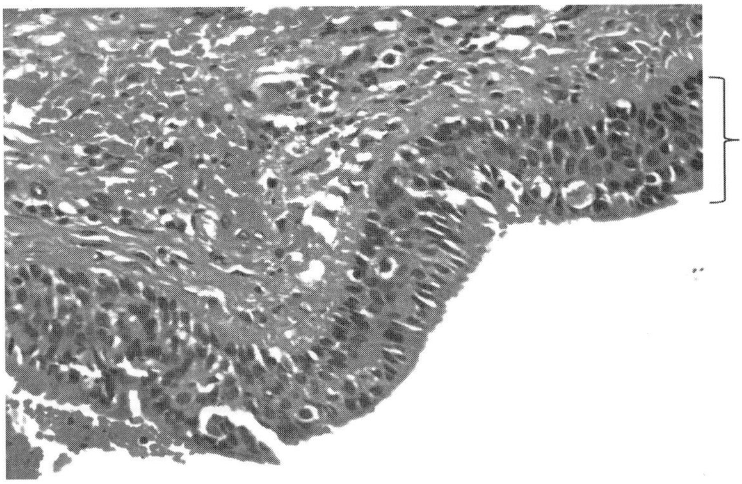

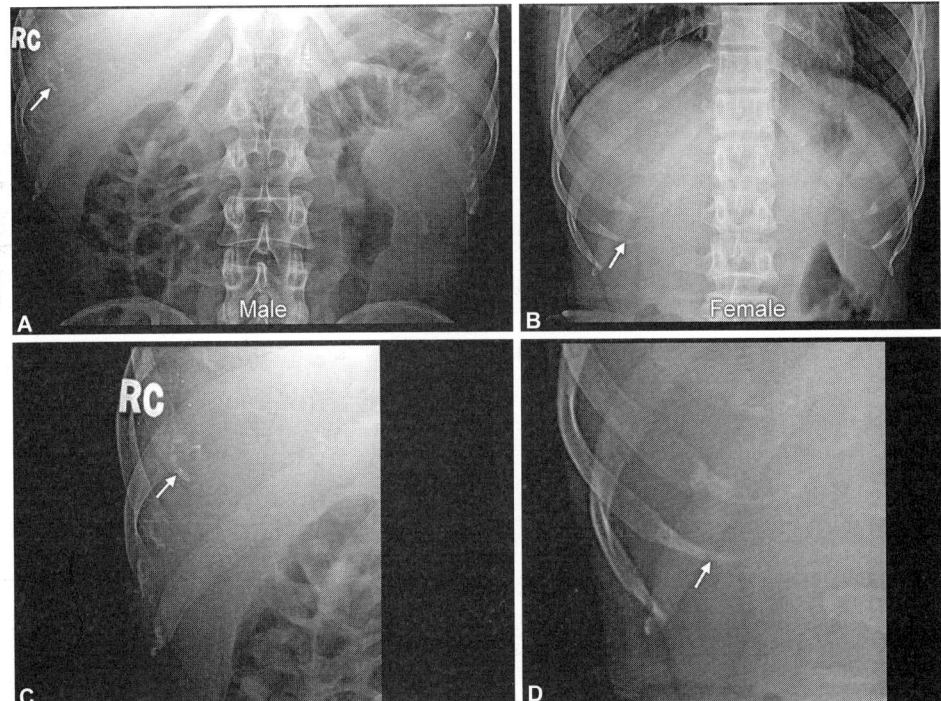

Fig. 8.12 Histopathological examination shows pseudostratified columnar epithelium (}) with fibrocollagenous tissue, the feature of a cyst wall *(For color version, see plate 4)*

Figs 8.13A to D X-ray lower chest shows costal cartilage calcification pattern of the lower ribs is that of a male and female

the age of 20 years in male and above the age of 16 years in females.

Pattern of calcification is peripheral (marginal) in males, it is mainly confined to the upper and lower margins of the costal cartilages **(Figs 8.13A to D)** and in female it is solid tongue-like protrusion of calcification, it central pyramidal (lingular) type of calcification with peak towards sternum. Costochondral calcification is marginal in males and central in female.

Dermoid Cysts

Dermoid cysts (or mature cystic teratomas) are benign germ cell tumors composed of mature epithelial elements, i.e. skin, hair, desquamated epithelium, and teeth **(Fig. 8.14)**. They have wider age distribution, but most commonly occur in age group of 16–55 years. Malignant dermoid cysts are rare and usually develop into squamous cell carcinoma in adults; in children it usually develops into endodermal sinus tumor.

Types of dermoid cysts are:
- Sequestration dermoids are caused when skin and skin structures become trapped during fetal development at the line of embryonic fusion. Common sites are forehead, head, root of nose and sublingual dermoid.
- Implantation dermoid occurs as epidermis gets buried into the deeper subcutaneous tissue due

to minor pricks or trauma, which causes reaction and cyst formation. Common sites are fingers, toes and feet. The inflammatory response may or may not be present and, in the cysts of long duration, calcification may be seen **(Figs 8.15 and 8.16)**.
- Teratomatous dermoid occurs in ovary, testis, retroperitoneum, and mediastinum.

Ultrasound (US) is the initial imaging investigation of choice. On US, they are smooth-walled cystic structure with varying internal composition depending upon mixture of epithelial elements. On CT, well-defined cystic appearance with fat content and calcification (e.g. tooth) is suggestive of a dermoid.

Guinea Worm

Calcified Guinea Worm

Guinea worm disease (Dracunculiasis) has been eradicated from Asia. In India, the last reported case was in July 1996 and on completion of three years of zero incidences, India was declared free from Guinea worm disease. In this case, infestation must have taken place before eradication. Transmission of dracunculiasis now occurs in only few African countries.

Man acquires infection by drinking water containing infected cyclops. In the stomach these cyclops are digested by gastric juice and the parasites are released. They penetrate the duodenal wall; migrate through viscera to the subcutaneous tissues of the various parts of the body. They grow into adults into 9–12 months. The female grows to a length of 55–120 cm, and the male is very short 2–3 cm. After infestation many of these parasites (usually gravid female, as male dies) emerge out through skin, while few of them are lodged in the subcutaneous tissues, die, get encapsulated and get calcified as string like appearance **(Figs 8.17 and 8.18)**. Upon contact with water, the female parasite releases up to one million, microscopic larvae which remain active in water for 3–6 days. They are picked up by small crustaceans called cyclops. The larvae require a period of about 15 days for development in cyclops, which is the intermediate host.

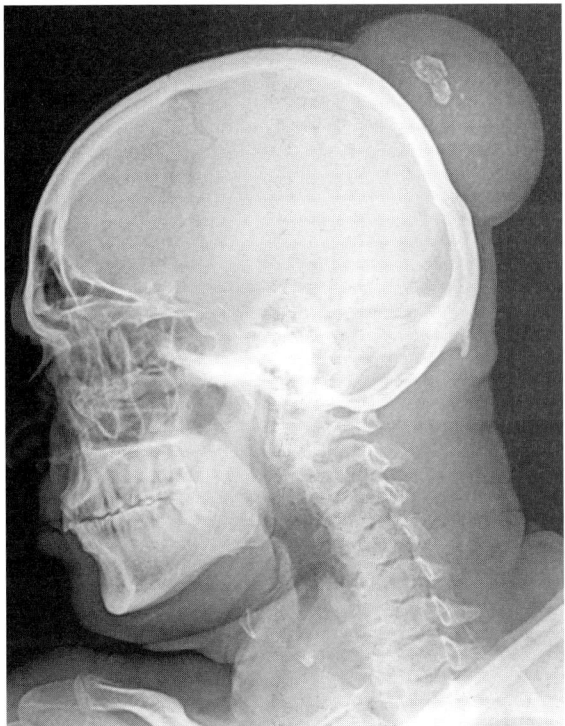

Fig. 8.14 X-ray lateral view head shows a dermoid cyst in the scalp posteriorly and in mid-line position with minimal scalloping of the vault, having a tooth like structure within. No intracranial extension is appreciated

Sarcoidosis

Sarcoidosis commonly develops thoracic lymphadenopathy and parenchymal lung opacities. Adenopathy almost always precedes pulmonary shadowing, but they are often present simultaneously. The chest radiograph is abnormal at some time in 90% of patients with sarcoidosis. In sarcoidosis there is bilateral symmetrical hilar enlargement involving both tracheobronchial and bronchopulmonary nodes. Bilateral hilar adenopathy in the correct clinical setting is considered as sufficient evidence of sarcoidosis and negate the need of biopsy, more so if they show presence of egg shell calcification **(Fig. 8.19)**.

Enlargement of other mediastinal nodes are rarely appreciated on the chest radiograph but may be seen on CT. If the hilar adenopathy is very asymmetrical or anterior mediastinal adenopathy is present alternative diagnosis should be considered. The involved lymph nodes may undergo calcification, when this calcification is in the periphery it is reffered as egg-shell calcification as seen in this case.

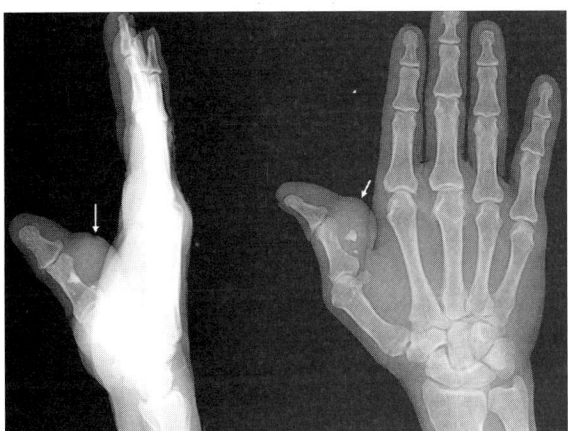

Figs 8.15 X-ray right hand, lateral and PA projections, shows an implantation dermoid on dorsal aspect overlying the proximal phalanx and metacarpal of the middle finger in its anteromedial aspect. It contains a nodule of calcification

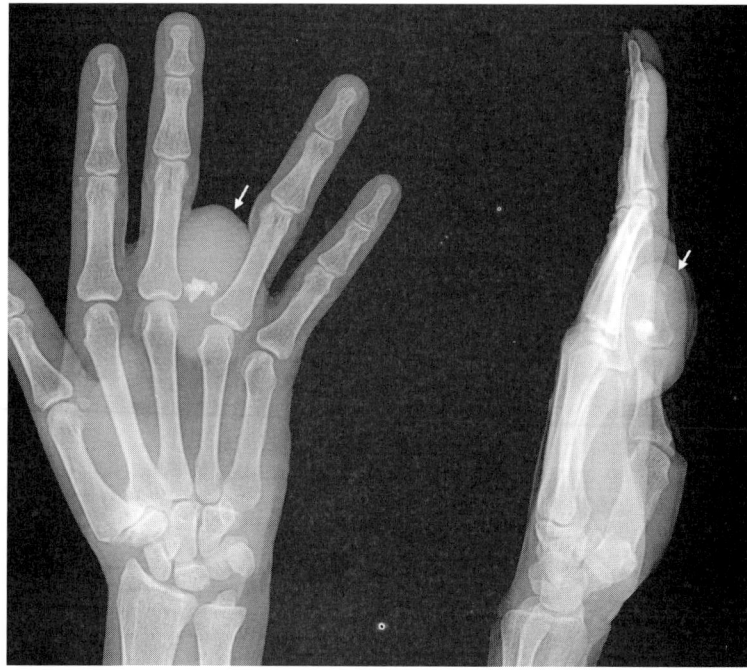

Figs 8.16 X-ray right hand, PA and lateral projections, shows an implantation dermoid on dorsal aspect overlying the proximal phalanx and metacarpal of the middle finger in its anteromedial aspect. It contains a nodule of calcification

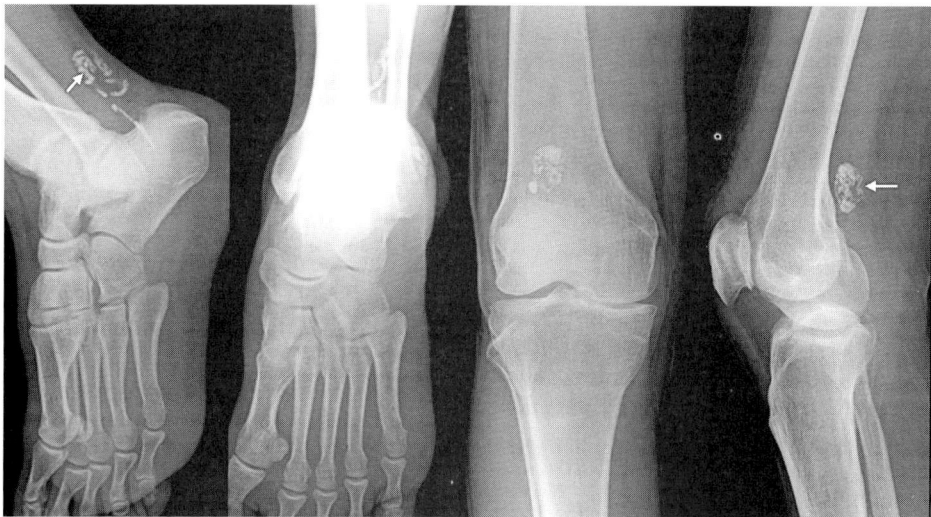

Fig. 8.17 X-ray chest shows calcified guinea worms as a high density string like calcification in the soft tissues of the right axilla and another string like calcified guinea worms in the soft tissues of the distal posterior aspect of thigh in the same patient

Other causes of bilateral hilar lymphadenopathy:
1. Infections like tuberculosis, mycoplasma, Whipple's disease
2. Lymphoma, carcinoma, mediastinal tumors
3. Organic dust diseases such as silicosis, berylliosis
4. Extrinsic allergic alveolitis such as bird fancier's disease
5. Less common causes such as Churg-Strauss syndrome, human immunodeficiency virus, extrinsic allergic alveolitis, pneumoconiosis, adult onset Still's disease.

Seminal Vesicle Calcification

The seminal vesicles are paired lobulated pouches, 5 cm in length but become atrophic with age. They lie on the posterior surface of urinary bladder. They run inferomedially into a thin duct and joins with the duct of the vas deferens to form the ejaculatory duct. The ejaculatory duct penetrates the prostate to enter the prostatic urethra on the verumontanum. Normal seminal vesicles are well appreciated on CT because of surrounding fat **(Figs 8.20 and 8.21)** and may show calcification in elderly and long standing diabetes.

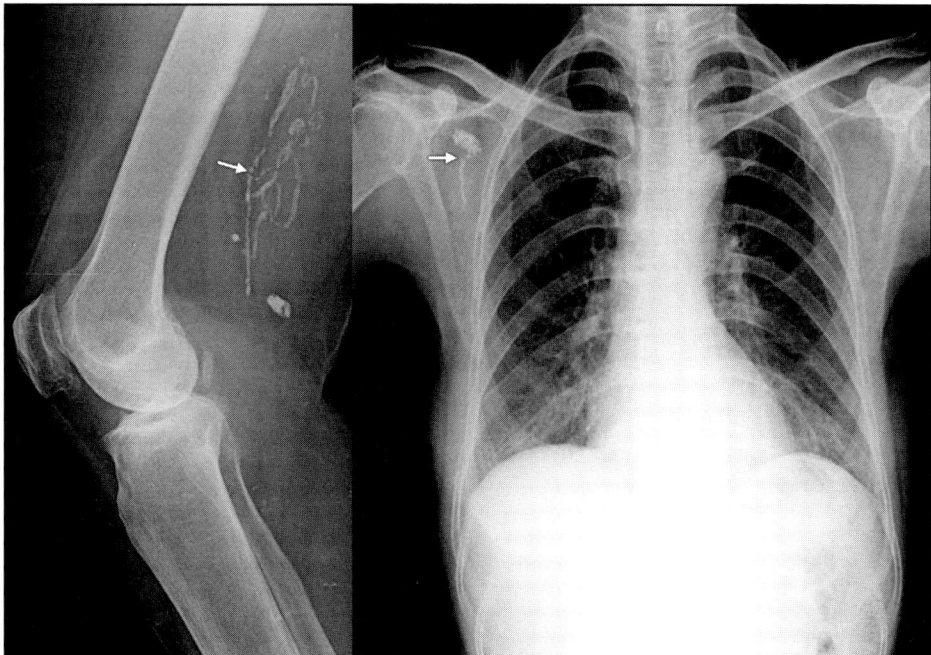

Fig. 8.18 X-ray knee lateral view shows calcified guinea worms as a high density string like calcification in the soft tissues of the posterior aspect of knee. Similar finding are seen in another patient, in the soft tissue of right axilla on PA view chest

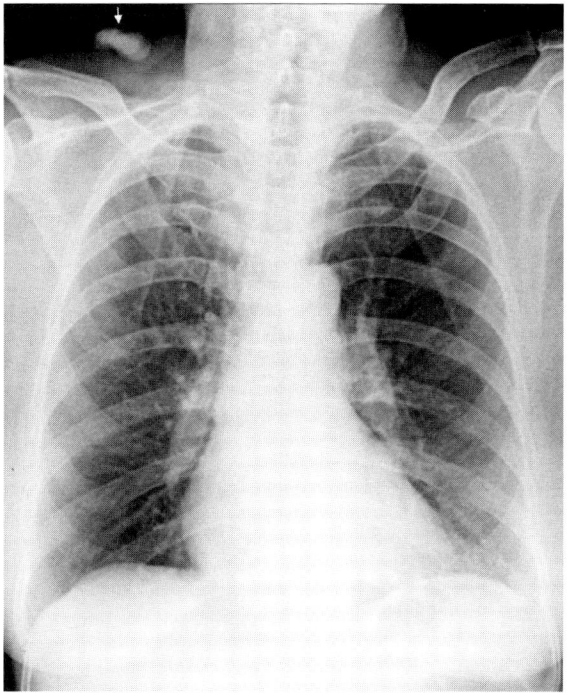

Fig. 8.19 X-ray chest shows multiple enlarged bilaterally symmetrical hilar lymph nodes which show peripheral or egg shell calcification

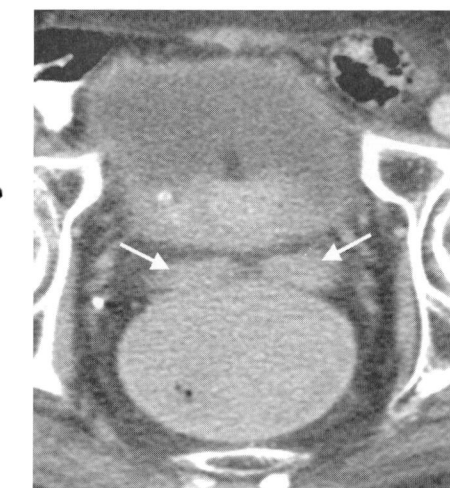

Fig. 8.20 CT pelvis shows normal seminal vesicles as moustache shaped structures

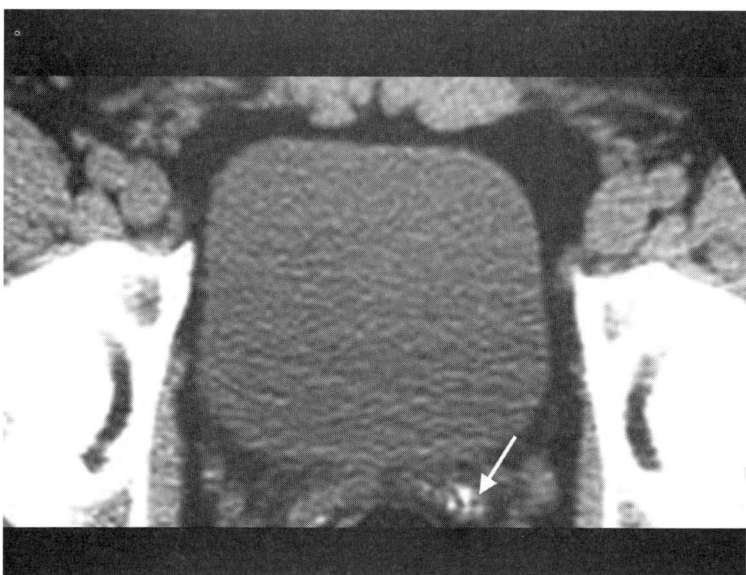

Fig. 8.21 CT pelvis shows calcification of both seminal vesicles in a case of long standing diabetes mellitus (arrow)

Calcification of the seminal vesicles is uncommon phenomenon. Calcifications appear more frequently in diabetic patients, it is more frequently visualized on CT. Other causes are seminal vesicle calcifications are diabetes mellitus, recurrent urinary tract infection and paraplegia with chronic infection.

Soft Tissue Calcification

Soft tissue calcification is frequently seen on conventional X-rays.

Soft tissue calcification is seen in pseudohypothyroidism **(Fig. 8.22A)**, it may also occur in thyroid adenomas **(Fig. 8.22B)**, carcinoma thyroid, tuberculous glands in the neck **(Fig. 8.22C)**, mediastinum or abdomen, neurofibromatosis **(Fig. 8.22D)**, fecalith **(Fig. 8.22E)**, bursa **(Fig. 8.22F)**, osteoarthritis **(Fig. 8.22G)**, synovial chondromatosis **(Fig. 8.22H)**, and calcification in damaged tendons like tendon achillis **(Fig. 8.22I)**.

Soft tissues calcification can be seen in some soft tissue tumors both benign and malignant. Arterial calcification is due to atheromatous change and is seen in the aortic arch abdominal aorta and iliacs frequent in the elderly. Wide spread arterial calcification may be seen in hyperparathyroidism. Other conditions with a high serum calcium such as chronic renal failure can give rise to calcification around joints. Scleroderma is associated with calcification in the digits. Gout shows calcified tophi in the soft tissues and dermatomyositis can give rise to calcification in the soft tissues.

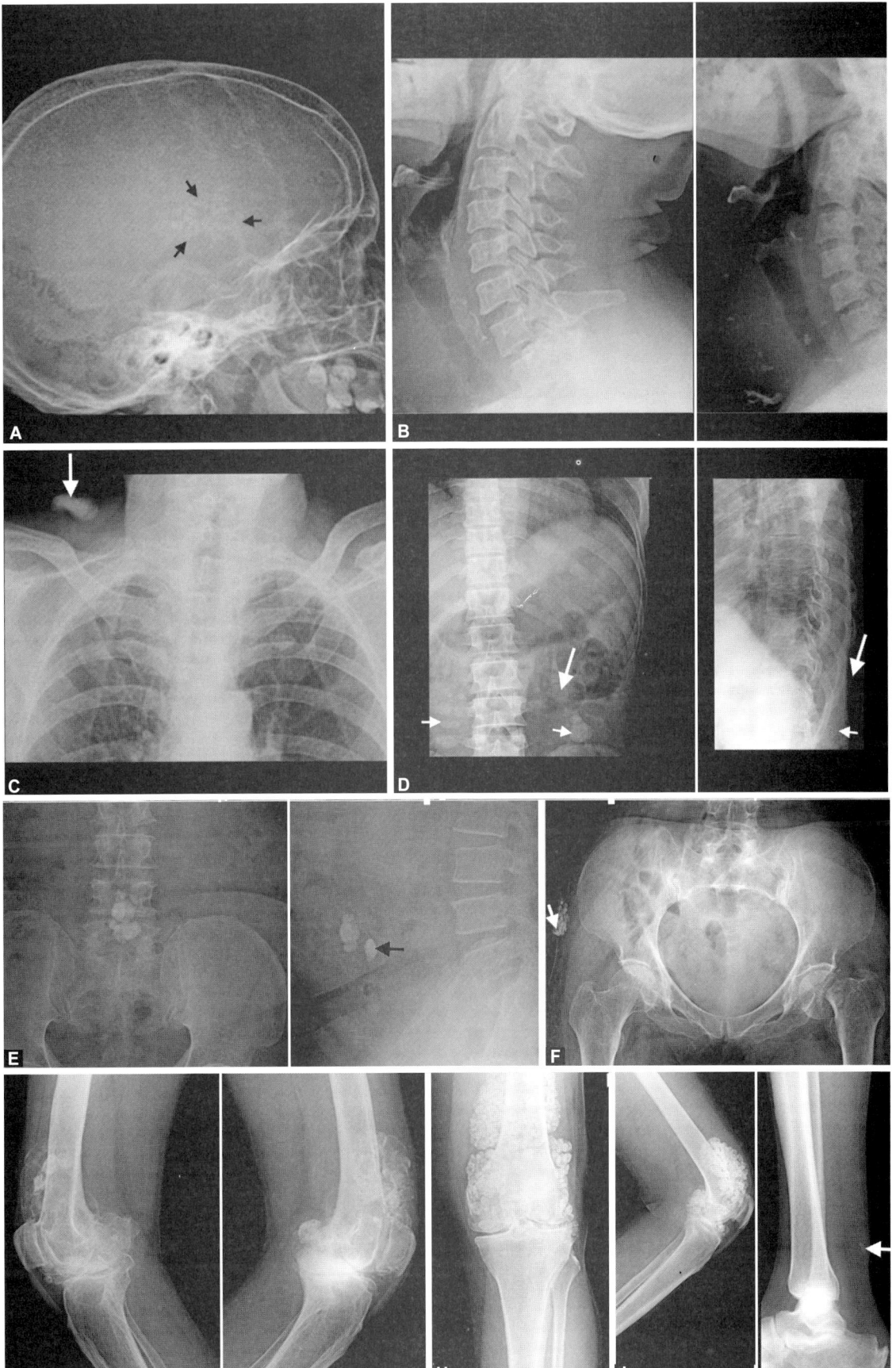

Figs 8.22A to I (A) X-rays show soft tissue calcification in pseudohypothyroidism; (B) Carcinoma thyroid; (C) Tuberculous glands in the neck; (D) Chest and abdominal neurofibromatosis (arrows); (E) X-rays show soft tissue calcification in (E) Fecalith; (F) Bursa; (G) Calcified loose bodies in osteoarthritis; (H) Synovial chondromatosis; (I) and in damaged tendo achilles

9
Breast

Breast Anatomy

The examination of the breast on mammography shows following normal anatomical structures:
- Skin
- Nipple and areola
- Fatty tissue
- The breast tissue proper and
- Blood vessels.

The skin appears as a thin, continuous, radiopaque rim of homogeneous density, 1 mm thick and readily visible against the radiolucency of the underlying subcutaneous premammary fatty tissue. If the breast is very dense the skin may not show up clearly even on a correctly exposed mammogram.

Nipple and Areola

The skin surrounding the nipple the areola can be up to 3–5 mm thick, with a central opacity, cylindrical in shape and of variable size and density, corresponding to the nipple. Posteriorly there is a triangular, heterogeneous trabecular area, the retroareolar region. Under normal conditions, the lactiferous ducts and sinuses are not seen.

Fatty Tissue

Varying amounts of fatty tissue may be present, forming anything from a thin subcutaneous layer to "islets" of various sizes that may occupy the whole breast, depending on the characteristics and age of the individual woman. The parenchymal cone is surrounded by fatty tissue which constitutes the premammary fat anteriorly and the retromammary fat posteriorly.

Breast Tissue Proper

The body of the mammary gland is roughly cone-shaped with the floor resting on the chest wall and the tip projecting towards the nipple. The shape and density of breast structures vary from individual to individual, and are influenced by specific sensitivity to hormonal stimuli, which affect relations between the various tissue components and hence the morphology of the breast.

Pectoralis Muscle

The pectoralis muscle is homogeneously radiopaque; it is located in front of the chest wall and is shaped like an upside-down triangle in the mediolateral oblique views.

Blood Vessels

Vessels are more readily visible in breasts that contain plentiful fatty tissue, and appear as thin ribbon-like opacities that may be more or less tortuous; vessel walls may be calcified giving typical "railwayline" images.

Normal breast tissue patterns or breast density on mammography is categorized into 4 groups (**Figs 9.1A to D**):

1. *The breasts are almost entirely fatty*: The breasts contain little fibrous and glandular tissue, which means the mammogram would likely detect anything abnormal.
2. *There are scattered areas of fibroglandular density*: There are a few areas of fibrous and glandular tissue in the breast.
3. The breasts are heterogeneously dense, which may obscure small masses the breast has more areas of fibrous and glandular tissue that are found throughout the breast. This can make it hard to see small masses.
4. The breasts are extremely dense, which lowers the sensitivity of mammography the breast has a lot of fibrous and glandular tissue. This can lead to missing some cancers.

Breast Imaging Reporting and Data System (BI-RADS)

Breast imaging reporting and data system (BI-RADS) developed by the American College of Radiology to describe mammogram findings and sorted into categories 0 through 6. This ensures a standard way of reporting and follows up of suspicious findings in mammograms.

BI-RADS 0: Need additional imaging evaluation and/or prior mammograms for comparison: When additional imaging studies are completed, a final assessment is made.

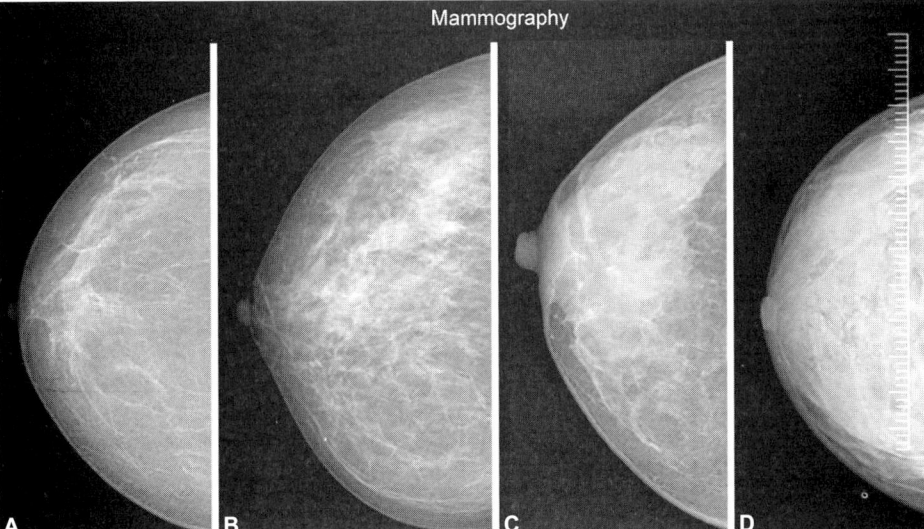

Figs 9.1A to D (A) Shows predominantly fatty breast with total absence of fibroglandular tissue. Only traces of the stromal network may remain (B) Breast shows Less adipose tissue, fibroglandular component gives it a "cobblestone" effect made up of small radiopaque nodular opacities measuring up to 3 mm in diameter (C) Fibroglandular structure. typical triangular fibroglandular configuration due to increased glandular component, clearly showing the tip of the triangle in the retroareolar region (D) Dense breast virtually no fatty tissue is present. The mammogram shows an intensely and uniformly radiopaque glandular and stromal component, in which the structures of the breast cannot be distinguished.

1. *BI-RADS 1: Negative*: There is nothing to comment on. There's no significant abnormality to report. The breasts are symmetrical and no masses, architectural distortion or suspicious calcifications are present.
2. *BI-RADS 2: Benign finding*: This is a normal assessment, but the interpreter chooses to describe a finding characteristically benign in appearances, and can be labeled with confidence such as benign calcifications, lymph nodes in the breast, calcified fibroadenomas fat-containing cysts, lipomas, galactoceles and mixed-density hamartomas. This ensures that others who look at the mammogram will not misinterpret the benign finding as suspicious. This finding is recorded in the mammogram report to help when comparing to future mammograms.
3. *BI-RADS 3: Probably benign finding*: The findings in this category have a very high chance of being benign, and should have less than a 2% risk of malignancy. It is not expected to change over the follow-up interval, since it is not proven benign, it is helpful to see if the area/lesion in question does change over time. If follow-up findings shows no change, the final assessment is changed to BI-RADS 2 (benign) and no further follow-up is needed. If a BI-RADS 3 lesion shows any change during follow-up, it will change into a BI-RADS 4 or 5 with suitable action to be taken.
4. *BI-RADS 4: Suspicious abnormality*: Biopsy should be considered: The findings that do not have the classic appearance of malignancy but have a wide range of probability of malignancy (2–95%).
5. *BI-RADS 5: Highly suggestive of malignancy: appropriate action should be taken*: It is reserved for findings that are classic breast cancers, with more than 95% likelihood of malignancy. Biopsy is very strongly recommended. A spiculated, irregular high-density mass, a segmental or linear arrangement of fine linear calcifications or an irregular spiculated mass with associated pleomorphic calcifications are examples of lesions that should be placed in BI-RADS 5.
6. *BI-RADS 6: known biopsy proven malignancy*: Appropriate action should be taken. It is reserved for lesions identified on the imaging study with biopsy proof of malignancy prior to definitive therapy. Mammograms may be used in this way to see how well the cancer is responding to treatment.

Breast Cysts

Breast cysts are fluid-filled sacs, round to oval lumps with distinct edges with texture like grapes, they are benign lesions and may be benign single or multiple. They are common in women before menopause, between ages 35 and 50, but can be found in women of any age. Breast cysts usually disappear after menopause, unless on hormone therapy. Breast cysts require no treatment unless a cyst is large and painful or otherwise uncomfortable. In that case, draining the fluid from a breast cyst can ease your symptoms. Simple cysts are the most common masses seen at mammography and result from dilatation and effacement of the terminal duct lobular unit (**Figs 9.2A to D**).

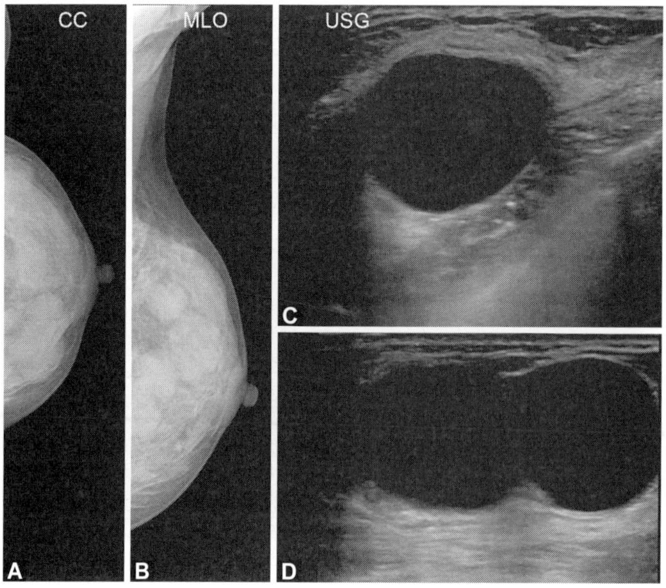

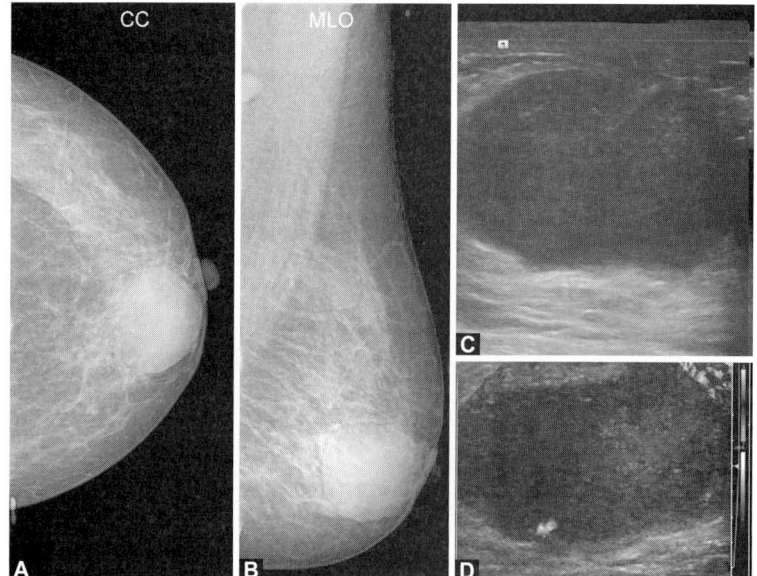

Figs 9.2A to D Patient came with complaint of multiple breast lumps since few years. Breast mammography shows dense parenchyma with multiple scattered indiscreet dense soft tissue opacities (BI-RADS 2). USG shows multiple anechoic lesions with posterior acoustic enhancement and lateral shadowing, largest measuring 32 × 15 mm. No evidence of internal echoes, septae or calcifications within the cysts

Figs 9.3A to D In patient with complaints of breast pain and antibiotic administration, mammography shows a well-defined soft tissue density mass with smooth margins in the outer lower quadrant of the left breast with no microcalcifications (A and B). No axillary lymphadenopathy seen. On ultrasound a well-defined heterogeneous mass with dense internal echoes and thick wall is seen in the outer lower quadrant of the left breast measuring 28 × 24 mm. It wider than taller (C). Color Doppler reveals peripheral vascularity (D) *(For color version, see plate 4)*

Antibioma

Cases of antibioma present with history of breast pain, tenderness and antibiotic administration for breast abscess, mammography findings are usually non specific and may include dense mass, distortion or skin thickening. Axillary lymphadenopathy may be enlarged. Ultrasound may show a heterogeneous, hypoechoic collection with dense echoes and septae with echogenic vascular rim and no vascularity within the collection **(Figs 9.3A to D)**. Imaging of antibioma are classified as BIRAD's II.

INTRAMAMMARY LYMPH NODE

Intramammary lymph nodes on mammography are seen as circumscribed oval or reniform structures with a central or peripheral lucency that represents fat within the hilum with following two criteria. Without exception the nodes are smoothly circumscribed and well-defined (BIRAD's III). These are low density lesions. If it is projected over the profile of the muscle, muscle is seen through the node. On ultrasonographic intramammary lymph nodes are seen as hypoechoic reniform lesion with well-defined margin. A hyperechoic central area resulting from the hilar fat may be seen. Sometimes a nearby blood vessel may be seen with some flow entering the hilum on color Doppler **(Figs 9.4A to C)**.

Fibroadenomas

Fibroadenomas are benign tumors of breast lobule and are composed of stromal and epithelial elements. Fibroadenoma is common in second and third decade of life. It is painless, firm in consistency and mobile and is referred as breast mouse. It is generally less than 5 cm in diameter. It occurs during developmental stage of breast, due to estrogen sensitivity. In about 10% cases it is multiple. If more than 5 cm, it is referred as giant fibroadenoma, however it has no malignant potential. Fibroadenomas on mammography are well circumscribed discrete masses which may have gentle lobulations and may present with popcorn calcifications **(Figs 9.5A and B)**. Ultrasound shows a well-circumscribed, round to ovoid lesion which may have gentle lobulations with generally uniform hypoechogenicity. Sometimes a *thin* echogenic rim-pseudocapsule may be seen. On elastography (a) El/B ratio of less than 1 (b) Elasticity score 3 or less (c) Strain ratio 3 or less suggest a benign lesion **(Figs 9.6A to D)**.

Treatment in women under 25 years, the fibroadenoma is not removed. Older women are subjected to excision biopsy, local recurrence is rare. In case of giant fibroadenoma, enucleation of complete tumor is done by cosmetic incision.

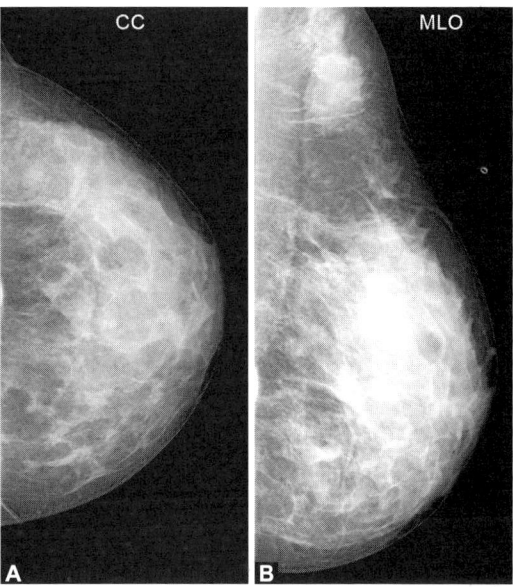

Figs 9.5A and B Mammography shows a well-defined isodense lesion in the region of the axillary tail of the left breast without skin puckering or nipple retraction

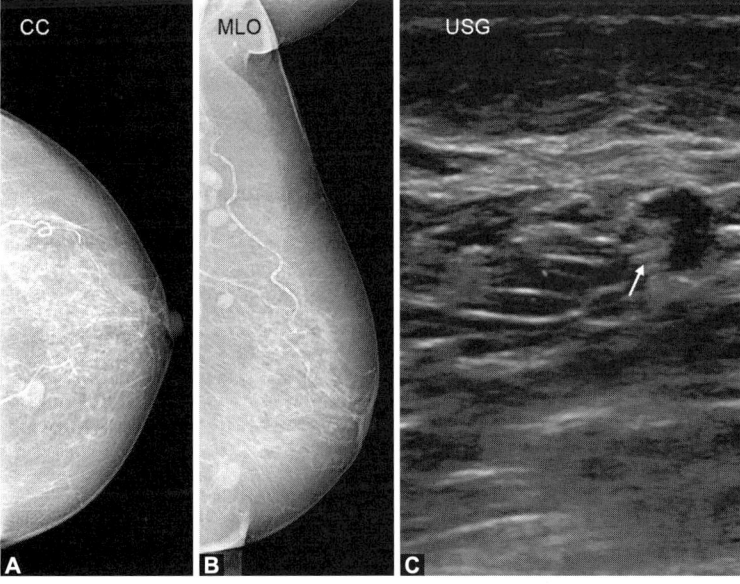

Figs 9.4A to C Mammographic shows a well-defined smoothly circumscribed low density lesion with a central lucency are seen in the inner lower quadrant along with axillary lymphadenopathy, multiple arterial calcifications are also seen (A and B). USG shows multiple enlarged axillary lymph nodes, largest measuring 32 mm (arrow). The fatty hila of the lymph nodes are preserved (C). Another small intramammary lymph node is seen in the inner lower quadrant of the left breast. No microcalcifications seen

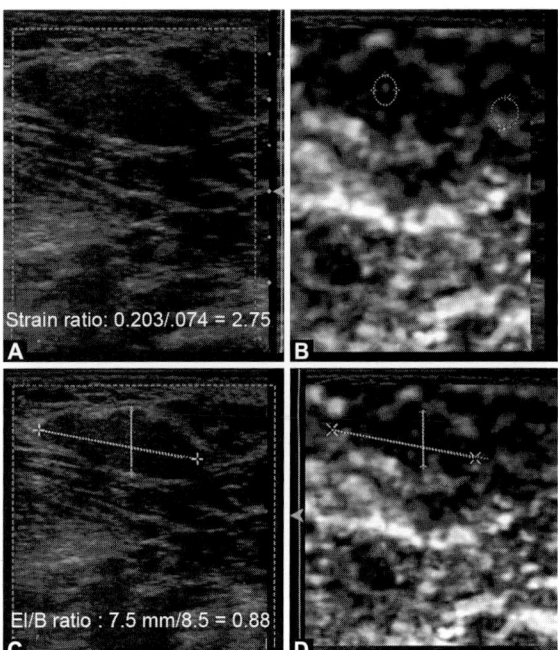

Figs 9.6A to D Ultrasonographic shows a well-defined oval, wider than taller isoechoic lesion having smooth margins with posterior acoustic enhancement and lateral shadowing is noted in the axillary tail of the left breast. The lesion appears hypovascular. Elastographic revealed EL/B ratio: 0.88, Elasticity score: 3 and Strain ratio: 2.75. Findings are of fibroadenoma in the left axillary tail (BIRAD's III)

GYNECOMASTIA

Gynecomastia is nonneoplastic enlargement of the male breast, it may be unilateral or bilateral. There is increase in glandular and stromal element in the enlarged breast. The ductal structure of the male breast is enlarged, elongated and branches out with ensheathing connective tissue. It has a bimodal prevalence first seen around the time of puberty, with a second peak beginning around age 50 years. Adolescence gynecomastia is often unilateral generally between ages of 12–15 years. Gynecomastia occurs in response to hormonal stimulation, mainly oestrogen, in men over 50 years of age is referred as senescent gynecomastia senescent gynecomastia is usually bilateral.

Mammography can show: (a) Nodular pattern in patients with gynecomastia for less than one year duration. Mammography reveals a nodular subareolar density. (b) Dendritic pattern in patients with gynecomastia for longer than one year duration. Mammograms show a dendritic subareolar density with posterior linear projections radiating into the surrounding tissue. (c) Diffuse glandular gynecomastia seen in patients receiving exogenous estrogen. Fan or Flame shaped centrally symmetric density is noted extending back from immediately beneath the nipple towards the upper outer quadrant of the breast **(Figs 9.7A to C)**.

Ideally there is no reason to perform ultrasound on a patient who has gynecomastia on mammography. However, ultrasonography will reveal an appearance similar to that seen in the developing preadolescent female breast bud. Differentials include pseudogynecomastia.

Phyllodes Tumor

Phyllodes or phyllodes tumor or cystosarcoma phyllodes tumors of the breast are uncommon, accounting for less than 1% of all breast tumors. Phyllodes tumors are extremely rare in men. The name "phyllodes," in Greek means leaflike. They can occur at any age. They can develop in people of any age. Phyllodes tumor is the most commonly occurring nonepithelial neoplasm of the breast. Most tumors are benign however their potential for malignancy should not be underestimated. They grow quickly, but rarely spread outside the breast. They are relatively large tumors and have a smooth, sharply demarcated texture and are freely movable **(Figs 9.8A to C)**.

The etiology of phyllodes tumors is unknown. They require surgery to reduce recurrence.

Carcinoma Breast

Breast elastography is a sonographic technique that provides additional characterization information on breast lesions over conventional sonography and mammography. This technique provides information on the strain or hardness of a lesion, similar to a clinical palpation examination. Two techniques are now available for clinical use: strain (compression-based elastography) and shear wave elastography. Initial evaluation of these techniques in clinical trials suggests that they may substantially improve the characterization of breast lesions as benign or malignant. This improvement may substantially reduce the number of benign biopsies performed. Elastography can be performed by several methods and is now available from several manufactures.

In the diagnostic evaluation of benign lesions, elastography improves diagnostic confidence and may in the future help to reduce the number of core biopsies. Features suggesting malignancy on elastography breast are EL/B mode ratio greater than 1, elasticity score of 4 or 5 and strain ratio of more than 3 **(Figs 9.9 and 9.10)**.

Carcinoma Breast with Metastases

Availability of baseline CT after mastectomy helps in the early identification of recurrent tumor which often becomes difficult by fibrosis after radiation, postoperative scar tissue, and poor surrounding fat. Regional lymph nodes and bones, including vertebrae should be carefully examined such that metastases

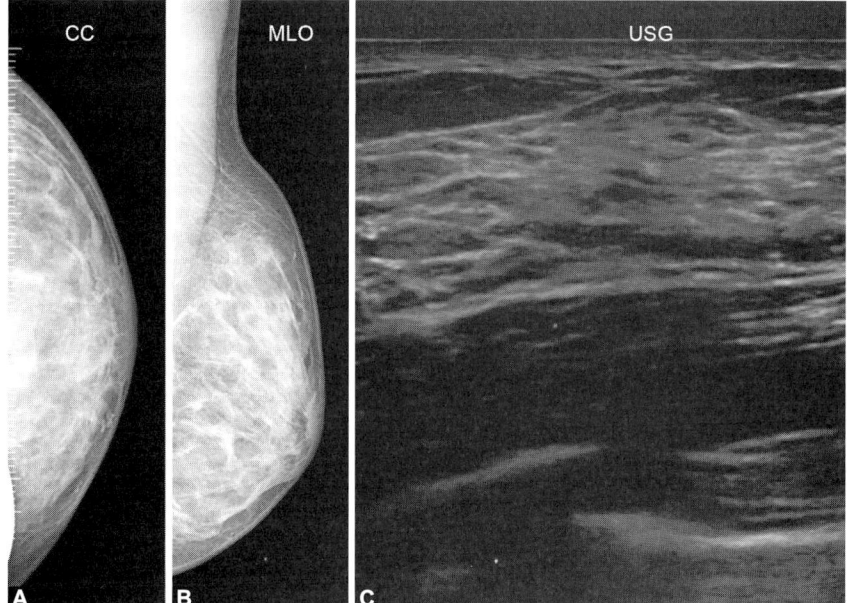

Figs 9.7A to C Mammography shows a fan shaped centrally symmetric density extending backwards from the nipple on the left side suggestive of diffuse glandular pattern of gynecomastia. No evidence of any spiculated mass lesion or microcalcifications. Ultrasound shows hyperechoic breast tissue in the subcutaneous plane on the left side. No focal solid cystic lesion or calcification seen

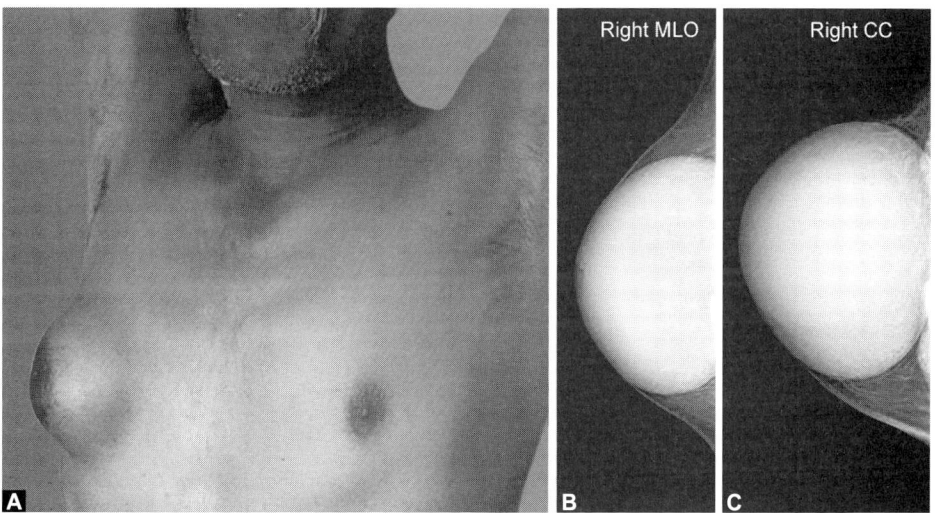

Figs 9.8A to C A 47 years old male with history of gradually increasing painless, firm, mobile, well-circumscribed, nontender swelling of right breast (A). Mammogram show a large dense encapsulated lesion with smooth margins, typical appearance of phyllodes tumor *(For color version, see plate 4)*

are not overlooked. In addition to mammography CT and MRI provide relevant useful information more so on postoperative status. Two postoperative are shown where CT **(Figs 9.11 and 9.12)** has been very informative.

Carcinoma in Situ

Carcinoma in situ (CIS) is an early form of carcinoma defined by the absence of invasion of surrounding tissues. It involves only the place in which it has begun and has not spread. It is an early-stage tumor. At CIS stage there is no mass lesion and the lesion is flat or follows the existing architecture of the organ. CIS is considered a precursor or incipient form of cancer that may, if left untreated long enough, transform into a malignant neoplasm. Carcinoma in situ is synonymous with high-grade dysplasia in most organs. It is usually treated much the same way as a malignant tumor.

Common sites for CIS are ductal carcinoma in situ (DCIS) of the breast, bladder, cervix, prostate, and Bowen's disease is squamous CIS of the skin.

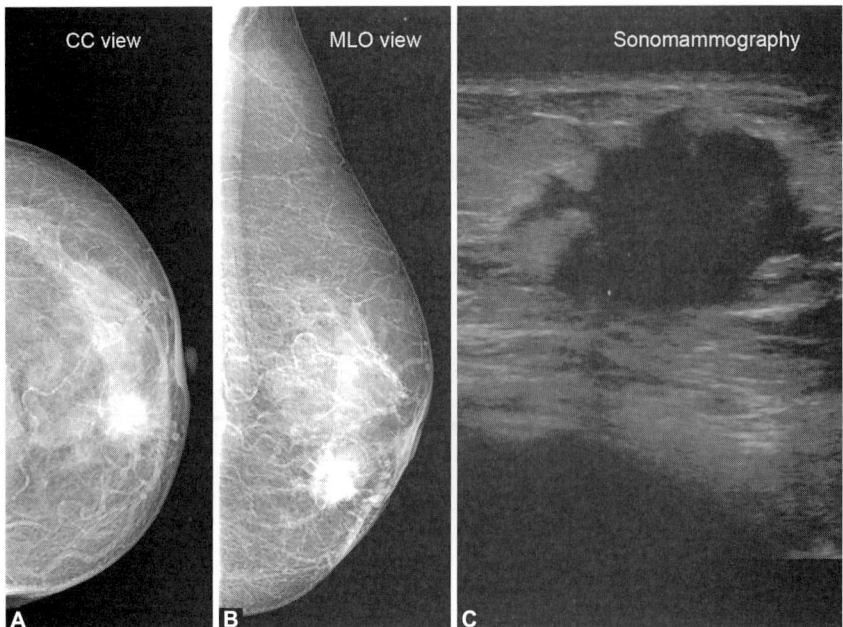

Figs 9.9A to C Mammography shows an irregular lesion with spiculated indistinct margins, focal asymmetry, and architectural distortion with few vascular calcifications

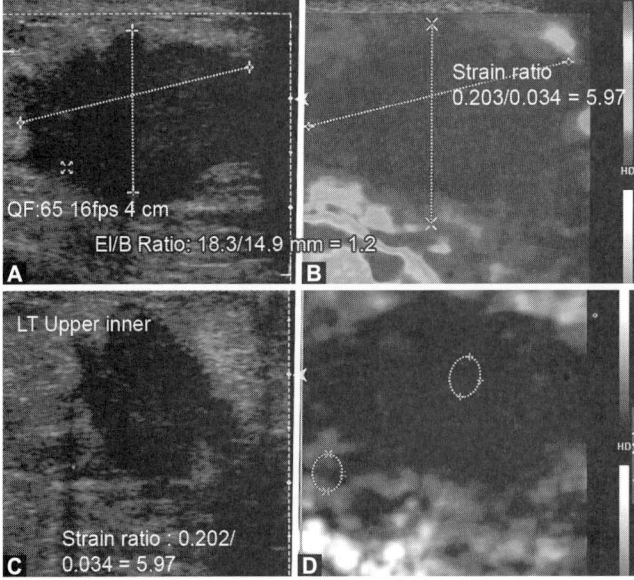

Figs 9.10A to D Breast ultrasonography shows heterogeneous, hypoechoic lesion with microlobulations or angulated margins. Elastography breast shows EI/B mode (elastography imaging B mode) ratio—1.2, strain ratio—5.97 and elasticity score—5 (not seen in figure). The lesion was categorized as BI-RADS 5 *(For color version, see plate 4)*

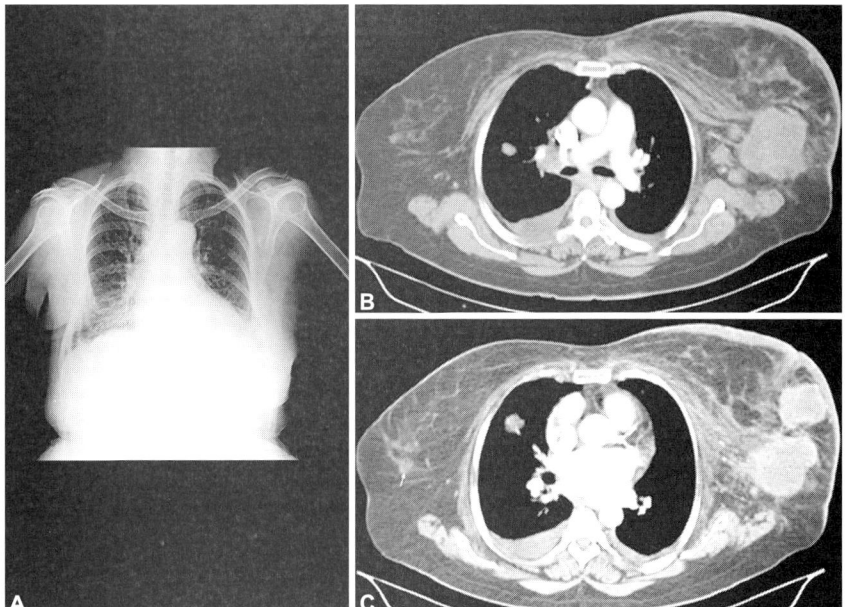

Figs 9.11A to C X-ray chest shows absence of right breast which has been surgically excised for carcinoma breast (A). Fifteen months after surgery CT scan done shows two large solid irregular marginated lesions seen in the left breast parenchyma, infiltrating into the adjacent fat and pectoralis muscles with thickening of the skin. Multiple enlarged axillary nodes are present (B and C). Right breast also shows two small nodular lesions in the parenchyma infiltrating into the adjacent fat (B). Left sides nipple was retracted (C). Multiple nodular metastatic lesions are seen in lungs, with bilateral pleural effusion. Sclerotic metastatic deposit was seen in the dorsal vertebral body(not seen in the figure)

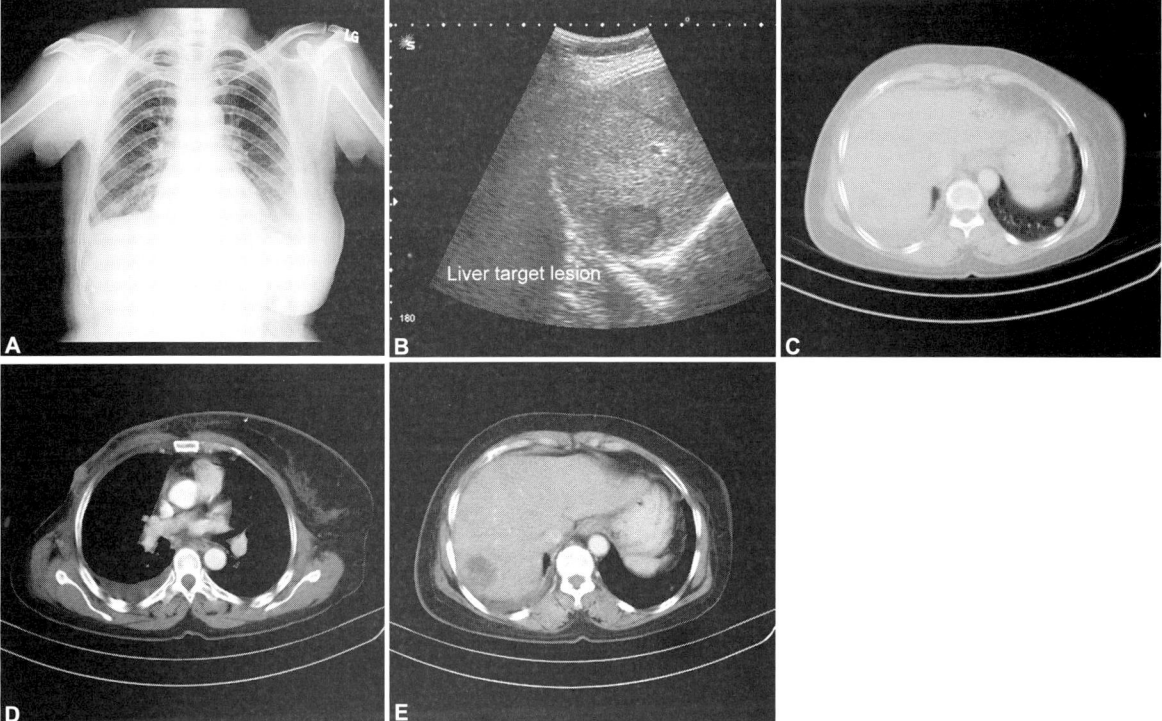

Figs 9.12A to E There is history of right mastectomy (chest PA view-A), patient developed complaints of breathlessness with recurrence of tumor in the right breast area in form of soft tissue nodules, well appreciated on CT (D). USG revealed a hypoechoic well-defined metastatic lesion in right lobe of liver (B), seen on CT as a peripherally enhancing hypodense lesion (C). CT chest shows multiple small metastatic nodules in the lungs (E) with right sided pleural effusion

10
Miscellaneous

Imaging in Sickle Cell Anemia

Sickle cell anemia (SCA) is rigid deformation of the cell caused by production of abnormal hemoglobin, which binds with other abnormal hemoglobin molecules within the red blood cell. Deformation impairs the ability of the cell to pass through small vascular channels; this result in sludging and congestion of vascular beds, followed by tissue ischemia and infarction. Infarction is common throughout the body in SCA, and it is responsible for the earliest clinical manifestation, the acute pain crisis, which results from marrow infarction. Such over a time insults result in medullary bone infarcts and epiphyseal osteonecrosis. White matter and gray matter infarcts are seen in the brain causing functional neurologic deficits and cognitive impairment.

In lung damage ranges from acute processes, such as pneumonia and acute chest syndrome (ACS), to chronic entities, such as pulmonary fibrosis. The radiographic findings of ACS is single or multiple areas of pulmonary consolidation. Abnormal chest radiographs show middle and lower lobe airspace disease more commonly than upper lobes. Pleural effusions are frequent and do not help differentiate infectious from ACS.

Skeletal complications of SCA include infarction and osteomyelitis. Bone marrow infarction is thought to be the underlying cause of most pain crises in SCA. On CT, an infarct initially manifests as disruption of the normal trabecular architecture and may be difficult to detect. As infarction progresses, it appears as circular area of decreased attenuation. MR imaging is the most sensitive, as it may show abnormality with a few days after the ischemic insult. Infarction appears as an area of high signal intensity on T2-weighted and inversion recovery images. Abnormal periosteal signal intensity and soft-tissue changes may also be seen at MR imaging, making differentiation between infarction and osteomyelitis difficult.

Hand-foot syndrome or dactylitis is the term used to describe painful, swollen hands and feet accompanied by fever. It is generally seen in children younger than four years of age and is rare after seven years of age. Following clinical manifestation of dactylitis, periostitis with subperiosteal new bone is typically evident. There is also cortical thinning, irregular attenuation of the medullary spaces, and an overall moth-eaten appearance of the involved bones of the hands and feet.

Osteomyelitis, although much less common than infarction, may be difficult to discriminate from infarction. MR imaging is the preferred modality for evaluating marrow. Osteomyelitis demonstrates abnormally elevated signal intensity in the marrow on T2-weighted and inversion recovery images. The edges of this abnormal-signal intensity area are typically ill-defined. The most sensitive and specific pulse sequence is T1-weighted, performed with fat saturation after administration of gadolinium.

Stroke, atrophy, and cognitive impairment are major consequences of SCA. Infarction in patients with SCA is an ischemic insult. Acute infarcts exhibit low signal intensity on T1-weighted images and high signal intensity on T2-weighted images. Between approximately 1 week and 1 month after onset, the infarcts become just slightly hypointense on T1-weighted images and remain high signal intensity on T2-weighted images. The chronic infarct exhibits low signal intensity on T1-weighted images and high signal intensity on T2-weighted images, developing better-defined margins and signs of focal atrophy. Infarcts demonstrate low attenuation areas on CT, becoming better defined and manifesting evidence of encephalomalacia with time.

The kidney in SCA has increased renal plasma flow and increased glomerular filtration rate. These changes are thought to arise from compensatory hypersecretion of prostaglandins with vasodilatory effects. The glomerulus is large and hyperfiltrating and as a result develops glomerulosclerosis. Capillary obliteration and medullary necrosis and fibrosis result, usually of the papillary tips and manifest as papillary necrosis. At US, the kidneys may display normal echogenicity may be mildly echogenic or show increased medullary echogenicity with normal cortical echogenicity. Over a time, the kidneys may shrink if renal failure ensues. Papillary necrosis is evident at excretory urography, when rounded collections of contrast material are seen pooling in areas of papillary loss.

The infarcted spleen is replaced by fibrosis, with calcium and hemosiderin deposition. Over a time, with infarction, the spleen becomes small, dense, and calcified. This calcification may be visible at radiography and CT. The infracted, fibrosed spleen has low signal intensity, regardless of MR imaging pulse sequence, secondary to ferrocalcinosis. Sequestration syndrome is another splenic complication of SCA. At imaging, the spleen is larger than expected. It appears heterogeneous at US, with multiple hypoechoic areas, which may be seen at the periphery. Low-attenuation peripheral areas are seen on CT. In adult, the spleen will show high signal intensity at T1- and T2-weighted MR imaging, compatible with hemorrhage.

Pycnodysostosis

Pycnodysostosis is a rare autosomal recessive bone dysplasia characterized by osteosclerosis and short stature. Pycnodysotosis is a lysosomal disorder due to genetic deficiency in Cathepsin K which has been mapped to chromosome 1q21. Cathepsin K is important for normal osteoclast function. It is also known as Maroteaux-Lamy disease.

Patient is short stature, predisposed to fractures, longitudinal striation of the nails and with relatively wide hands and feet. The head is large, with a bird-like appearance of the face because of small facial bones with narrow mandible. The cranial sutures and fontanelles are widened and remain open. Distal part of the clavicle is absent. There is hypoplasia of the distal phalanges and absence of the ungual process, spina bifida is generally present

On imaging bone show increased density and narrowed medullary cavities and the tubular bones are more delicate, but normal in shape. The parietal bones frequently show wormian bones formation. The mastoids may be nonaerated. The paranasal sinuses and maxillary bones are. Hypoplasia of the mandible with almost total disappearance of the mandibular angle. There is poor dental formation, with a double row of teeth, permanent teeth usually appear on schedule. The orbital rims may be dense. Aplasia of the terminal phalanges of the hands and feet is seen. With shortening of other phalanges, metacarpals and metatarsals. There may be aplasia or hypoplasia of clavicle. The vertebrae are dense and of the infantile type. There may be spondylolysis, of the 5th lumbar component. The pelvis may show shallow acetabulum with increase in the angulation of the acetabulum.

Solitary Dense Vertebra

Increased density or osteosclerosis of the spongiosa of the vertebral bodies is observed in various diseases. The sclerosis may sometimes be diffuse and give the impression of an "ivory vertebra" as the spongiosa is replaced by homogeneous bony mass. In other cases, the spongiosa is atrophic with only increased prominence of the trabeculae or it is replaced by dense, spotty, irregular masses of bone. The radiographic finding of a solitary dense sclerotic vertebral body retaining normal size and contour without alteration in adjacent intervertebral disc spaces is the ivory vertebra sign. Various conditions are responsible for ivory vertebra. In adults, the most common include metastatic carcinoma, lymphoma, postradiation necrosis, and infection and Paget disease. Less common are chordoma, primary sarcomas, renal osteodystrophy, osteopetrosis pycnodysostosis, myelofibrosis, and fluorosis.

Radiographically, the vertebra is dense, sclerotic with possible involvement of the posterior elements. Adjacent intervertebral disc spaces are preserved. Lumbar vertebrae are more commonly involved. Computed tomography (CT) shows the sclerotic change involving most if not all of the affected vertebral body. Magnetic resonance imaging (MRI) shows decreased marrow signal intensity on T1-weighted sequences with mildly increased signal on fluid-sensitive sequences. Bone scan may show increased radionuclide uptake. Elevated SUV levels in PET examination are seen with neoplasm, fracture, and other metabolically active processes, such as infection.

Rib Notching

Rib notching is a radiologic sign where the surface of the rib is deformed. It can be unilateral or bilateral and can affect the superior or inferior surface of the rib. It can involve single rib or multiple ribs.

The differential diagnosis differs according to whether the notching is on the inferior or superior surface and unilateral or bilateral. It is also important to differentiate true rib notching from pseudo notching. Pseudo rib notching is irregular cortical thickening of the ribs as seen in tuberous sclerosis.

Causes of superior and inferior rib notching: Inferior rib notching may be seen in a wide variety of conditions and generally results from enlargement of some element of the neurovascular bundle. With coarctation the first and second intercostal arteries and ribs are not affected because they arise proximally from the costocervical trunk. Notching on the posterolateral inferior aspect of the ribs typically affects the 3rd to 9th ribs and reflects increased collateral flow through intercostal arteries at this site **(Table 10.1)**. The lower ribs are not affected unless the lower abdominal aorta is also involved. A preductal coarctation does not produce rib notching.

Bone Infarct

Bone infarct refers to a necrotic focus in the metaphyseal or diaphyseal regions, whereas osteonecrosis indicates the presence of ischemic cellular death of bone and bone marrow. Ischemic necrosis generally applies to areas of epiphyseal or subarticular involvement. Bone infarcts can be subdivided into four zones:
a. Central zone of cell death
b. Zone of ischemic injury
c. Zone of active hyperemia, and
d. Normal tissue.

Table 10.1 Causes of rib notching

Inferior rib notching	Superior rib notching	Causes of unilateral rib notching	Bilateral rib notching

• Enlarged collateral vessels
 – Coarctation of the aorta
 – Interrupted aortic arch
 – Subclavian artery obstruction
   - Takayasu disease
   - Blalock-Taussig shunt: involves only upper 2 rib spaces
 – AVM of the chest wall
 – SVC obstruction with enlarged venous collaterals
	• Enlarged collateral vessels
	 – Coarctation of the aorta
	 – Interrupted aortic arch
	 – Subclavian artery obstruction
	   - Takayasu disease
	   - Blalock-Taussig shunt: involves only upper 2 rib spaces
	 – AVM of the chest wall
	 – SVC obstruction with enlarged venous collaterals
	• Neurogenic tumors
	 – Schwannoma (usually single)
	 – Neurofibromatosis type 1 (rarely can be superior if neurofibroma is very large)
		• Coarctation of aorta proximal to left subclavian artery: Right sided rib notching
		• Coarctation of the aorta with an aberrant right subclavian artery: Left sided rib notching. Occurs when the aberrant right subclavian artery arises after the coarctation
		• Subclavian artery stenosis: Ipsilateral to the side of stenosis
		• Blalock-Taussig shunt: Ipsilateral to side of shunt. Due to division of all the branches of the first part of the subclavian artery performed during shunt creation
		• Neurofibromatosis of the intercostal nerves
		• Vascular malformations of the thoracic wall: Enlarged intercostal veins cause rib notching
		• Superior vena cava obstruction: Due to development of collateral channels to the inferior vena cava via the intercostal veins
			• Bilateral Blalock–Taussig shunt
			• Coarctation distal to both subclavian arteries

A mnemonic intended to assist remembering causes of superior rib notching is PORN-MCh: P polio, O osteogenesis imperfecta, R restrictive lung disease, N neurofibromatosis, M Marfans syndrome, C connective tissue disease, H hyperparathyroidism, and for mnemonic for inferior rib notching is C-PAST: C coarctation of aorta, P pulmonary oligemia, A aortic thrombosis, S subclavian obstruction, T Tausig Blalock obstruction

In sickle cell anemia, diaphyseal infarction of larger tubular bones, the proximal aspect of the femur is common. Radiographically, bone infarction appears initially as a linear radiodense shadow adjacent to the cortex, which may extend along the entire shaft. Subsequently, the cortex becomes thickened. A bone within bone appearance is seen, which is diagnostic of osteonecrosis, is seen beneath the cortical bone. Other bones that may be infarcted include those of the pelvis, spine and thorax. Increased radiodensity of bone and a coarsened trabecular pattern are typical. In addition, epiphyseal infarcts in sickle cell anemia may involve the capital femoral epiphysis, leading to an appearance simulating that of Legg-Calvé-Perthes disease (LCPD). Focal lucency and sclerosis, subchondral linear or curvilinear radiolucent shadows, collapse, and fragmentation are evident in involved epiphyses.

MR imaging (**Figs 10.1A to C**) is a very sensitive method for the early diagnosis of ischemic necrosis of bone. It appears to be more sensitive in this regard than standard bone scintigraphy.

Fibrous Dysplasia

Fibrous dysplasia is a benign disorder characterized by a tumor-like proliferation of fibro-osseous tissue. The cause of fibrous dysplasia is unknown. Fibrous dysplasia is usually found in the proximal femur, tibia, humerus, ribs, and craniofacial bones in decreasing order of incidence. Usually, only one bone is involved (monostotic fibrous dysplasia). Less often, multiple bones are involved (polyostotic fibrous dysplasia). The polyostotic form is generally more severe and is discovered earlier. This form can involve as few as two bones in the same limb or multiple bones throughout the skeleton. Males and females are equally affected by the disorder. Cases are usually diagnosed within the first three decades of life. It is usually asymptomatic, though pain and swelling may accompany the lesion.

Polyostotic fibrous dysplasia is known to have multiple associations with other disorders. The combination of polyostotic fibrous dysplasia, precocious puberty, and cafe au lait spots is called McCune Albright's syndrome. The association of fibrous dysplasia and soft tissue tumors has been given the name Mazabraud's syndrome. Other endocrine abnormalities including hyperthyroidism, Cushing's disease, thyromegaly, hypophosphatemia, and hyperprolactinemia have been associated with fibrous dysplasia.

Radiographically, fibrous dysplasia appears as a well circumscribed lesion in a long bone with a ground glass or hazy appearance of the matrix. There is a narrow zone of transition and no periosteal reaction or soft tissue mass. The lesions are normally located in the metaphysis or diaphysis with occasional focal thinning of the overlying cortex due to scalloping from

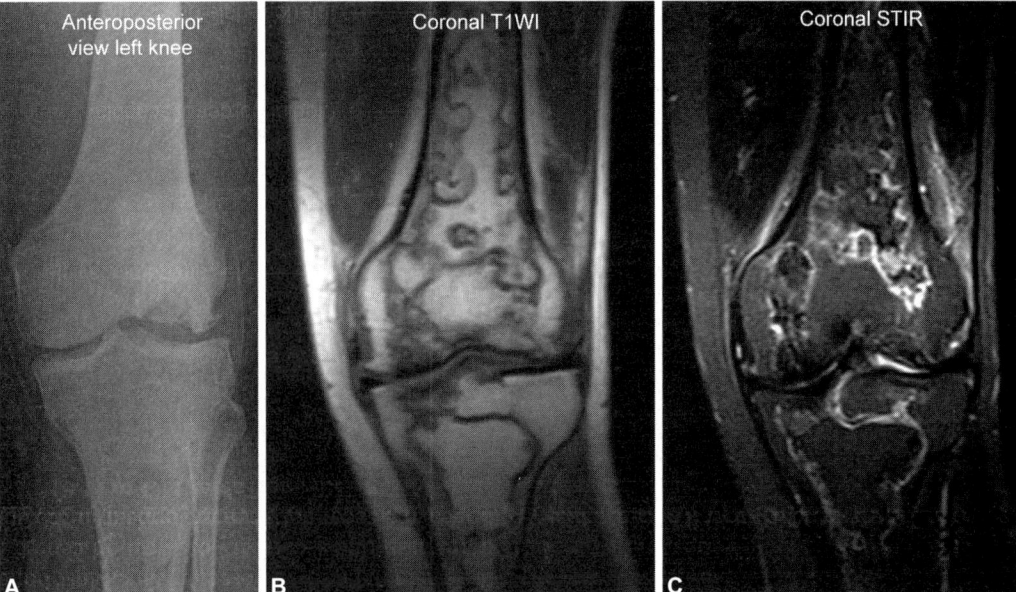

Figs 10.1A to C X-ray left knee AP view (A) shows fracture of the articular surface of lateral femoral condyle. T1WI (B) and STIR images (C) show multiple geographic hyperintense lesions in the epiphysis, metaphysis and diaphysis of femur and tibia. The infarcts have sharply defined serpentine borders of low signal intensity on proton density imaging. Subchondral fracture in the lateral femoral condyle is seen

within. The radiological appearance can also be cystic, pagetoid, or dense and sclerotic. Repeated fractures through lesions in the proximal femur can result in the formation of a shepherd's crook deformity. MRI is helpful in delineating the extent of the lesion (**Figs 10.2 and 10.3**) and identifying possible pathological fractures and also sarcomatous change within the lesion. The lesions shows heterogeneous intermediate signal on T1W images and heterogeneously low signal on T2W images but may have regions of higher signal. Post contrast T1W images show heterogeneous contrast enhancement. Bone scans demonstrate increased tracer uptake on Tc^{99} bone scans.

Kienböck's Disease

Kienböck's disease is osteonecrosis of the carpal lunate bone that often follows a history of trauma. It is more common in adults but is occasionally seen in children, typically athletic adolescents and particularly gymnasts. The patient may experience progressive pain, swelling and disability. On radiographs the lunate may have a normal architecture and density initially, although a linear or compression fracture may be present. Later the lunate bone becomes denser than the other carpal bones and eventually the entire lunate may collapse and fragment. Complications include scapholunate dissociation and secondary degenerative joint disease. The two features of the lunate that may predispose this bone to injury and subsequent osteonecrosis are its vulnerable blood supply and its fixed position in the wrist, which leads to stress.

MR imaging shows initial decreased signal on T1 and increased signal on T2-weighted or STIR sequences reflecting edema. Later there will be decreased signal or signal void on T1 and T2-weighted sequences reflecting bone death or sclerosis (**Figs 10.4A to D**), this signal void may be limited to the med body of the lunate. There may be an associated synovitis seen best on intravenous contrast-enhanced fat suppressed T1-weighted sequences.

Avascular Necrosis Scaphoid

Avascular necrosis (AVN) or osteonecrosis frequently affects the proximal pole of the scaphoid bone after trauma to this region; the distal pole is less likely to undergo necrosis. Sometimes this condition is not apparent on radiographs until 4–8 weeks after injury. Delayed fracture union or nonunion, collapse of the necrotic segment, and secondary degenerative joint disease may complicate this process. Diagnosis may be facilitated by MR imaging or scintigraphy. A spontaneous osteonecrosis of the scaphoid, or Preiser's disease, has also been reported. The radiographic findings resemble those of Kienböck's disease.

MR imaging shows initial decreased signal on T1 and increased signal on T2-weighted or STIR sequences (**Figs 10.5A and B**) images reflecting edema. Later develop decreased signal or signal void on T1- and T2-weighted sequences reflecting bone death or sclerosis.

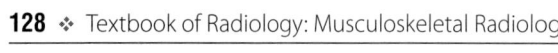

Figs 10.2A to F CT topogram (A) reveals diffuse thickening of calvarium. Axial CT (B) reveals diffuse thickening of calvarium, skull base with ground glass appearance. Sagittal T1W (C), sagittal coronal and axial T2-weighted images (D to F) shows diffuse thickening of calvarium, skull base and maxillofacial bones

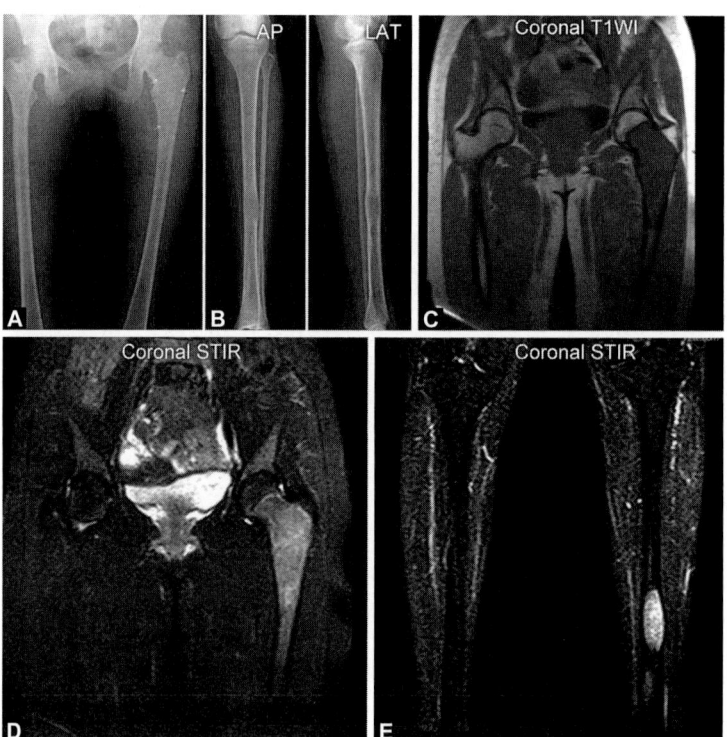

Figs 10.3A to E Fifteen-year-old female patient presented with complaint of left leg pain since seven months. X-ray of both hips and thigh AP (A) view shows expansile trabeculated lytic lesion in left femoral metadiaphysis causing expansion of medullary cavity with thinning of cortex. X-ray left leg including knee joint, AP and lateral view (B) shows expansile lytic lesion seen in distal third shaft of tibia causing expansion of medullary cavity and thinning of cortex. T1W coronal image shows iso to hypointense lesion in meta-diaphyseal region of left femur causing expansion of medullary cavity and thinning of cortex. Coronal STIR image (D) shows the lesion as hyperintense. STIR coronal (E) image of left thigh shows hyperintense lesion in distal third of left tibia causing expansion of medullary cavity and thinning of cortices. These findings suggest diagnosis of polyostotic fibrous dysplasia

Miscellaneous ❖ 129

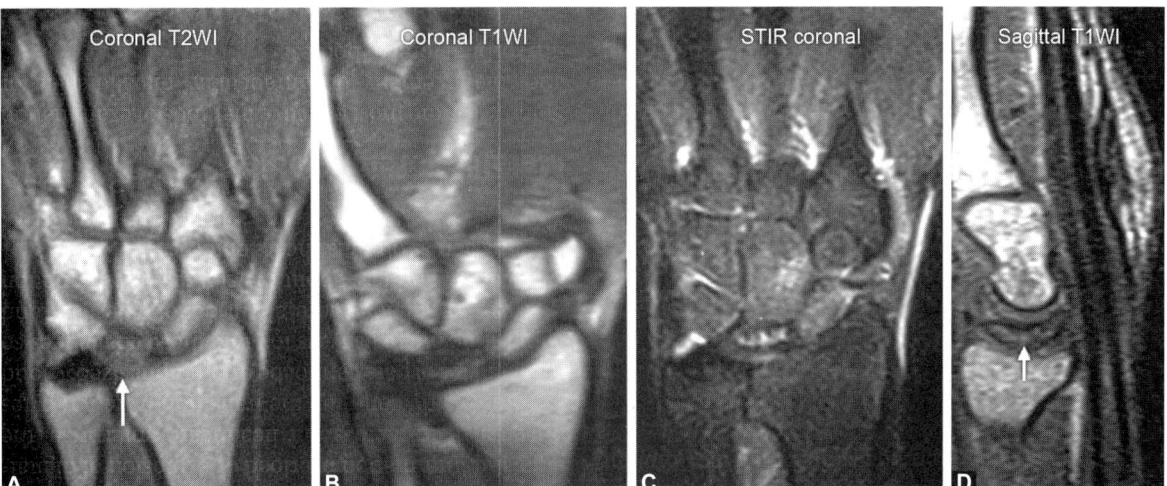

Figs 10.4A to D A 20-year-old male patient with history of wrist pain on MR shows abnormal hyperintense signal with marrow edema on coronal T2WI (A) and STIR (C) in lunate bone, appearing hypointense on coronal T1WI (B) and sagittal T1WI (D) Findings are suggestive of Kienböck's disease

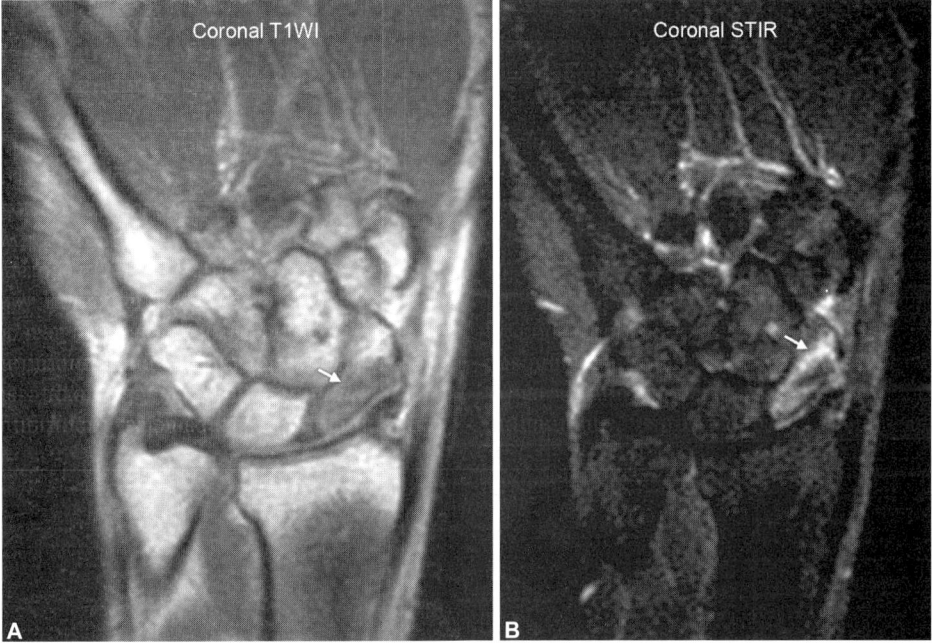

Figs 10.5A and B Coronal T1W image (A) reveals hypointense signal in the scaphoid appearing hyperintense on coronal STIR (B) image features consistent with AVN scaphoid

Hyperostosis Frontalis Interna

Etiology of hyperostosis frontalis interna is unknown, it is benign overgrowth of the inner table of the frontal bone. It is seen commonly seen in older females. It is bilateral and symmetrical, and may extend to parietal bones. The skull thickening is generally sessile rarely nodular, and may be focal or diffuse **(Figs 10.6A to E)**. It does not extend across the midline at the sagittal suture. It has no differential diagnosis. However, if there is variation in imaging from above, following should be considered: Paget's disease, fibrous dysplasia, sclerotic metastases and meningioma.

Renal Osteodystrophy

The group of musculoskeletal abnormalities associated with all pathologic features of bone in patients with chronic renal failure and is referred as renal osteodystrophy. This includes: (a) Osteomalacia in adults and rickets in children (b) hyperparathyroidism (c) Soft-tissue calcifications (d) Osteosclerosis (e) Soft tissue calcifications and vascular calcifications. In this there is primary retention of phosphate by abnormal kidneys results in hyperphosphatemia, which causes hypocalcemia, resulting in secondary hyperparathyroidism. Therefore, the spectrum of

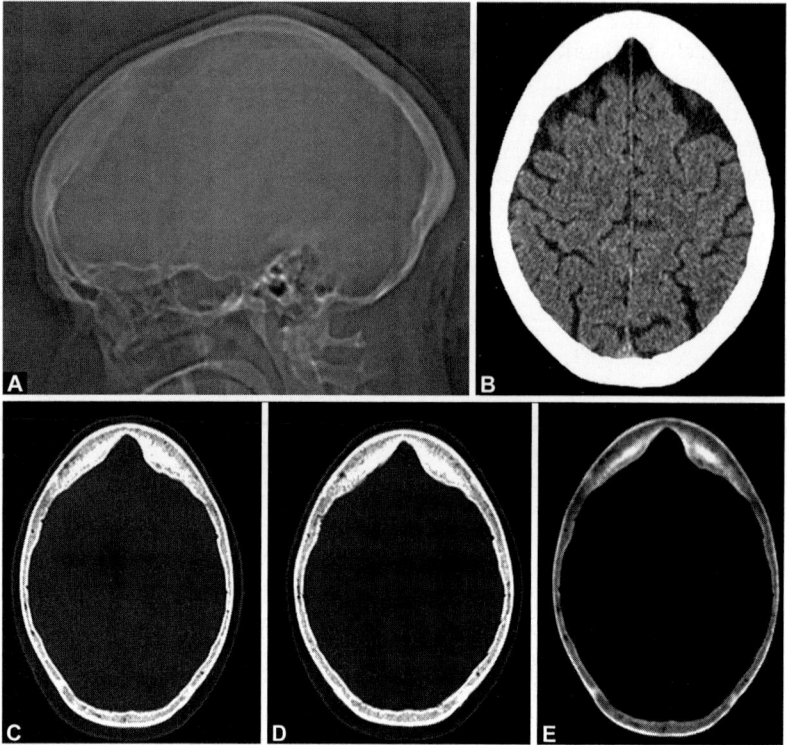

Figs 10.6A to E Incidental finding of hyperostosis frontalis interna in a 62-year-old female on scanogram (A) and CT axial sections on different windows (B to E)

clinical and radiographic findings in renal osteodystrophy may be a manifestation of any of these disorders.

Clinical Features

Renal osteodystrophy often present with nonspecific signs and symptoms like weakness, bone pain. Presentation varies markedly with age. Adults may present with findings of osteomalacia, where as children show growth retardation. Similarly complications depend on the patient's age. The most common is fracture, which may be insufficiency fractures through osteomalacic bone or pathologic fractures through brown tumors or amyloid deposits. Dialysis patients may experience carpal tunnel syndrome, osteomyelitis, septic arthritis, and osteonecrosis. Renal transplant patients may experience osteonecrosis, tendinitis, tendon rupture, and fracture.

On imaging: (a) osteopenia is often seen early in the course of the disease (b) Thinning of cortices and trabeculae (c) Salt and pepper appearance of skull (d) Subperiosteal resorption: characteristic subperiosteal resorption may be seen on radial aspects of middle phalanges of index and long fingers.

Rugger-jersey spine seen as sclerosis of the vertebral body and its end plates. Demineralization is usually subperiosteal, however it may involve joint margins, endosteal, subchondral, subligamentous areas, and cortical bone. Soft tissue calcification when seen can be well appreciated. Amyloid deposition in and around joint erosion be looked for. There may be fractures.

Ozone Therapy

Back pain affects a large percentage of world's population. It is a very disturbing symptom and the most common etiology is herniated disc lesion, which needs treatment with least invasive procedure. The newer modality for treating it is use of intradiscal oxygen-ozone therapy. In 1998 Muto and Avella suggested intradiscal injection of ozone for disc herniation under CT guidance, this was followed by successful outcome reported by many European centers.

Ozone is a tri-atomic oxygen molecule (O_3), with a different molecular structure than oxygen. Ozone is produced from pure medical grade oxygen with the help of high voltage electrical discharge. Medical ozone is a mixture of oxygen and ozone of different concentration. It is always freshly prepared on site (in a special generator) for immediate administration. Most of its actions are due to the active oxygen atom liberated from breaking down of ozone molecule. Besides its action as bactericidal, fungicidal, virucidal agent, it activates cellular metabolism, modulates the immune system and increases and activates body's own antioxidants.

In case of prolapsed inter-vertebral disc: Ozone's action is due to the active oxygen atom liberated from it, and attaches with the proteoglycan bridges in the nucleus pulposus causing its degradation. They are broken down and are no longer capable of holding water. This causes dehydration and resorption of the disc hernia. As a result disc shrinks and mummified and there is decompression of nerve roots. Ozone has analgesic and anti-inflammatory effects as it modifies mediators of inflammation and pain.

The protocol involves a 22 gauge 12 cm long needle is introduced by percutaneous route, needle through needle into the affected disc, using the tunnel view under fluoroscopic guidance. The position of the needle is confirmed by AP and lateral view of the spine and 3–7 mL of oxygen-ozone mixture at a concentration of 30 µg/mL is injected into the center of the disc by ozone resistant syringe over a period of 15–20 seconds.

Benefits of ozone nucleolysis treatment: It is a minimally invasive treatment with a negligible cost and rare side effects. It has no contraindications and it does not require hospitalization. It produced an improvement of the clinical, biochemical parameters and on imaging. Cervical disc lesions need less ozone therapy sessions (2–4 sessions) to eliminate the pain, compared to lumbar disc lesions which need between 6 and 10 sessions to obtain the results.

Ozone nucleolysis is a percutaneous procedure almost devoid of serious complications with high success rate of nearly 90% and with a low recurrence rate. An attenuation of the symptoms, and resumption of daily activities in over 80 % of patients.

Geode

Geode is a defined lytic lesion in the periarticular area. The term geode is borrowed from a geology meaning a rounded pocket of gas in a mineral specimen. Geode is seen as a cyst or cystic erosion in a bone end. Cyst is a cavity lined with epithelium. However geode or subchondral bone cysts are not necessarily lined with epithelium.

Geode formation takes place possibly when synovial fluid is forced into the subchondral bone, causing a cystic collection of joint fluid, or following a bone contusion, in which the contused bone forms a cyst. Geodes are seen in (a) rheumatoid arthritis (b) degenerative joint disease (c) avascular necrosis and (d) calcium pyrophosphate dihydrate crystal deposition disease.

Subchondral radiolucencies are frequently without cavitation and uniformly without an epithelial lining. Subchondral bone cysts may result from pressure or stress on articular cartilage and subchondral bone, leading to synovial fluid intrusion. Bone cysts frequently occur in association with joint space loss and bone eburnation; communication with the joint cavity may or may not be present **(Figs 10.7A to D)**. Geodes are common in many types of articular

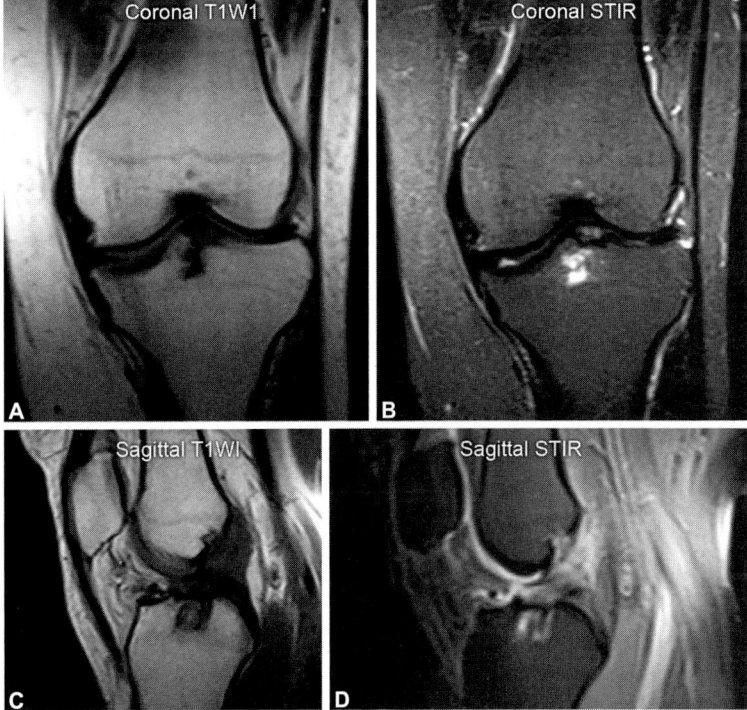

Figs 10.7A to D Subarticular T1WI (A) shows hypointense lesion measuring 6 mm just beneath. The tibial spine appearing hyperintense on STIR image (B). Subarticular geode appearing hypointense on sagittal T1W image (C) and hyperintense on STIR images (D)

diseases particularly osteoarthritis, rheumatoid arthritis and osteonecrosis. Geodes rarely cause problems by themselves but are often misdiagnosed leading to unnecessary biopsy might be performed on the basis of the differential of an epiphyseal lesion.

Magnetic Susceptibility Artifact

Magnetic susceptibility is tendency of material to become magnetized when placed in magnetic field. Caused by material with large differences in susceptibility create local disturbance in magnetic field resulting in nonlinear changes of resonant frequency, which in turn creates image distortion and signal changes leading to signal void in image.

Ferromagnetic metal artifacts show up as characteristic geometric distortion with a region of near zero signal intensity adjacent to a bright region. Removal of the metal object eliminates this type of artifact. Patient related extrinsic type magnetic susceptibility artifact is caused by the internal fixating metallic implant **(Figs 10.8A to D)**.

Cloud Computing

Cloud computing is a term that involves delivering hosted services over the internet. Computing power is stored in the cloud and one can use what one need when one needs it, and when done with it, it gets released back to the cloud. The goal of cloud computing is to allow users to take benefit from all of these technologies, without the need for knowledge or expertise with each one of them. It aims to cut cost, and help the users focus on their core activity instead of being impeded by IT obstacles. The origin of the term *cloud computing* is not clear. The expression *cloud* is used in science for a large conglomeration of objects that visually appear from a distance as a cloud. Cloud computing has created virtualization. Virtualization is an operating system, a server, a storage device or network resources. Virtualization software allows a physical computing device to be electronically separated into one or more virtual devices, each of which can be easily used and managed to perform computing task.

The power of cloud computing for radiology, particularly for its large content storage and an online digital low-cost platform, may just look at the media and entertainment (M and E) industry which have huge ever-growing libraries of digital media in petabytes **(Table 10.2)**, they need to archive for infinity and stream on-demand. The imaging department of the future in general will have to deal a lot more intelligently with data. Being on the edge of data and information overload or explosion of digital-imaging realm across our healthcare enterprise, the need to swiftly continue the transition from terabytes to petabytes of data cannot be over emphasized. Cloud computing offers us ways to tame these challenges so that we are talking more about actionable data and knowledge, and less about the storage of information systems across our healthcare enterprise.

Metallic Foreign Bodies

Spiral CT is the most effective methods of examination and management of intraocular, maxillofacial or intraorbital foreign bodies.

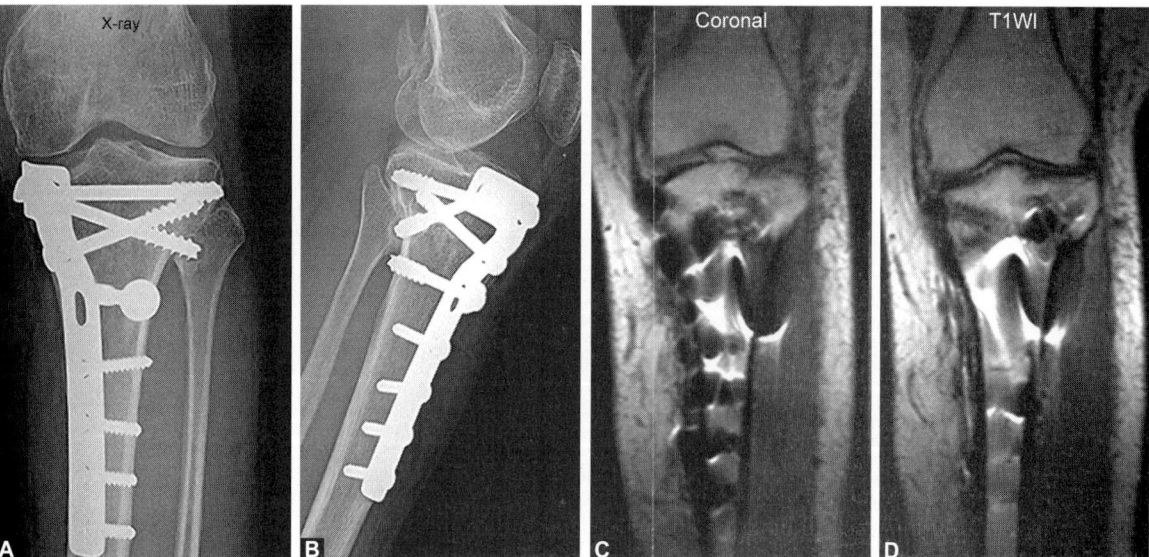

Figs 10.8A to D X-ray left leg anteroposterior (AP) and lateral views leg (A and B), tibia shows internal fixating metallic implant and coronal MR T1WI (C and D) shows susceptibility artifact caused by the internal fixating metallic implant

Table 10.2 How big is petabyte and other data storage units in "Globally inter connected database" by Julian Bunn

Unit	Bytes	Equivalent space
Byte	8 Bits	A single character
Kilobyte	1000	A short story
Megabyte	1 000 000	A small novel or a 3.5 inch floppy disk
Gigabyte	1 000 000 000	A pickup truck filled with paper or a movie at TV quality or 10 meters of shelved books
Terabyte	1 000 000 000 000	10 Terabytes equal to the printed collection of the US Library of Congress
Petabyte	1 000 000 000 000 000	2 Petabytes equal to all US academic research libraries
Exabyte	1 000 000 000 000 000 000	5 Exabytes equal to all words ever spoken by human beings
Zettabyte	1 000 000 000 000 000 000 000	
Yottabyte	1 000 000 000 000 000 000 000 000	
Xenottabyte	1 000 000 000 000 000 000 000 000 000	
Shilentnobyte	1 000 000 000 000 000 000 000 000 000 000	
Domegemegrottebyte	1 000 000 000 000 000 000 000 000 000 000 000	

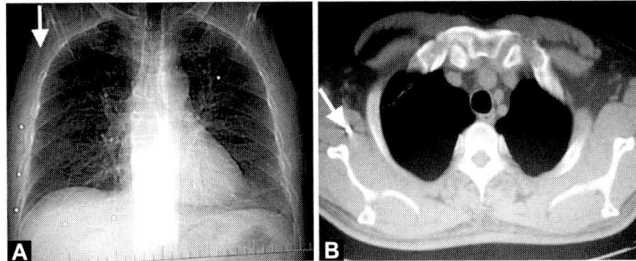

Figs 10.9A and B (A) X-ray chest shows multiple radio-opaque metallic density foreign bodies (about 7), these are 12 Bore gun pellets scattered over the chest, majority appear in the chest wall. (B) Axial CT section shows a pallet (CT value 3112 HU) in the anterolateral aspect of right subscapularis muscle (arrow)

As it is a continuous scanning of a volume of the patients body during table movement, there is no section lost due to uneven breathing of the patient from one section to another, and can be achieved quality reconstruction in different planes. CT chest provides the exact location and count of the foreign bodies **(Figs 10.9A and B)**, and show if there is an associated fracture.

11
Ossification Centers

Ossification is the first area of a bone which starts to ossify, the point where ossification commences is termed as ossification center. There are two types of ossification centers: (a) The primary ossification center is the first area of a bone to start ossifying. It appears during prenatal development in the central part of each developing bone. In long bones the primary centers occur in the shaft and in other it occurs usually in the body of the bone. Usually bones have one primary center as in all long bones. Few bones like hip and vertebrae have multiple primary centers. (b) The secondary ossification center is the area of ossification that appears after the primary ossification center, most secondary ossification center appear during the postnatal and adolescent years. Most bones have more than one secondary ossification center. In long bones, the secondary centers appear in the epiphysis **(Figs 11.1 to 11.6 and Tables 11.1 to 11.6)**.

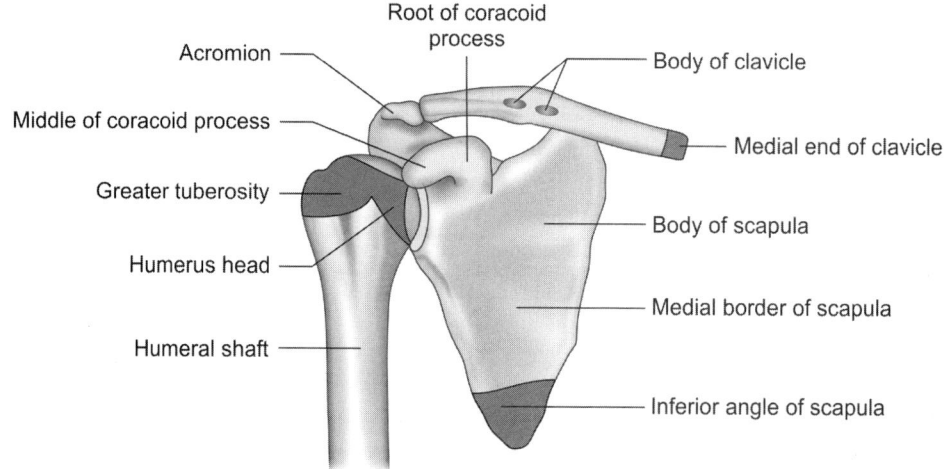

Fig. 11.1 Shoulder joint

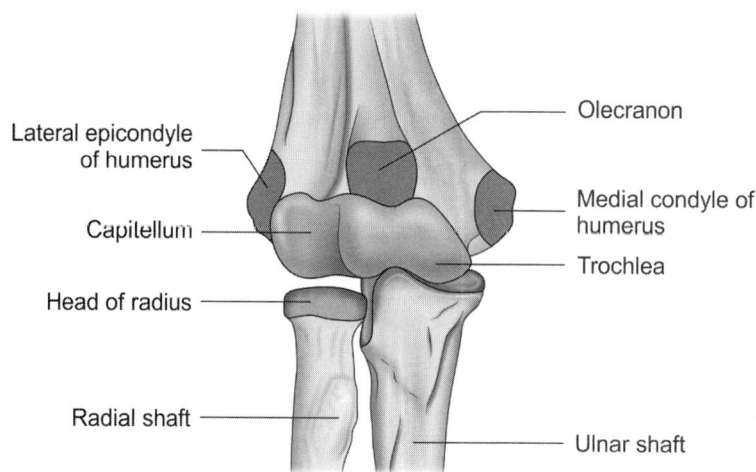

Fig. 11.2 Elbow joint

Ossification Centers ❖ **135**

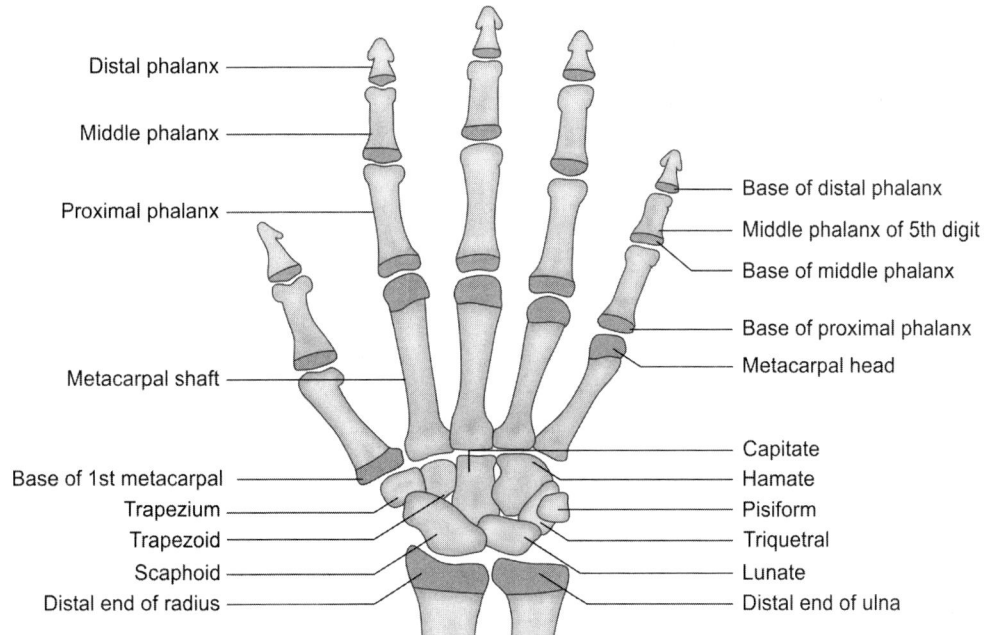

Fig. 11.3 Wrist and hand

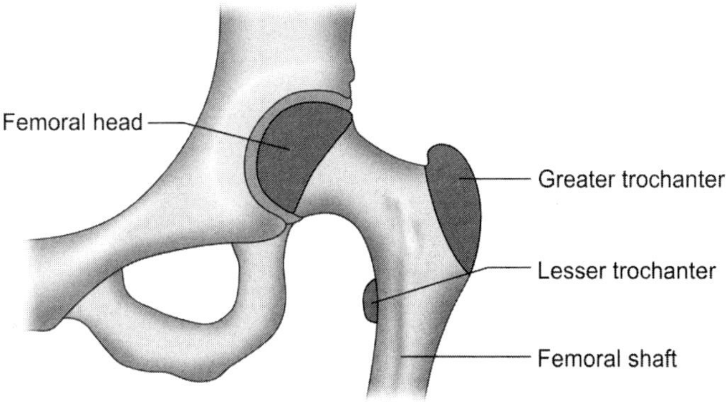

Fig. 11.4 Hip joint

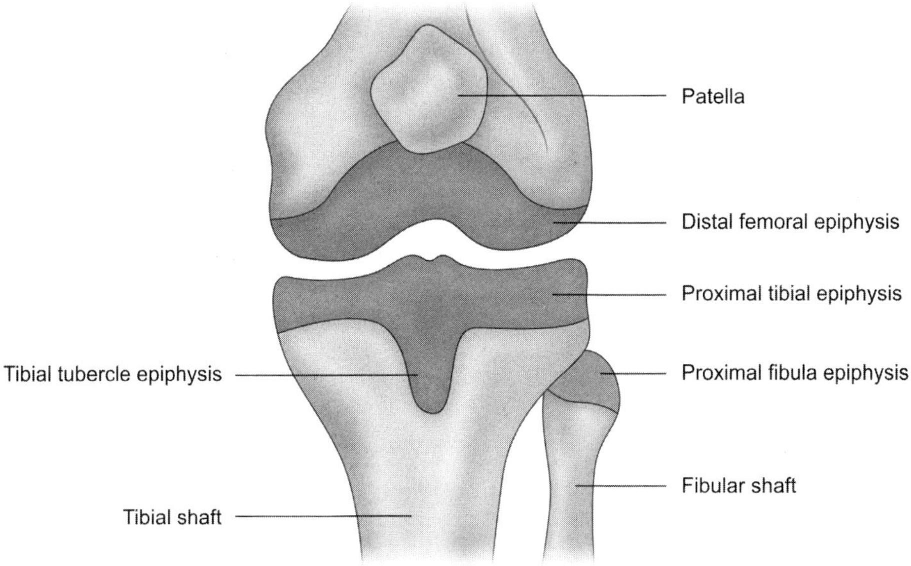

Fig. 11.5 Knee joint

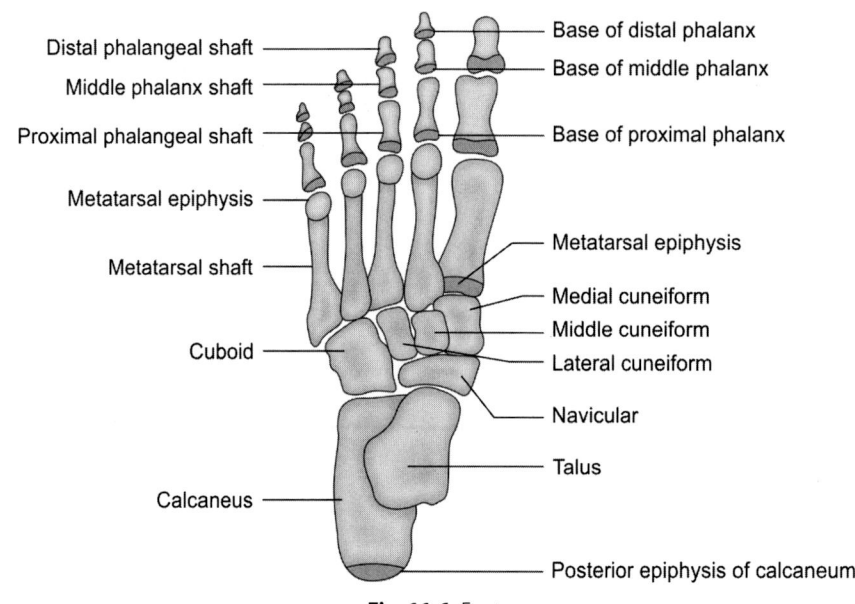

Fig. 11.6 Foot

Table 11.1 Shoulder joint

Bones	Ossification	
Body of scapula	8th week of fetal life	
Body of clavicle (two centers)	5th and 6th week of fetal life	
Shaft of humerus	8th week of fetal life	
Epiphysis	Appearance	Fusion
Head of humerus	1 year	
Greater tuberosity	3 years	
Lesser tuberosity	5 years	
Acromion process	15–18 years	25th year
Middle of coracoid process	1 year	15th year
Root of coracoid process	17th years	25th year
Inferior angle of scapula	14–20 years	22–25th year
Medial border of scapula	14–20 years	22–25th year
Medial end of clavicle	18–20 years	25th year

Table 11.2 Elbow joint

Bones	Ossification	
Radial shaft	8th week of fetal life	
Ulnar shaft	8th week of fetal life	
Epiphysis	Appearance	Fusion
Lateral epicondyle	10–12 years	17–18 years
Medial epicondyle	5–8 years	17–18 years
Capitellum	1–3 years	17–18 years
Head of radius	5–6 years	16–19 years
Trochlea	11th year	18th year
Olecranon process	10–13 years	16–20 years

Table 11.3 Wrist and hand

Bones	Ossification	
Capitate	4 months	
Hamate	4 months	
Triquetral	3 years	
Lunate	4–5 years	
Trapezium	6 years	
Trapezoid	6 years	
Scaphoid	6 years	
Pisiform	11 years	
Metacarpals	10th week of fetal life	
Proximal phalanges	11th week of fetal life	
Middle phalanges	12th week of fetal life	
Distal phalanges	9th week of fetal life	
Middle phalanx of 5th digit	14th week of fetal life	
Epiphysis	**Appearance**	**Fusion**
Lower end of radius	1–2 years	20th year
Lower end of ulna	5–8 years	20th year
Metacarpal heads	2.5 years	20th year
Base of proximal phalanges	2.5 years	20th year
Base of middle phalanges	3 years	18–20th years
Base of distal phalanges	3 years	18–20th years
Base of 1st metacarpal	2.5 years	20th year

Table 11.4 Hip joint

Bones	Ossification	
Proximal femoral shaft	7th week of fetal life	
Epiphysis	**Appearance**	**Fusion**
Femoral head	1 year	18–20 years
Greater trochanter	3–5 years	18–20 years
Lesser trochanter	8–14 years	18–20 years

Table 11.5 Knee joint

Bones	Ossification	
Tibial shaft	7th week of fetal life	
Fibular shaft	8th week of fetal life	
Patella	5 years	
Epiphysis	**Appearance**	**Fusion**
Proximal tibia	At birth	20th year
Tibial tubercle	5–10 years	20th year
Proximal fibular	4th year	25th year
Distal femur	At birth	20th year

Table 11.6 Foot

Bones	Ossification	
Calcaneus	6th month of fetal life	
Talus	6th month of fetal life	
Navicular	3–4 years	
Cuboid	At birth	
Lateral cuneiform	1 year	
Middle cuneiform	3 years	
Medial cuneiform	3 years	
Metatarsal shafts	8th–9th week of fetal life	
Phalangeal shafts	10th week of fetal life	
Epiphysis	*Appearance*	*Fusion*
Metatarsals	3 years	17–20 years
Proximal phalangeal base	3 years	17–20 years
Middle phalangeal base	3 years	17–20 years
Distal phalangeal base	5 years	17–20 years
Posterior calcaneal	5 years	At puberty

Index

Page numbers followed by *f* refer to figure and *t* refer to table.

A

Abscess, subperiosteal 33
Acromioclavicular
  degeneration 48
  joint 48, 50*f*
    osteoarthritis 48
Acro-osteolysis 27, 30, 43
Acro-osteosclerosis 30
Adamantinoma 72, 79
Addison's disease 24
Adipocytic tumors 102
Albers-Schönberg disease 2
Algodystrophy 18
Allergic alveolitis, extrinsic 112
Amebiasis 43
Ameloblastoma 89
Amyloidosis 83
Aneurysmal bone cyst 28, 72, 73, 78*f*
Angiolipoma 102
Angiomatoid fibrous histiocytoma 103
Angiomatosis 103
Angiomyofibroblastoma 102
Angiomyolipoma, extra-renal 102
Angiosarcoma 72
Anticonvulsant therapy 22
Aorta, coarctation of 126
Aortic
  aneurysm 43
  arch 126
Apert syndrome 31
Aponeurotic fibroma 102
Arcuate popliteal ligament 59
Areola 116
Arterial calcifications, multiple 119*f*
Arthritis 41
  infectious 37
  inflammatory 29, 32
  noninfective inflammatory 41
  psoriatic 27, 41, 44
  septic 36, 36*f*, 37, 58, 83
  tuberculous 36, 50
Arthrogryposis 30
Arthropathy
  neurogenic 71
  psoriatic 27
Atypical lipomatous tumor 102
Avascular necrosis 10, 18, 34, 56, 127
  scaphoid 127

B

Baker's cyst 106
Barton's fracture 15, 16*f*
Basal cell nevus syndrome 30
Beckwith-Wiedemann syndrome 30
Biconcave vertebrae 25
Bifid sternum, congenital 10
Biliary cirrhosis 43
Bird Fancier's disease 112
Blalock-Taussig shunt 126
Blood vessels 116
Body fibromatosis 102
Bone
  cyst, solitary 89
  density 84*f*
  dysplasia 30
  formation 43
  infarct 125
  island 11
  marrow replacement 24
  primary lymphoma of 98
  proximal segment of 15
  reaction 84*f*
  sarcomas 72
  scan 56
  scintigraphy 33
  tumors 72
    malignant 72*t*
    TMN classification of 73*t*
    WHO classification of 72
Bow tie sign 65
Bowel, neoplasms of 43
Breast 116
  anatomy 116
  cysts 117
  imaging reporting and data system 116
  lumps, multiple 118*f*
  pain 118*f*
  tissue 116
  ultrasonography 122*f*
Brodie's abscess 33, 34
Bronchiectasis 43
Bucket handle tear 65

C

Café au lait spots 126
Caffey's disease 42
Calcific densities 31
Calcium
  deficiency 24
  pyrophosphate dehydrate 30
Callus formation 12, 14*f*
Calvarial hyperostosis 26
Camurati-Engelmann disease 43
Carcinoma 112
  breast 120, 123*f*
  in situ 121
  thyroid 115*f*
Cardiovascular disorder 43
Carpal tunnel syndrome 15
Carpenter syndrome 31
Cartilage
  and osteogenic bone tumors, WHO classification of 72*t*
  tumors 72
Celiac sprue 43
Cell death, central zone of 125
Cellular angiofibroma 102
Cellulitis 40
Chauffeur's fracture 16, 16*f*
Chest 5
  syndrome, acute 124
  wall hamartoma 72
Chondroblastoma 72
Chondroid lipoma 102
Chondroma 72
  periosteal 72
Chondromatosis 76
  multiple 72
  synovial 72
Chondromyxoid fibroma 29, 72
Chondro-osseous tumors 103
Chordoma 72
Churg-Strauss syndrome 112
Cirrhosis, hepatic 43
Clavicle
  body of 136
  medial end of 136
Clear cell myomelanocytic tumor 103
Cleidocranial dysostosis 4
Codman's angle 32
Collagen vascular disease 27, 30
Collateral ligament 63
  normal lateral 65*f*
  normal medial 64*f*
Colle's fracture 14, 15, 15*f*
  complications of 15
Compartment syndrome 15, 17
Coracoid process, middle of 136
Cortex, buckling of 17
Costal cartilage calcification 109
Cruciate ligament 59, 63
  anterior 19, 63
  posterior 63, 65
Crystal deposition disease 30
Cushing's syndrome 24
Cyst
  bronchogenic 43
  dentigerous 89
  dermoid 110, 111*f*
  ganglion 50
  paralabral 49
  parameniscal 67, 69*f*

D

Dactylitis 31
Dermatomyositis 27, 30, 31
Dermoid cysts, types of 110
Diabetes 24, 30
  mellitus 27, 114
Diabetic osteomyelitis 33
Diaphyseal
  aclasis 76
  infarction 126
Distal
  fragment, dorsal displacement of 15*f*
  radioulnar joint, dislocation of 14*f*
Dorsal chip radius fracture 14
Double posterior cruciate ligament sign 65, 66

Down's syndrome 30, 31
Ductal carcinoma *in situ* 121
Dysplasia
  epiphysealis capitis femoris 10
  osteofibrous 72
  ectodermal 30
  fibrous 6, 43, 72, 86, 126

E

Eccentric multiloculated osteolytic lesion 80*f*
Ectopic hamartomatous thymoma 103
Ectrodactyly ectodermal dysplasia cleft lip syndrome 1
Ehlers-Danlos syndrome 30
Elastofibroma 102
Elbow joint 134*f*, 136*t*
Ellis-Van Creveld syndrome 31
Embryonal rhabdomyosarcoma 102
Empyema 43
Enchondroma 28, 72
Endocarditis, bacterial 43
Endosteal cellular proliferation 12
Epidermolysis bullosa 27
Epiphyseal dysplasia, multiple 3, 5*f*, 30
Epithelioid fibrosarcoma, sclerosing 102
Erdheim-Chester disease 72
Erythrocyte sedimentation rate 40
Escherichia coli 33, 37
Esophagus, neoplasms of 43
Ewing's sarcoma 32, 72, 94, 96
Extensor pollicis longus, rupture of 15

F

Fallen fragment sign 74
Fat
  embolism 17
  stripes, displacement of 16
Fatty tissue 116
  proliferation of 4*f*
Felty's syndrome 70
Femur, distal 137
Fibroadenomas 119
Fibroblastoma, desmoplastic 102
Fibrodysplasia ossificans progressiva 7
Fibroglandular tissue 117*f*
Fibroma
  desmoplastic 72
  non-ossifying 28
  nuchal type 102
Fibromatosis
  colli 102
  desmoid type 102
Fibromyxoid sarcoma, low grade 102
Fibromyxoma, odontogenic 90
Fibrosarcoma 72
  adult 102
  infantile 102
Fibrous dysplasia, polyostotic 87, 126
Fibula, distal 18
Fibular collateral ligament 59
Fine needle aspiration 33
Fingertip calcifications 31
Flipped meniscus sign 65
Fluorodeoxyglucose 38

Fluorosis 26, 32, 125
Foot 136*f*, 138*t*
Fracture 16
  avulsion 12, 13*f*, 16, 20, 49*f*
  carpal 21
    bone 14
  comminuted 12, 13*f*, 16
  complete 12, 12*f*, 16
  complications of 17
  fatigue 18
  healing of 12, 32*f*
  incomplete 12, 12*f*, 16
  linear 12, 16
    transverse 12*f*
  occult 12, 16
  patterns of 12
  proximal humerus 14
  scaphoid 14, 15*f*, 21
  segmental 12, 13*f*, 16
  stress 18
  transverse 12

G

Galeazzi fracture 14, 14*f*
Gardner fibroma 102
Gastrointestinal disorders 43
Genitourinary tract infection 33
Giant cell
  angiofibroma 102
  tumor 29, 72, 77
    diffuse-type 102
Glenohumeral
  joint 46
    ligaments of 46
  ligament lesion
    bony humeral avulsion of 50
    humeral avulsion of 50
Glenoid labrum
  ovoid mass 50
  tear 50
Gluten sensitive enteropathy 43
Gout 29
Gracilis muscles 98*f*, 105*f*, 106*f*
Granulation tissue 51
Greater tuberosity 20*f*, 49*f*, 136
  avulsion of 47
Guinea worm 111
Gynecomastia 120
  diffuse glandular pattern of 121*f*

H

Haemophilus influenzae 33
Hairline fracture 12, 13*f*, 16
Hamartoma, fibrolipomatous 80, 105
Hand-foot syndrome 124
Heart disease
  congenital 5*f*
  cyanotic congenital 43
Hemangioma 72, 78
  epithelioid 103
Hematoma formation 12
Hemophilia 10
Hereditary multiple exostoses 30, 76
Heterogeneous hyperintense soft tissue mass 85*f*
High-grade surface osteosarcoma 92, 95

Hill-Sachs lesion 47
Hip
  dislocation, congenital 2, 3*f*
  joint 52, 53*f*-55*f*, 135*f*, 137*t*
    anatomy 52
Hodgkin's disease 30, 97
Holt-Oram syndrome 5, 5*f*
Homocystinuria 24
Human
  immunodeficiency virus 112
  leukocyte antigen 40
Humerus
  head of 136
  shaft of 136
  supracondylar fracture of 14*f*
Hunter's syndrome 8
Hurler's syndrome 8, 30
Hyalinizing spindle cell tumor 102
Hyperostosis frontalis interna 129
Hyperparathyroidism 24, 27, 30, 31, 129
Hyperthyroidism 24
Hypertrophy 43
Hypervitaminosis A 32
Hypophosphatasia 28

I

Idiopathic avascular necrosis 10
Infection 32, 112
  hematogenous spread of 58
Inflammatory
  bowel disease 43
  myofibroblastic tumor 102
Intercondylar notch sign 65
Intercostal nerves, neurofibromatosis of 126
Intra-articular oblique fracture 16*f*
Ischemic
  fasciitis 102
  injury, zone of 125
Ivory vertebra 125

J

Jaundice, obstructive 43
Joint 46
  effusion 17
  lesions 72
  sacroiliac 39*f*
  synovial 41
Juvenile
  chronic arthritis 30
  hyaline fibromatosis 102
  rheumatoid arthritis 10

K

Kaposi sarcoma 103
Keratoconjunctivitis 70
Keratocyst, odontogenic 89
Kienböck's disease 127
Kissing contusions 66
  classification of 67
Klebsiella 33
Knee
  joint 58, 60*f*-62*f*, 79*f*, 135*f*, 137*t*
    anatomy 58

ligaments of 59
posterior aspect of 113f

L

Langerhans cell histiocytosis 72
Legg-Calvé-Perthes disease 10, 126
Leiomyoma 72
Leiomyosarcoma 72, 101
Leprosy 27, 30
Lipoblastoma 102
Lipofibromatosis 102
Lipoma 72, 78, 101, 102
  pleomorphic 102
Lipomatosis 102
Liposarcoma 72, 98, 102, 105
  mixed-type 102
  pleomorphic 102
  round cell 102
Liver
  abscess 43
  neoplasms of 43
Lorry driver fracture 16f
Lung
  abscess 43
  tumors 43
Lymph node
  intramammary 119
  regional 73
Lymphadenopathy 71
Lymphangioma 103
Lymphoma 12, 112
  malignant 72
  osseous 96

M

Macrodystrophia lipomatosa 3, 103
Macroglobulinemia 82
Madelung's deformity 1, 2f, 30
Marble bone disease 2
Maroteaux-Lamy syndrome 9
Mature cystic teratomas 110
Mazabraud's syndrome 126
McCune Albright's syndrome 89, 126
Meckel-Gruber syndrome 31
Mediastinal tumors 43, 112
Mesenchymal chondrosarcoma 103
Mesenchymoma, malignant 103
Mesothelioma 43
Metacarpal sign 30
Metaphyseal chondroplasia 28
Meyer dysplasia 10
Mid shaft humerus, fracture of 14f
Monostotic fibrous dysplasia 126
Monteggia fracture dislocation 14
Morning stiffness 71
Morquio's disease 8
Morquio's syndrome 30
Mucopolysaccharidoses 7
Multifocal osteosarcoma 92, 96
Muscle, sternocleidomastoid 79f
Mycobacterium tuberculosis 37
Mycoplasma 112
Myelofibrosis 125
Myelolipoma, extra-adrenal 102

Myeloma
  multiple 24, 81, 83
  sclerosing 83
  solitary 83
Myelomeningocele 27, 30
Myoepithelioma 103
Myofibroblastic
  sarcoma, low grade 102
  tumors 102
Myofibroma 102
Myofibromatosis 102
Myolipoma 102
Myositis 40
  ossificans 17, 102
Myxedema 43
Myxofibrosarcoma 101, 102
Myxoid
  chondrosarcoma, extra-skeletal 103
  liposarcoma 102
Myxoma
  intramuscular 103
  juxta-articular 103

N

Nasolabial cyst 109
  bilateral 109f
Natowicz syndrome 9
Necrotizing fasciitis 40
Neonatal osteomyelits 34
Nerve, lipomatosis of 102
Neuroectodermal tumors 72
Neurofibromatosis 31
Nipple 116
  retraction 119f
Nodular fasciitis 102

O

Obstructive pulmonary disease,
    chronic 43
Organic dust diseases 112
Osteoarthritis 29
  premature 34
Osteoarthropathy, hypertrophic 42,
    43, 43t
Osteoblastoma 72
Osteochondral lesion 90f
Osteochondritis 37
  dissecans 90
Osteochondroma 72, 75
Osteochondromatosis 37
Osteodystrophy, renal 24, 125, 129,
    130
Osteogenesis imperfecta 24
Osteoid osteoma 54, 72, 74
Osteomalacia 23f, 24, 24t, 25, 129
Osteomyelitis 10, 32, 37, 69, 83, 124
  acute 33
  chronic 34, 35f
  vertebral 33
Osteopenia 29
Osteopetrosis 2, 3f
  pycnodysostosis 125
Osteophyte 25, 58f
  formation 50f
Osteoporosis 24, 24t
  periarticular 41

Osteosarcoma 32, 72, 90-92, 95
  central 92
  classic 92
  conventional 92
  extra-osseous 92, 96
  extra-skeletal 103
  juxtacortical 94
  periosteal 92, 95
  telangiectatic 92, 93
Osteosclerosis 129
Ozone therapy 130

P

Pachydermoperiostosis 27, 30
Paget's disease 43, 73, 96, 125
Pain
  ankle 19f
  wrist 129f
Paranasal sinuses 26
Paraneoplastic syndromes 24
Parosteal osteosarcoma 92, 94
Pectoralis muscle 116
Pelvis 5
Periosteal reaction
  causes of 32
  types of 32
Periostitis 32, 43
Perthes' disease 10
Phalanges, distal 137
Phyllodes tumor 120
Pigmented villonodular synovitis
    37, 69, 84
Plasma cell
  myeloma 72
  tumor 81
Plasmacytoma 82, 83
  solitary 83
Plexiform fibrohistiocytic tumor 102
Pneumoconiosis 112
Pneumonia 17
POEMS syndrome 83
Poland syndrome 31
Polyarteritis nodosa 43
Polyarthritis 42
Polycythemia 43
Porphyria 30
Pott's puffy tumor 33
Primitive neuroectodermal tumor 103
Prognathism 26
Proliferative
  fasciitis 102
  myositis 102
Protein deficiency 24
Proximal tibial epimetaphysis 92f
Pseudoarthrosis, development of 36f
Pseudohypoparathyroidism 30
Pseudohypothyroidism 115f
Psoriasis 30
Puberty, precocious 126
Pulmonary osteoarthropathy,
    hypertrophic 32
Pycnodysostosis 27, 125

R

Radial fracture, non-articular 15f
Radiation therapy 24

Radius
  head of 136
  lower end of 137
Raynaud's disease 27, 30, 31
Raynaud's phenomenon 30
Reiter's syndrome 41, 42
Retiform hemangioendothelioma 103
Rhabdoid tumor, extra-renal 103
Rhabdomyoma 102
Rhabdomyosarcoma
  alveolar 102
  pleomorphic 102
Rheumatoid
  arthritis 24, 29, 30, 37, 41, 42, 69
  nodules 71
  vasculitis 71
Rib notching 125
  causes of 126t
Rickets 22, 28
  renal 23
Rotator cuff tears 52
Rugger-Jersey spine 130

S

Sacrococcygeal teratoma 99
Sacroiliitis 38, 44
Sanfilippo's disease 8
Sarcoidosis 27, 30, 43, 111
Sarcoma
  epithelioid 103
  fibroblastic 102
  intimal 103
  osteogenic 32
  synovial 103
Scapholunate dissociation 21
Scapula
  body of 136
  inferior angle of 136
  medial border of 136
Schmorl's nodes 25
Scleroderma 27, 30, 31
Sclerosis 84f
Scurvy 24
Seminal vesicle calcification 112
Septic arthritis, pyogenic 37
Seronegative spondyloarthropathy 41
Shock 17
Short-rib polydactyl syndrome 31
Shoulder
  discharging sinus 37f
  dislocation 49
  joint 46, 46f-48f, 90, 90f, 134f, 136t
    anatomy 46
  pain 50f

Sickle cell
  anemia 30, 124, 126
  disease 33
Simple bone cyst 74
Sjögren's syndrome 70
Skeletal anomalies and dysplasia,
    congenital 1
Skin 116
Sly syndrome 9
Small cell osteosarcoma 92, 94
Smith's fracture 15, 15f
Smooth muscle tumors 72
Soft tissue 31, 101, 113f
  abscess 40
  calcifications 109, 114, 129
  calcifications 129
  chondroma 103
  clear cell sarcoma of 103
  giant cell tumor of 102
  sarcomas 101
  swelling 16, 71
  tumors 126
    WHO classification of 102t
Spinal anomalies, multiple 5f
Spindle cell 102
Spinoglenoid
  cyst 49, 51f
  notch 51f
Spondylitis, ankylosing 41, 44
Sprengel deformity 3, 4f
Staphylococcus aureus 32, 37
Streptococcus pneumoniae 37
Subchondral bony erosions 44
Subchondral collapse 57f
Subclavian artery 126
  obstruction 126
  stenosis 126
Sudeck's atrophy 18
Sudeck's osteodystrophy 15
Supraspinatus tendon 53f
  partial tear of 49
Swelling
  postreduction 15
  symmetric 71
Syphilis, congenital 37
Syringomyelia 27, 30
Systemic lupus erythematosus 30, 31

T

Takayasu disease 126
Tallus chondroblastoma 77
Tarsal bones 18
Tendon sheath
  fibroma of 102
  giant cell tumor of 102

Thoracolumbar junction 9f
Thromboangiitis obliterans 30
Thromboembolism 17
Thyrotoxicosis 43
Tibia, distal articular surface of 90f
Tibial
  condyles 68f
  plasmacytoma 82
  tubercle 137
Trapezium 137
Trauma 12, 32
Treponema pallidum 37
Trisomy 13 31
T-score, interpretation of 25t
Tuberculosis 112
  intestinal 43
  pulmonary 43
Tumor 10
  fibrogenic 72
  fibrohistiocytic 102
  fibrous 102
  hematopoietic 72
  lipogenic 72
  malignant 90, 93, 101
  myomelanocytic 103
  neurogenic 106, 126
  notochordal 72
  ossifying fibromyxoid 103
  osteogenic 72
  pleural 43
Turner's syndrome 30

U

Ulcerative colitis 43
Ulna, lower end of 137

V

Van Buchem disease 43
Venereal Disease Research Laboratory
    Test 37
Vinyl chloride poisoning 27
Vitamin D deficiency 22
Volkmann's ischemia 17

W

Werner's syndrome 30
Whipple's disease 112

X

Xerostomia 70

Z

Z-score 25